Rehabilitation
of the
Coronary Patient

Rehabilitation of the Coronary Patient

EDITED BY

Nanette Kass Wenger, M.D.
Professor of Medicine (Cardiology)
Emory University School of Medicine
Director, Cardiac Clinics
Grady Memorial Hospital
Atlanta, Georgia

Herman K. Hellerstein, M.D.
Professor of Medicine
School of Medicine
Case Western Reserve University
Physician, Chief Cardiology Outpatient Department
University Hospitals of Cleveland
Cleveland, Ohio

A WILEY MEDICAL PUBLICATION

John Wiley & Sons

New York / Chichester / Brisbane / Toronto

Library of Congress Cataloging in Publication Data:

Main entry under title:

Rehabilitation of the coronary patient.

(A Wiley medical publication)
Includes index.
1. Coronary heart disease—Prevention.   2. Cardiovascular patient—Rehabilitation.   3. Cardiovascular
patient—Rehabilitation—Social aspects.   4. Heart—
Infarction—Prevention.   I. Wenger, Nanette K.
II. Hellerstein, Herman K. [DNLM: 1. Myocardial
infarct—Rehabilitation.   WG300.3 R345]

RC685.C6R44   616.1′2   78-12531
ISBN 0-471-93369-4

Printed in the United States of America

10 9 8 7 6 5 4 3 2 1

To Julius Wenger, M.D.,
and
Mary Hellerstein, M.D.

Contributors

Ezra A. Amsterdam, M.D.
Associate Professor of Medicine
Section of Cardiovascular Medicine
University of California School of
  Medicine
Davis, California

Nina T. Argondizzo, R.N., M.A.
Assistant Dean and Assistant Profes-
  sor
Division of Continuing Education
Cornell University–New York Hos-
  pital School of Nursing
New York, New York

Henry Blackburn, M.D.
Professor and Director
Laboratory of Physiological Hygiene
School of Public Health
Professor of Medicine
University of Minnesota Medical
  School
Minneapolis, Minnesota

C. Gunnar Blomqvist, M.D., Ph.D.
Professor of Medicine and Physiology
University of Texas Health Science
  Center
Southwestern Medical School
The Pauline and Adolph Weinberger
  Laboratory for Cardiopulmonary
  Research
Dallas, Texas

Ned H. Cassem, M.D.
Associate Professor of Psychiatry
Harvard Medical School
Chief, Consultation-Liaison Service
Massachusetts General Hospital
Boston, Massachusetts

Sydney H. Croog, Ph.D.
Professor of Behavioral Sciences and
  Psychiatry
Department of Behavioral Sciences
  and Community Health
University of Connecticut Health
  Center
Farmington, Connecticut

Barry A. Franklin, Ph.D.
Assistant Professor of Medicine
School of Medicine
Case Western Reserve University
Cleveland, Ohio

Peter L. Frommer, M.D.
Deputy Director, National Heart,
  Lung and Blood Institute
Bethesda, Maryland

Thomas P. Hackett, M.D.
Eben S. Draper Professor of Psychi-
  atry
Harvard Medical School
Chief of Psychiatry
Massachusetts General Hospital
Boston, Massachusetts

William L. Haskell, Ph.D.
Co-Director, Stanford Cardiac Rehabilitation Program
Division of Cardiology
Stanford University Medical School
Palo Alto, California

Herman K. Hellerstein, M.D.
Professor of Medicine
School of Medicine
Case Western Reserve University
Physician, Chief Cardiology Outpatient Department
University Hospitals of Cleveland
Cleveland, Ohio

Michael Lesch, M.D.
Magerstadt Professor of Medicine
Northwestern University Medical School
Director, Section of Cardiology
Northwestern Memorial Hospital
Chicago, Illinois

Robert I. Levy, M.D.
Director, National Heart, Lung and Blood Institute
Bethesda, Maryland

Dean T. Mason, M.D.
Professor and Chairman
Section of Cardiovascular Medicine
University of California School of Medicine
Davis, California

John Naughton, M.D.
Dean, School of Medicine
The State University of New York at Buffalo
Buffalo, New York

Eugene R. Passamani, M.D.
Division of Heart and Vascular Diseases
National Heart, Lung and Blood Institute
Bethesda, Maryland

Elliot L. Sagall, M.D.
Assistant Clinical Professor of Medicine
Harvard Medical School
Instructor in Legal Medicine
Boston College Law School
Boston, Massachusetts

Edmund H. Sonnenblick, M.D.
Professor of Medicine
Chief, Division of Cardiology
Albert Einstein College of Medicine
New York, New York

Nanette Kass Wenger, M.D.
Professor of Medicine (Cardiology)
Emory University School of Medicine
Director, Cardiac Clinics
Grady Memorial Hospital
Atlanta, Georgia

Preface

One of the most exciting features of the rehabilitative approach to the cardiac patient during the past decade has been the establishment of its validity and its acceptance and progressive incorporation into the mainstream of traditional medical care.

We have witnessed the increasing use of exercise testing to evaluate objectively function and responses to various types of therapy and the subsequent institution of exercise training programs to improve the patient's functional capacity. Equally significant attention is currently being focused on the psychosocial factors affecting the patient after myocardial infarction, since these factors often contribute more to disability than physiologic impairment. Patient, public, and professional educational efforts have begun, appropriately, to emphasize that most patients after myocardial infarction and after aortocoronary bypass surgery can and should return to their customary normal or near-normal lifestyle. Aortocoronary bypass surgery has also received increasing acceptance as a sound method of rehabilitation.

The rehabilitative approach should begin at the onset of illness and remain as a continuing feature in the long-term care of the patient; however, the initiation and coordination of rehabilitation efforts must be the responsibility of the patient's primary physician, although he may utilize the knowledge, skills, techniques, and services of a variety of medical consultants and health care professionals to implement the actual rehabilitative processes.

The important components of myocardial infarction rehabilitative programs include physical activity, functional evaluation, prescriptive training, patient and family education, and psychosocial and vocational counseling.

This book is designed to provide background information about the physiologic, medical, and social problems associated with myocardial infarction, to present insight into the scientific bases for rehabilitation programming, and to furnish a detailed description of a realistic rehabilitative approach to the patient after myocardial infarction. It is hoped that the primary care physician and other members of the health team will find the presentations helpful in improving the care of their patients who have sustained a myocardial infarction or who have undergone aortocoronary bypass surgery. The clinical advent of coronary atherosclerotic heart disease is overwhelming because of the residual functional impairment, both physiologic and psychologic. Appropriate attention is directed to the recognition, assessment, prevention, and management of this impairment.

Several currently developing methods are not included in this book because their practical application to rehabilitation, although promising, is not yet established. These methods include isotopic myocardial imaging scanning, radionuclide cineangiography, ventricular systolic intervals, psychologic (quiz) stress testing, etc.

In the text, the terms *heart attack* and *myocardial infarction* are used synonymously and the terms *heart patient* and *cardiac patient* are used interchangeably. The individual identified as a *myocardial infarction patient* or a *coronary patient* is considered to have coronary atherosclerotic heart disease. Finally, *primary care physician* designates the individual responsible for the continuing care of the patient; this individual may be an internist, cardiologist, family physician, etc.

It is our hope that the readers will share our view that the health sciences are entering the dawn of the scientific era of rehabilitation, which encompasses basic and clinical sciences and humanism.

We would like to express our gratitude to Betty Martin for the administrative coordination of the text; she served as liaison among editors, authors, and publisher, shepherding the myriad of details required for the coordination of a multiauthored book. Special appreciation goes to Julia Wright for verifying references, typing manuscripts, responding to authors' concerns, and working with Betty Martin in the proofreading and correction of galleys. Special thanks also go to Vera Husselman, Charline Hutton, and Elaine Shaw for typing chapters. And we give sincerest appreciation to John Wiley & Sons, particularly John de Carville, Ruth Wreschner, and Margery Carazzone for their ongoing encouragement, help, and expertise.

We would also like to thank the specialists who contributed to this text. They are leaders in their respective fields of endeavor and have painstakingly summarized the newest knowledge in each area, emphasizing scientific background information and application to patient care.

Nanette Kass Wenger, M.D.
Herman K. Hellerstein, M.D.

Contents

1   Coronary Heart Disease: An Overview   1
    Eugene R. Passamani, Peter L. Frommer, and Robert I. Levy

2   Alterations of Cardiac Structure and Function in Myocardial Infarction   19
    Michael Lesch and Edmund H. Sonnenblick

3   Guidelines to Patient Management   29
    Ezra A. Amsterdam and Dean T. Mason

4   Early Ambulation After Myocardial Infarction: Rationale, Program
        Components, and Results   53
    Nanette Kass Wenger

5   The Potential for Preventing Reinfarction   67
    Henry Blackburn

6   Patient and Family Education   117
    Nina T. Argondizzo

7   Clinical Exercise Physiology   133
    C. Gunnar Blomqvist

8   Exercise Testing and Prescription   149
    Herman K. Hellerstein and Barry A. Franklin

9   Design and Implementation of Cardiac Conditioning Programs   203
    William L. Haskell

10 Psychologic Aspects of Rehabilitation After Myocardial Infarction   243
    Thomas P. Hackett and Ned H. Cassem

11 Social Aspects of Rehabilitation After Myocardial Infarction:
        A Selective Review   255
    Sydney H. Croog

12   Legal Aspects of Rehabilitation After Myocardial Infarction   269
     Elliot L. Sagall

13   Vocational Aspects of Rehabilitation After Myocardial Infarction   283
     John Naughton

14   Community Resources for Rehabilitation of the Myocardial
        Infarction Patient   295
     Nanette Kass Wenger

     Glossary   305

     Index   321

1
Coronary Heart Disease: An Overview

Eugene R. Passamani, M.D.

Peter L. Frommer, M.D.

Robert I. Levy, M.D.

Diseases of the heart and blood vessels have accounted for slightly more than 50% of all deaths in the United States in recent years, and two-thirds of these deaths have resulted from ischemic heart disease. During the past decade there has been a substantial decrease in the death rate due to ischemic heart disease, but it remains the cause of death for approximately 650,000 persons annually, twice the number of deaths related to malignant neoplasms and more than three times the number due to cerebrovascular diseases, the second and third leading causes of death (1).

The incidence and prevalence of coronary heart disease are less well known. It has been estimated that 1.25 million persons experience myocardial infarction each year. Nearly two-thirds of these attacks have occurred in individuals who ostensibly have been healthy prior to their attacks. It has been estimated that 3.9 million Americans have chronic coronary heart disease (2).

A particularly disquieting aspect of the statistics relating to coronary heart disease concerns the high attack rate and high death rate among persons middle-aged and younger who presumably are at the height of their productive and creative capacities. It has been estimated that 475,000 persons each year under 65 years of age have their first coronary attacks; there are 160,000 deaths due to ischemic heart disease each year in this age group. Indeed, coronary heart disease is the leading cause of death for women over 55 years of age and for men over 40 years of age.

Death due to coronary heart disease has been an accompaniment of the human condition for hundreds and probably thousands of years, but the attack rate appears to have increased substantially in the twentieth century, particularly in young and middle-aged men. Coronary heart disease death rates vary not only with the passage of time but also geographically (3), as can be seen in Figure 1.

1

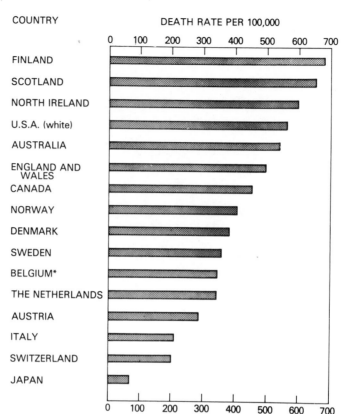

Figure 1. Death rates for coronary heart diseases in 16 countries, 1973, males, age 45–64 years. Data from Tables 2 and 7 in World Health Statistics Annual, 1976, W.H.O. Asterisk indicates 1972 data.

Moreover, migration from a nation enjoying a low coronary death rate (e.g., Japan) to one with a high rate (e.g., the United States) appears to result in an intermediate risk of coronary death (4). These variations in coronary death rate geographically and temporally make it likely that nongenetic factors are quite influential in the genesis of this disorder, in addition to the recognized genetic predisposition.

Excellent epidemiologic studies in recent years have demonstrated large differences in the propensity to develop coronary heart disease among ostensibly healthy middle-aged Americans; these differences in predisposition are strongly correlated with a number of personal characteristics or risk factors. The most important risk factors appear to be cigarette smoking, hypercholesterolemia, hypertension, age, and male sex (5–7). Risk factors can also be applied to the prediction of recurrent events in patients with coronary heart disease; additional clinical measurements, including the number of infarcts experienced, the presence of angina, the occurrence of congestive heart failure, the appearance of the resting electrocardiogram, and the severity of coronary arterial disease as demonstrated by arteriography, sharpen the predictive power of the more traditional risk factor profile (8–13).

Thus there exist substantial variations in coronary heart disease attack rates among various populations of men and women with and without symptomatic coronary heart disease. These differences can be observed either by comparing coronary morbidity and mortality of populations living in different nations or by observing the experiences of individuals within a population. Some, but not all, of the variation can be explained by risk factor differences. Risk factors and their relative importances are similar but not identical in various parts of the world, which indicates complex interrelationships among known risk factors and perhaps risk factors yet to be discovered.

On the basis of these observations a number of hypotheses have been constructed suggesting that various modifications in life-style may prevent or postpone the onset of coronary heart disease and, when applied to patients with symptomatic coronary disease, may decrease the severity of symptoms and delay death.

A brief overview of coronary heart disease will be presented, with particular emphasis on the public health challenge it presents.

ATHEROSCLEROTIC PROCESS

Arteriosclerosis is a family of degenerative processes occurring in the walls of arteries; these nearly always are concomitants of aging in persons in the United States. Atherosclerosis is one of several different types of arteriosclerosis; it is related to the deposition of blood fats, primarily cholesterol, in the intima of large and medium-size arteries. In the vast majority of individuals this process begins in the first or second decade of life, whether or not they are destined to develop clinically manifest arterial disease (14). The earliest easily discernible lesion is a fatty streak. This is an intimal thickening composed of increased amounts of cellular and intercellular materials and increased intracellular lipid. In various individuals, indeed in some societies, progression beyond the stage of the fatty streak is rare. In others, however, some if not all fatty streaks grow in size and evolve in makeup through a fibrous plaque stage, ending as a complex atherosclerotic lesion that significantly compromises or totally occludes the lumen of the affected artery. The details concerning which fatty streaks evolve, the time course, and the mechanism or mechanisms involved remain obscure, although blood lipid infiltration, recurrent surface thrombosis, and intralesional hemorrhage are all likely candidates. The process favors certain parts of the arterial tree and certain segments of arteries within each part of the arterial tree. Eventually symptoms may develop referable to the heart, brain, kidney, lower extremities, and intestines, depending on which arteries happen to be involved.

The most important and least well understood processes involved in the genesis of atherosclerotic lesions are operative after the development of fatty streaks in the first decade of life and before the onset of clinical ischemic symptoms in the third and later decades. The presence of symptoms, regardless of the organ system involved, is the clinical correlate of extensive, far-advanced, end-stage arterial disease. The long, subclinical developmental phase is the result of many factors, including extensive reserve arterial blood delivery capacity, slow growth of atherosclerotic lesions, and the existence of compensatory mechanisms such as collateral circulation that may develop pari passu with the progressive atherosclerotic luminal encroachment.

Human atherosclerotic lesions, particularly the late complex lesions, probably arise as a result of multiple causes acting and interacting over lengthy periods of time. Inability to detect the nascent stages of atherosclerosis and monitor its progression effectively in man has seriously hampered attempts to study the etiology and pathogenesis of this disorder and has forced the use of indirect methods of detection.

The epidemiologic model has been used to study the genesis of human atherosclerosis (particularly coronary atherosclerosis) with some vigor and success in recent years. This involves meticulous collection of baseline biologic data on large population samples. The study populations are observed for varying numbers of years, and the incidences of coronary attacks are noted. This research has resulted in identification of a number of risk factors that are easily measured and that either singly or in aggregate appear to identify groups of individuals with widely varying propensities toward the development of coronary heart disease (15).

RISK FACTORS

Cigarette smoking, hypercholesterolemia, and hypertension are the major coronary heart disease risk factors. Each is present in a substantial portion of the adult population; each exerts a powerful independent influence on coronary attack rates, particularly in younger coronary victims; and each can to some degree be modified. Other risk factors of variable prevalence, strength, and ease of modification include age, male sex, glucose intolerance, obesity, physical inactivity, hyperuricemia, family history (genetics), soft water consumption, and personality type (16). It should be noted at the outset that an absence of identifiable risk factors by no means guarantees an individual immunity from coronary heart disease; conversely, the presence of some or all of these risk factors by no means makes it inevitable. Furthermore, the relative importance of each risk factor depends on the population to which it is applied. Finally, clear demonstration of pathophysiologic mechanisms and rigorous proof of cause and effect have not been forthcoming for any of the risk factors, although much progress has been made in the past several decades.

As was noted previously, coronary attack rates climb with age, so that coronary heart disease becomes the leading cause of death in men after age 40 years and in women after age 55 years. The reason behind this age-related increase is unclear. Which of the myriad male–female differences is responsible for male predominance, particularly in younger victims, is not yet understood, although many hypotheses exist.

It is clear that individuals with glucose intolerance ranging in degree from an elevation in postprandial blood glucose level to a requirement for insulin face an increased risk for arterial disease that is not explained entirely by the often associated lipid disorders, obesity, and hypertension. Although basement membrane thickening is a vascular disorder observed exclusively in patients with diabetes, atherosclerosis in diabetics (coronary and otherwise) is not distinct from that seen in nondiabetics, except that the 10-year grace period usually afforded women in terms of age of onset of coronary artery disease is not observed in diabetics. It is not clear that rigorous control of glucose metabolism has any effect on the rate of development of atherosclerosis in diabetics.

Individuals with hyperuricemia appear to be at increased risk of coronary attack. The mechanism underlying this observation is quite obscure, and it may involve a linkage between hyperuricemia and other risk factors.

Obesity and physical inactivity appear to be related to coronary heart disease. Methodologic problems involved in examining these variables in epidemiologic studies have resulted in mixed reports regarding the strength of their association with coronary attacks. The correlation may in part rest on their association with the three major risk factors.

Families share not only genes but also many risk factors, which makes interpretation of this important association difficult. Behavioral patterns and various social parameters are associated with premature coronary heart disease, although problems with precise definitions and measurement continue to exist. A most intriguing inverse relationship between water hardness and coronary attack rate is currently the subject of intense research activity. All three of these potentially important risk factors require further clarification.

Smokers have a risk of death 1.7 times that of the nonsmoking population. This is demonstrated by a dose–response curve: men smoking less than 10, 10–19, 20–39, and more than 40 cigarettes per day have mortality ratios of 1.4, 1.7, 1.9, and 2.2, respectively. Mortality ratios between smokers and nonsmokers, as well as heavy and light smokers, are magnified in the younger age groups. The surgeon general's report identified coronary heart disease as the prime contributor to this excess mortality among smokers, followed closely by lung cancer (17). The coronary attack rate (16) is graphically portrayed in Figure 2. Other reports have confirmed these data (18–20). The particularly strong correlation with sudden death noted in Figure 3 (16) was confirmed in a recent report (21).

Several things are abundantly clear: cigarette smoking is not inherently a human requirement; smoking augments the risk of death via a variety of causes, led by coronary heart disease, followed closely by lung cancer, chronic bronchitis, and emphysema, as well as a plethora of other neoplasms; cessation of smoking results in a decrease in the risk of death.

The specific mechanisms behind the increased risk of coronary artery disease in smokers are unclear, although a number of constituents of tobacco smoke, including nicotine and carbon monoxide, have important cardiovascular actions. The importance of cigarette smoking as a predictor of coronary heart disease depends on the population observed, and presumably this is due to the mix of other risk factors present overall.

The risk of coronary heart disease rises progressively with blood cholesterol levels from the lowest to the highest values noted in the population (22). This observation has been confirmed repeatedly, not only within the United States but also in an international study on the epidemiology of cardiovascular disease in which the 5-year incidences of coronary heart disease were correlated with mean population cholesterol levels (6). The influences of various cholesterol levels on 10-year coronary attack rates are displayed in Figure 4 (16).

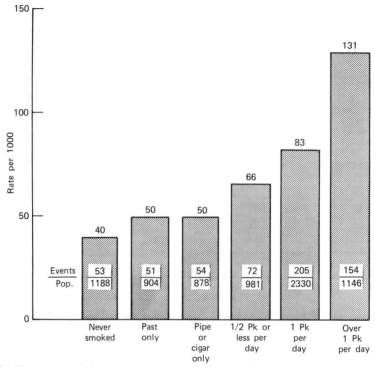

Figure 2. Cigarette-smoking status at entry and age-adjusted rates of first major coronary event for white males age 30–59 years at entry. National Cooperative Pooling Project. Rates for 10 years of follow-up adjusted by age to the U.S. white male population, 1960. (Reprinted from "Arteriosclerosis," a Report by the National Heart and Lung Institute Task Force on Arteriosclerosis, National Institutes of Health, vol II, June 1971, DHEW Publicaton No. NIH 72-219, p 81.)

The population of individuals with elevated lipid concentrations can be divided into several subgroups on the basis of measurements of lipid-protein aggregates of lipoproteins (23). One of these subgroups, type II hyperlipoproteinemia, appears to be inherited in some cases in an autosomal dominant fashion; the risk of coronary attack and death among affected relatives as compared with normal family members is sobering. It was found that among male heterozygous relatives with type II hyperlipoproteinemia 16% and 52% experienced fatal or nonfatal coronary heart disease by the ages of 40 years and 60 years, respectively; the proportions in normal male relatives were zero and 12.7%. The higher attack rate among female relatives with type II hyperlipoproteinemia becomes apparent by age 50 years, with 19% and 8% of those affected and unaffected, respectively, experiencing their first coronary attacks by this age; at age 60 years the disparity in attack rates increases, with 32% of type II relatives and 10% of normal relatives experiencing coronary heart disease (24). Homozygous individuals have approximately double the cholesterol levels of their heterozygote parents, and they die in the first and second decades of life of coronary heart disease (23).

It has been clearly demonstrated that diet therapy that restricts both cholesterol and saturated fat results in a significant decrement in serum cholesterol (25). This effect can be enhanced by drug therapy (26). The issue whether

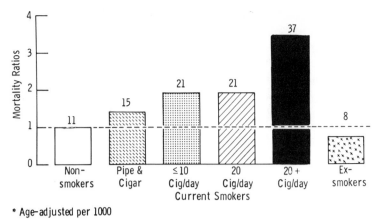

(National Cooperative Pooling Project, A.H.A., 1970)

Figure 3. Mortality ratios and death rates (age-adjusted per 1000) for sudden coronary death in men age 30–59 years by type of smoking and number of cigarettes. National Cooperative Pooling Project, A.H.A., 1970. (Reprinted from "Arteriosclerosis," a Report by the National Heart and Lung Institute Task Force on Arteriosclerosis, National Institutes of Health, vol II, June 1971, DHEW Publication No. NIH 72-219, p 87.)

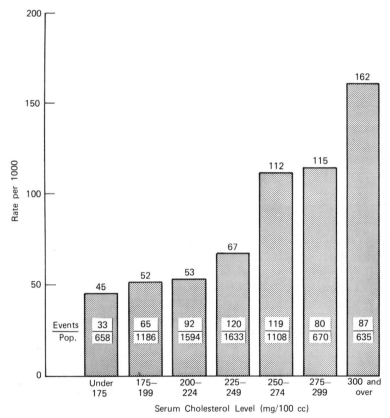

Figure 4. Serum cholesterol level at entry and age-adjusted rates of first major coronary event for white males age 30–59 years at entry. National Cooperative Pooling Project. Rates for 10 years of follow-up adjusted by age to the U.S. white male population, 1960. (Reprinted from "Arteriosclerosis," a Report by the National Heart and Lung Institute Task Force on Arteriosclerosis, National Institutes of Health, vol II, June 1971, DHEW Publication No. NIH 72-219, p 53.)

cholesterol-lowering regimens will postpone or prevent coronary heart disease or improve the course of the disease in patients with symptomatic coronary disease has not been settled. Our current inability to detect and measure accurately early coronary atherosclerosis has prevented study of the effects of cholesterol lowering on this important stage in the natural history of the disorder. Moreover, in patients with symptomatic coronary heart disease in whom monitoring of the progression of arterial disease may be possible with arteriography, it is plausible that cholesterol-lowering regimens may be less efficacious.

The effects of cholesterol-lowering regimens in subjects with type II hyperlipoproteinemia who do not have symptomatic coronary heart disease are currently being investigated in a national clinical trial. The results of this effort, which will be forthcoming in the next 5–10 years, will be important in guiding medical therapy not only for patients with type II hyperlipoproteinemia but also for those with less severely elevated cholesterol levels commonly observed in the general population. In the meantime, it would seem prudent to advise moderate restriction of dietary saturated fat and cholesterol.

Hypertension, systolic or diastolic, is associated with a significant increase in coronary attack rate, as can be seen in Figure 5 (16). A large collaborative trial recently demonstrated the utility of blood-pressure-lowering regimens in preventing death (27, 28). Although a decrement in ischemic heart disease mortality was observed in the treated group, it did not reach statistical significance. However, given the rather small sample size, it was unlikely that a significant effect would have been seen. Because of the significant decrease in total mortality following treatment, a trial designed to demonstrate the effect of antihypertensive treatment on coronary mortality (at least in subjects with significant hypertension) probably will never be done; in fact, it would seem unethical. Two questions remain unanswered: What absolute level of blood pressure is deleterious and should therefore be treated? Should other aspects of an individual's risk profile be taken into account in deciding whether to institute antihypertensive therapy?

Despite the simplicity of the diagnosis, in many hypertensive persons in the United States the diagnosis has not been made. It has been estimated that recent educational campaigns have reduced the unrecognized proportion of hypertensives to 40%. Even among recognized hypertensives only a minority are receiving adequate therapy, although in the vast majority of individuals treatment is easily administered, quite effective, and free of major toxic side effects.

The effects of combined major risk factors and estimates of prevalence are displayed in Figure 6 (5). The following eloquent summary of the risk factor connection remains accurate (5):

> Converging lines of epidemiological, clinical and experimental evidence, both animal and human, support the judgment that the relationship between the risk factors, particularly the major risk factors—i.e., hypercholesterolemia, cigarette smoking, hypertension—and the development of coronary heart disease is probably causal. This should not be interpreted as implying that the evidence on this matter is conclusive. Nevertheless, the data strongly indicate that to a considerable degree coronary heart disease in the United States, particularly in the under 60 age group, results principally from the impact of these three widely prevalent risk factors. This critically important conclusion rests on the following foundations: Confirmatory

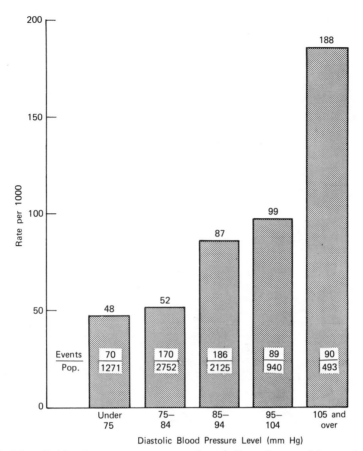

Figure 5. Diastolic blood pressure at entry and age-adjusted rates of first major coronary event for white males age 30–59 years at entry, National Cooperative Pooling Project. Rates for 10 years of follow-up adjusted by age to the U.S. white male population, 1960. (Reprinted from "Arteriosclerosis," a Report by the National Heart and Lung Institute Task Force on Arteriosclerosis, National Institutes of Health, vol II, June 1971, DHEW Publication No. NIH 72-219, p 75.)

data are available from many sources of the epidemiologic associations; these associations persist when confounding variables are taken into account; the associations are strong and consistent; they are in accord with findings from other research disciplines and are biologically plausible in terms of reasonable pathogenetic mechanisms and concepts of multifactorial etiology relating apparent cause and disease. Alternative hypotheses to account for the associations do not fit the majority of observations to date.

A large collaborative trial has been instituted to determine whether a preventive program aimed at reducing blood pressure and blood cholesterol, as well as eliminating or reducing cigarette use, will result in a decrease in coronary attack rate in middle-aged men. The recruitment phase of this trial was recently concluded, and the results should be forthcoming in several years.

The occurrence of premature coronary attacks in the absence of known risk factors means that other influences not yet characterized are operating and must

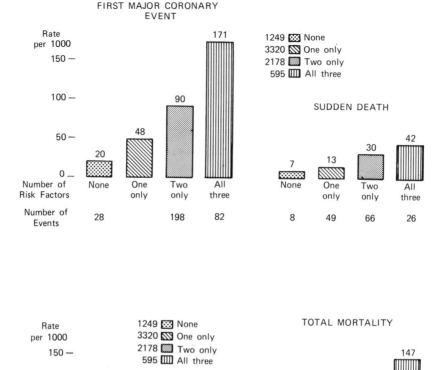

Figure 6. National Cooperative Pooling Project. Hypercholesterolemia, hypertension, cigarette smoking, and 10-year age-adjusted rates per 1000 men for the following: any major coronary event, sudden death (upper graphs); all coronary heart disease deaths and death from all causes (lower graphs). Any major coronary event includes nonfatal myocardial infarction, fatal myocardial infarction and sudden death due to coronary heart disease. U.S. white males, age 30–50 years at entry; all rates age-adjusted by 10-year age groups to the U.S. white male population, 1960. Cutoff points: serum cholesterol ≥ 250 mg/dl; diastolic blood pressure ≥ 90 mm Hg; any use of cigarettes at entry. (Reprinted from the Inter-Society Commission for Heart Disease Resources Report on "Primary Prevention of the Atherosclerotic Diseases," published in *Circulation* 42:A-68, 1970.)

be identified. For example, the recent demonstration of an association between oral contraceptive use and coronary attacks in middle-aged women may have revealed a new risk factor (29, 30). Furthermore, clear pathophysiologic ties between the major risk factors and coronary atherosclerosis are lacking; interactions among the major risk factors are even less well understood. These and other questions about the genesis of coronary atherosclerosis must be answered before a comprehensive and specific program to prevent coronary heart disease can be mounted. However, on the basis of what is already known, it would seem proper to recommend cessation of cigarette smoking. Aggressive diagnosis and therapy of hypertension must be undertaken. Dietary therapy and, if need be, drug therapy of hypercholesterolemia would also appear to be useful; however, in the absence of any demonstration of efficacy in the prevention of morbidity and mortality, this would seem to be not nearly as pressing as cessation of smoking and treatment of hypertension. Moderate, prudent exercise and attainment of ideal body weight should also be strongly considered.

CLINICAL ASPECTS

It has become axiomatic that the onset of symptoms, whether angina, myocardial infarction, or sudden cardiac death, is indicative of far-advanced coronary atherosclerotic involvement of at least one and generally two or all three of the major coronary arteries. The reasons for this are several. Arterial narrowing must be substantial before it, rather than arteriolar tone, limits blood flow. Collaterals may develop and ameliorate the effects of the stenosis. Finally, there appears to be marked variation in perception of ischemic symptoms on the part of patients with coronary heart disease.

First coronary events, including the onset of angina pectoris, fatal and non-fatal myocardial infarction, and sudden cardiac death, occur each year in probably more than 1 million individuals with previously silent but advanced coronary atherosclerosis. The events occurring in a "healthy" person with unsuspected coronary artery disease that precipitate death, myocardial infarction, or angina are unknown, but presumably they involve worsening of arterial obstruction, at least in part. Furthermore, it should be pointed out that intimate knowledge of the extent and degree of coronary atherosclerosis is not very useful in predicting which of the three major coronary symptoms or combinations thereof any given patient will experience. It can be predicted that the more advanced the coronary arterial lesions, the more likely it is that symptoms of some kind will be present.

Angina pectoris is a name that was applied to transient ischemic cardiac chest pain by Heberden; his article was entitled "Some Account of a Disorder of the Breast" and was published in 1772. The diagnosis is made by taking a medical history, which must reveal midsternal or left arm discomfort that is precipitated by some form of stress and that may be relieved in 5–10 min by removal of the stress. The clinician Heberden described it in the following fashion in 1768 (31):

> There is a disorder of the breast, marked with strong and peculiar symptoms, considerable for the kind of danger belonging to it, and not extremely rare, of which I do not recollect any mention among medical authors. The seat of it, and sense of

strangling and anxiety with which it is attended may make it not improperly be called angina pectoris.

Those who are afflicted with it, are seized, while they are walking, and more particularly when they walk soon after eating, with a painful and most disagreeable sensation in the breast, which seems as if it would take their life away, if it were to increase or to continue; the moment they stand still, all this uneasiness vanishes. In all other respects the patients are at the beginning of this disorder perfectly well, and in particular have no shortness of breath, from which it is totally different.

It has been estimated that approximately one-third of persons experiencing the onset of clinical coronary heart disease do so by developing angina pectoris (32). The diagnosis is in large part dependent on history alone, since few, if any, attendant physical or electrocardiographic findings are present at rest. Angina is the "softest" of the clinical categories of coronary heart disease; prevalence estimates of numbers of patients with coronary heart disease are probably quite conservative because of delay and reluctance on the part of patients with angina to seek medical consultation, as well as misclassification of patients with angina. Both physician and patient may be reluctant to accept a diagnosis of angina unless the history is quite typical. Many cases of atypical angina are misdiagnosed, since the location, quality of pain, precipitating factors, and perhaps most important the ability of the patient to describe symptoms all may vary a good deal.

Myocardial infarction can be defined as ischemic myocardial necrosis; it is typically manifest by a history of prolonged chest pain followed by evolutionary changes noted in the electrocardiogram and elevations of serum enzyme concentrations. The necrosis is the result of nearly absolute oxygen deprivation in the myocardium and local metabolic sequelae. Approximately one-half of individuals developing coronary heart disease do so by experiencing a myocardial infarction (32). Myocardial infarction was first clearly described by Herrick in 1912; he emphasized the relationship between thrombosis of the coronary artery and subsequent myocardial necrosis (33). Although this is a topic of some debate, the proximate cause of the severe myocardial oxygen supply–demand disparity in the majority of myocardial infarctions is probably closure or sudden worsening of stenosis of a major coronary artery.

Unstable angina pectoris is a syndrome intermediate in severity between stable angina and acute myocardial infarction. This clinical spectrum reflects an underlying myocardial oxygen supply–demand disparity. The factors leading to either side of the spectrum are obscure and probably depend ultimately on the severity of underlying coronary atherosclerotic changes.

For 15–25% of individuals developing coronary heart disease, their first symptom is their last. Sudden cardiac death has been variously defined: death occurring instantaneously or death occurring as long as 24 hr after onset of symptoms. More than 60% of coronary heart disease deaths occur outside the hospital, and for many purposes this constitutes a rough but convenient definition of sudden cardiac death. Furthermore, depending on one's definition of suddenness and on the population studied, it has been estimated that 40–60% of sudden cardiac deaths have occurred in individuals who had not previously carried a diagnosis of coronary heart disease but who doubtless for years had been afflicted with asymptomatic coronary atherosclerosis. The mechanism in the majority of cases is probably ventricular fibrillation. A modern emergency care system can resuscitate some fraction of these victims; however, it is evident that effective prevention of sudden cardiac death must be accomplished if coronary mortality rates are to be reduced. This depends ultimately on prevention of coronary atherosclerosis or, failing that, on interruption of whatever mechanism or mechanisms convert chronic coronary heart disease into an abrupt catastrophic event.

As was noted previously, a major obstruction to gaining an understanding of coronary atherosclerosis and instituting effective early therapy has been the lack of precise diagnostic tools. Clearly the traditional medical weapons of history, physical examination, and routine laboratory work lack sufficient sensitivity and specificity, since many individuals with far-advanced coronary artery disease are classified as normal, and, conversely, angina will occasionally be diagnosed in a patient without actual heart disease.

The electrocardiogram and even the stress electrocardiogram lack the sensitivity and specificity that would make them useful in identifying early coronary artery disease in the general population (34, 35). Patients with far-advanced coronary artery disease that is demonstrated angiographically not infrequently have normal stress electrocardiograms (lack of sensitivity); moreover, some individuals with clearly normal or near normal coronary arteriograms occasionally have positive stress tests (lack of specificity). Although exercise testing does not have sufficient diagnostic reliability to be used in study of the pathogenesis of coronary atherosclerosis, it can be useful in conjunction with other diagnostic information, and it also provides valuable information referable to exercise tolerance.

The development and application of coronary angiography by Sones and by Judkins in the late 1950s were major advances. It appears that, as compared with examination of pathologic specimens, coronary arteriography in general underestimates the degree of luminal narrowing (37–39). Nevertheless, it represents something like a "gold standard" against which tools developed in the future will be measured. Because of the expense and the slight risk of the procedure, it cannot be applied to mass screening of healthy populations. However, it is quite helpful in management of patients with symptomatic coronary heart disease, allowing precision in diagnosis, prognosis, and selection of therapeutic alternatives. It is also useful in identifying subjects with chest pain syndromes not due to coronary atherosclerosis.

The development of a simple, inexpensive, and noninvasive test that could be used to identify with high specificity and sensitivity those individuals with early coronary atherosclerosis and measure the lesions precisely would be exceedingly useful in the study and treatment of coronary disease. Just as coronary arteriography has placed the treatment of individuals with ischemic heart disease on a much more rational and objective footing, a precise noninvasive measurement of coronary atherosclerosis in asymptomatic individuals would allow more rapid confirmation or refutation of the risk factor hypotheses and obviate the argument for a shotgun approach to primary prevention presently advocated by some.

Therapy for the acute aspects of myocardial infarction has changed a good deal in the past several decades. The advent of the coronary care unit and the concept of care involved therein have led to prevention of a substantial fraction of electrical deaths in the wake of myocardial infarction. It now appears that both early survival and late survival after myocardial infarction are exquisitely dependent on the amount of remaining viable myocardium; furthermore, it appears that death of myocardium during the episode has a temporal dispersion such that various pharmacologic and mechanical maneuvers within 24 hr of onset may preserve tissue that would otherwise be lost (39). This is currently an area of intense research activity that may lead to significant prolongation of life in patients sustaining myocardial infarction.

Management of angina pectoris involves risk factor modification and relief of the frequency and severity of attacks of angina. The former includes measures such as weight loss, cessation of smoking, and prudent exercise, as well as the specific measures noted previously. The latter involves use of drugs such as nitroglycerin and propranolol; it appears that both, by a variety of mechanisms, reduce myocardial oxygen supply–demand disparities and are quite effective in reducing symptoms. Equal in importance to these "therapeutic measures" is the compassionate and knowledgeable advice of the physician in teaching the patient how to live with his disease and in relieving the anxiety elicited with each attack of angina, often the most disagreeable feature of the attack. However, some patients continue to have frequent and severe angina in the face of these regimens. Surgical therapy is effective in relief of chest pain in substantial numbers of patients refractory to medical therapy.

Surgical therapy for coronary heart disease has had a long and colorful history, beginning with cervical sympathectomy at the turn of the century, continuing through pericardial poudrage, coronary sinus ligation and perfusion, and internal mammary artery ligation and implantation, and culminating in 1967 with aorto-coronary saphenous vein bypass grafting and direct internal mammary coronary anastomosis. Good reviews of this topic have recently been published (40, 41).

Experience accumulated to date indicates that bypass surgery in selected patients results in relief of chest pain in 80–90% of survivors and that 60–70% become pain-free. However, 1–5% of patients accepted for operation die during or shortly after the procedure, and 5–15% experience perioperative myocardial infarction. The range of these statistics is dependent on the clinical state of the patient, the severity of the coronary artery disease, and the skill and experience of the surgical team. Other factors must also be considered. For example, arterial occlusion may occur more rapidly in coronary arteries that have been surgically manipulated (42). Furthermore, the known placebo effect of surgery (43, 44) makes interpretation of chest pain relief difficult in the absence of more objective parameters such as prevention of death and prevention of recurrent myocardial infarction.

Several large clinical trials are now being conducted to compare medical management and surgical management of patients with coronary heart disease. The results should be forthcoming in the next decade. It would appear that coronary bypass surgery, at the very least, is a useful palliative procedure in patients with severe angina and is also indicated in patients with life-threatening left main coronary artery lesions. At present, the indications for its use in other clinical anatomic subgroups remain unclear.

SUMMARY

Coronary heart disease has progressed since the turn of the century from a relatively rare and largely unknown disorder to become the leading cause of death in the United States and other developed countries. An indictment of man's ecology (in the most general sense of the word) has been fashioned to explain this, based on epidemiologic, clinical, and laboratory evidence. It may well be that man, in his adjustment to modern life, has developed a number of bad habits, including smoking cigarettes, eating foods that contain excessive amounts of calories and saturated fats, neglecting physical activity, and participating in a highly stressful emotional environment. One or all of these items, as well as others, may soon be convicted of having a causal relationship to coronary atherosclerosis and thus to coronary heart disease with its immense burden of morbidity and mortality. A new emphasis on education and prevention in the traditional health care delivery system will be required before the findings of basic and clinical research can have an effect in helping to reduce coronary attack rates and death rates. The cost of such a venture, although substantial, is dwarfed by the cost of therapy for individuals with far-advanced lesions, not to mention the personal and social costs associated with premature coronary deaths.

Advances are occurring rapidly in the management of patients with angina pectoris and myocardial infarction. Improved therapies for patients with clinically manifested coronary artery disease necessarily have much more limited goals. Nevertheless, substantial improvements in the quality and quantity of life are possible with current therapy.

Primary prevention or, failing that, postponement of coronary heart disease is a most challenging and difficult problem, but at the same time it offers the reward, if it can be effected, of a major increase in life expectancy for the U.S. population and improved quality of life as well. It is a worthy goal and one that seems within reach.

REFERENCES

1. Monthly Vital Statistics Report, Provisional Statistics Annual Summary for the United States, 1974, Vol 23, No 13, May 30, 1975, pp 21–22

2. Coronary Heart Disease in Adults, United States 1960–1962. National Health Survey, Vital and Health Statistics, Series 11, No 10. US Department of Health, Education, and Welfare, Public Health Service, Washington, DC, 1965

3. Moniyama IM, Stamler J, Krueger DE: *Cardiovascular Diseases in the United States*. Harvard University Press, Cambridge, Mass, 1971, p 110

4. Ibid, pp 291–294

5. Primary prevention of the atherosclerotic diseases. *Circulation* 42:A-55, 1970

6. Keys A (ed): Coronary heart disease in seven countries. *Circulation* 41 (Suppl. I), 1970

7. Gordon T, Sorlie P, Kannel WB: Coronary Heart Disease, Atherothrombotic Brain Infarction, Intermittent Claudication—A Multivariate Analysis of Some Factors Related to Their Incidence: Framingham Study, 16-Year Follow-up. Section 27, US Government Printing Office, Washington, DC, 1971

8. Coronary Drug Project Research Group: The prognostic importance of the electrocardiogram

after myocardial infarction: Experience in the coronary drug project. *Ann Intern Med* 77:677, 1972

9. Coronary Drug Project Research Group: Prognostic importance of premature beats following myocardial infarction: Experience in the coronary drug project. *JAMA* 223:1116, 1973

10. Coronary Drug Project Research Group: Factors influencing long-term prognosis after recovery from myocardial infarction—Three year findings of the coronary drug project. *J Chronic Dis* 27:267, 1974

11. Burggraf GW, Parker JO: Prognosis in coronary artery disease: Angiographic, hemodynamic and clinical factors. *Circulation* 51:146, 1975

12. Humphries JO, Kuller L, Ross RS, et al: Natural history of ischemic heart disease in relation to arterio-graphic findings: A twelve year study of 224 patients. *Circulation* 49:489, 1974

13. Moberg CH, Webster JS, Sones FM Jr: Natural history of severe proximal coronary disease as defined by cineangiography (200 patients, 7 year follow-up). *Am J Cardiol* 29:282, 1972

14. McMillan GC: Development of arteriosclerosis. *Am J Cardiol* 31:542, 1973

15. Gordon T, Kannel WB: Coronary Risk Handbook. American Heart Association Monograph, 1973

16. Arteriosclerosis, Vol 2. A Report by the National Heart and Lung Institute Task Force on Arteriosclerosis. DHEW publication (NIH) 72-219. National Institutes of Health, Bethesda, 1971

17. Smoking and Health Report of the Advisory Committee to the Surgeon General of the Public Health Service. DHEW publication 1103, PHS No 110, US Department of Health, Education, and Welfare, Washington, DC, 1964

18. Doyle JT, Dawber TR, Kannel WB, et al: The relationship of cigarette smoking to coronary heart disease. The second report of the combined experiences of the Albany, New York, and Framingham, Mass. studies. *JAMA* 190:886, 1964

19. Auerbach O, Hammond EC, Garfinkel L: Smoking in relation to atherosclerosis of the coronary arteries. *N Engl J Med* 273:775, 1965

20. Strong JP, Richards ML, McGill IDJ, et al: On the association of cigarette smoking with coronary and aortic athero-sclerosis. *J Atheroscler Res* 10:303, 1969

21. Kannel WB, Doyle JT, McNamara PM, et al: Precursors of sudden coronary death. Factors related to the incidence of sudden death. *Circulation* 51:606, 1975

22. Kannell WB, Castelli WP, Gordon T, et al: Serum cholesterol, lipoproteins, and the risk of coronary heart disease. The Framingham study. *Ann Intern Med* 74:1, 1971

23. Frederickson DS, Levy RI: Familial hyperlipoproteinemia. In Stanbury JB, Weingaardon J, Frederickson DS (eds): *The Metabolic Basis of Inherited Diseases* (ed 3). McGraw-Hill, New York, 1971

24. Stone NJ, Levy RI, Frederickson DS, et al: Coronary artery disease in 116 kindred with familial type II hyperlipoproteinemia. *Circulation* 49:476, 1974

25. National Diet-Heart Study Research Group: The National Diet-Heart Study Final Report. *Circulation* 33(Suppl I), 1968

26. Levy RI, Frederickson DW, Shulman R, et al: Dietary and drug treatment of primary hyper-lipoproteinemia. *Ann Intern Med* 77:267, 1972

27. Veterans Administration Cooperative Study Group on Antihypertensive Agents: Effects of treatment on morbidity in hypertension: Results in patients with diastolic blood pressure averaging 115 through 129 mmHg. *JAMA* 202:1028, 1967

28. Veterans Administration Cooperative Study Group on Antihypertensive Agents: Effects of treatment on morbidity in hypertension: II. Results in patients with diastolic blood pressure averaging 90 through 114 mmHg. *JAMA* 213:1143, 1970

29. Mann JI, Vessey MP, Thorogood M, et al: Myocardial infarction in young women with special reference to oral contraceptive practice. *Br Med J* 2:241, 1975

30. Mann JI, Inman WHW: Oral contraceptives and death from myocardial infarction. *Br Med J* 2:245, 1975

31. White PD: The historical background of angina pectoris. *Mod Concepts Cardiovasc Dis* 43:109, 1974

32. Ross RS: Surgery in ischemic heart disease—Angina pectoris and myocardial infarction. *Disease-a-Month* July 1972, pp 1–31

33. Herrick JB: Clinical features of sudden obstruction of the coronary arteries. *JAMA* 59:2015, 1912

34. Froelicher VF, Yanowitz F, Thompson A, et al: The correlation of coronary angiography and the abnormal electrocardiographic response to maximal treadmill exericse in 76 asymptomatic men. *Circulation* 48:597, 1973

35. Borer JW, Brensike JF, Redwood DR, et al: Limitations of the electrocardiographic response to exercise in predicting coronary artery disease. *N Engl J Med* 283:367, 1975

36. Vlodaver Z, Frech R, Vantassel RA, et al: Correlation of the antemortem coronary arteriogram and postmortem specimen. *Circulation* 47:162, 1973

37. Grondin CM, Dyrda I, Pasternac A, et al: Discrepancies between cineangiographic and postmortem findings in patients with coronary artery disease and recent myocardial revascularization. *Circulation* 49:703, 1974

38. Schwartz JN, Kong Y, Hacket DB, et al: Comparison of angiographic and postmortem findings in patients with coronary artery disease. *Am J Cardiol* 36:174, 1975

39. Braunwald E: Protection and function of the ischemic myocardium. *Circulation* (Suppl: II) 52:1, 1975

40. Dunkman WB, Perloff JK, Kastor JA, et al: Medical perspectives in coronary artery survey—A caveat. *Ann Intern Med* 81:817, 1974

41. Mundth ED, Austen WG: Surgical measures for coronary heart disease. *N Engl J Med* 293:13–19, 75–80, 124–130, 1975

42. Griffith LSC, Achuff SC, Conti CR, et al: Changes in intrinsic coronary circulation and segmental ventricular motion after saphenous-vein coronary bypass graft surgery. *N Engl J Med* 288:589, 1973

43. Cobb LA, Thomas GI, Dillard DH, et al: An evaluation of internal-mammary-artery ligation by a double blind technique. *N Engl J Med* 260:1115, 1959

44. Dimond EG, Kittle CF, Crockett JE: Comparison of internal mammary artery ligation and sham operation for angina pectoris. *Am J Cardiol* 5:483, 1960

2

Alterations of Cardiac Structure and Function in Myocardial Infarction

Michael Lesch, M.D.

Edmund H. Sonnenblick, M.D.

Myocardial ischemia exists whenever the oxygen demands of the heart exceed the myocardial oxygen supply. Differential diagnosis of ischemic heart disease covers a broad range, encompassing situations such as anemia and hypertrophy, wherein the physiologic oxygen demands of the heart may exceed the ability of even a normal coronary circulation to provide adequate perfusion, as well as situations wherein intrinsic disease of the coronary arteries (arteritis, embolus, atherosclerosis) prevents any increased perfusion. In the present discussion the term *myocardial ischemia and infarction* will be used only in the context of coronary atherosclerosis in human disease or acute coronary ligation in experimental animals. Moreover, the issue whether infarction can occur in the absence of acute thrombosis will not be addressed in detail. The accrued evidence indicates that when infarction occurs in the absence of complete obstruction of a coronary artery, it occurs in the context of severe coronary atherosclerosis during a period of significant hemodynamic stress (hypotension, tachycardia), with subendocardial distribution. Since there is no evidence that the basic pathologic alterations that occur in acute subendocardial infarction are distinguishable in kind from those occurring with transmural infarction, these two forms of infarction will be considered as identical biologic phenomena that differ only in topography and extent.

The effects of myocardial ischemia on cardiac function and structure are variable; they depend to a significant degree on the duration and severity of the ischemic state. Transient degrees of minor ischemia can temporarily alter the contractile behavior of the affected zone of myocardium without resulting in permanent alterations in structure or function. In this situation the ischemic state induces transient physiologic dysfunction, but not cell death, since oxygenation is still adequate to maintain the basal degree of cellular metabolism required

19

to ensure viability but is inadequate to meet the needs for contractile element function. If the region of myocardium involved is large enough, the patient may experience transient symptoms of acute left ventricular failure, such as severe shortness of breath due to pulmonary congestion. A major unresolved problem concerns the mechanism by which mild transient ischemia causes contractile activity to cease. Laboratory experiments have demonstrated that ischemic tissue will neither conduct an action potential nor contract at a time when adenosine triphosphate stores are still well maintained. It is clear that an insufficient amount of high-energy phosphate is not the factor immediately responsible for the abnormality of contractile element function that characterizes ischemia. Therefore, abnormalities in energy use, rather than depletion of energy stores, are believed to be responsible for this dysfunction. Current thinking suggests that the calcium gating mechanism that regulates alternate activation and deactivation of the myosin-actin interaction and is responsible at the molecular level for contraction and relaxation at the tissue level is highly sensitive to ischemia and fails early in the course of ischemic insult.

In contrast to transient ischemia, severe permanent ischemia not only results in the deterioration of physiologic function that is characteristic of is-chemic muscle but also affects cellular homeostasis to such a degree that myo-cardial cell death invariably follows. These extreme examples of *mild transient ischemia* and *total permanent ischemia* serve to illustrate the variability of response that an ischemic event may induce. Precise information about the functional and structural consequences of prolonged and/or repetitive periods of intermediate degrees of ischemia is unavailable. In this chapter, therefore, discussion will be limited to description of the structural and functional abnormalities resulting from an ischemic episode of sufficient severity to induce tissue necrosis.

PATHOLOGY OF ACUTE MYOCARDIAL INFARCTION

Site of Infarction

Myocardial infarction is to a great extent a disease of the left ventricle and interventricular septum. The infarct may be transmural or subendocardial, extensive or focal, limited to the distribution of a single coronary vessel or involving the distribution of multiple vessels, depending on the interplay of factors such as the degree of coronary atherosclerosis, the site or sites of coro-nary atherosclerosis, the rapidity with which the precipitating event develops and the status of the collateral circulation. Whenever the coronary blood supply becomes limited, the greatest decrease occurs in the subendocardial area, as compared with the more superficial layers of the ventricular wall. The greatest degree of myocardial infarction is also found in the subendocardial region, with extension toward the epicardium.

Until recently, infarction of the right ventricle was believed to be distinctly unusual. Recent studies have demonstrated that the right ventricle may become infarcted when right coronary artery occlusion results in extensive infarction of the posterior wall involving the posterior aspect of the interventricular septum. Some investigators have contended that the incidence of right ventricular in-farction may be even higher than that estimated from autopsy studies, since no specific electrocardiographic findings for right ventricular infarction have been identified, and thus minor degrees of right ventricular infarction may go unnoticed.

It has been estimated that atrial infarction occurs in 15–20% of patients with myocardial infarction. At one time the right atrium was believed to be the exclusive site of atrial infarction, since it was postulated that the thin-walled left atrium could obtain adequate oxygenation to prevent cell death by diffusion from oxygenated left atrial blood. However, recent pathologic studies have indicated that either the left or right atrium may be the site of infarction. Although electrocardiographic criteria for the diagnosis of atrial infarction exist, autopsy studies have clearly demonstrated that the electrocardiogram does not have sufficient sensitivity to yield an accurate assessment of the incidence of atrial infarction.

Gross Pathologic Changes

Myocardial ischemia that is sudden in onset, severe in degree, and more than 15–30 min in duration leads to myocardial necrosis. It is not known if a lesser degree of ischemia that is gradual in onset and of longer duration will result in myocardial cell death, nor is it known if the type of cell death so produced is identical to that created by acute ischemia. Consequently the description of gross pathologic changes contained herein relates only to infarction resulting from acute ischemia, as defined in autopsy studies of patients dying following infarction or in animal studies using coronary ligation as the means to create infarction.

Little or no gross anatomic change is noted within the first 24 hr following the acute episode, although the infarcted area may be somewhat pale and swollen as compared to adjacent normal tissue. By the second day the infarcted myocardium has a purple color and appears hemorrhagic, even though hemorrhage is not usually demonstrable. Serofibrinous exudate is noted at this time on the pericardial surface if the infarction is transmural and extends to the epicardium. The hemorrhagic appearance disappears within 48 hr, and by the third or fourth day the infarcted area assumes a grayish white color that may be outlined by a reddish band at the periphery.

As the acute inflammatory stage (0–4 days) gradually evolves into the phase of early healing (8–12 days), the infarcted area loses volume and appears depressed as thinning of the infarct becomes prominent. By 2 weeks, formation of scar tissue begins, and the infarcted area is gradually replaced by a hard, firm collagenous scar in the following weeks. The time required for this final stage of healing is variable, depending primarily on the size of the infarct. Small infarcts may be completely healed by 3 weeks, whereas larger infarcts take 6 weeks or longer to complete the healing process. As scar tissue replaces muscle and the scar contracts, thinning of the infarcted area becomes more apparent.

Microscopic Pathologic Changes

Acutely infarcted myocardium retains a normal histologic appearance for approximately 12–18 hr following the onset of acute ischemia. At this point, capillary dilatation, congestion, and eosinophilic changes in the muscle fibers become apparent, and the beginning of a leukocytic infiltrate can be discerned.

Nuclei of the muscle cells become pyknotic at this time, somewhat before a similar process is noted in the nuclei of the epithelial and connective tissue cells. By 24–36 hr the process of leukocyte infiltration into the infarct has been completed, and this peak inflammatory response is characterized by fragmentation of fibers, granular and hyaline degeneration, and gross uneven staining of myofibers. The cross-striations of the muscle fibers become blurred but do not disappear as the process of ischemic necrosis progresses. The period from 4 to 8 days is distinguished by the gradual disappearance of the inflammatory reaction (i.e., polymorphonuclear cells) as muscle breakdown continues and invading macrophages remove necrotic muscle. At the end of the early acute inflammatory stage (6–8 days) a healing process at the edge of the infarct becomes apparent as fibroblasts and capillaries begin to proliferate. The subsequent course of histologic healing features gradual removal of the entire mass of infarcted muscle by macrophages and slow replacement of this tissue with granulation tissue and collagen. The infarcted muscle becomes friable during this phase in proportion to the degree to which transudated fluid from neighboring vessels dissects into the degenerating muscle. Remnants of necrotic muscle remain visible, and pigment granules that stain positively for iron are noted both within and outside the macrophages. These granules presumably represent old hemorrhage. If the epicardium has been involved and pericarditis has resulted from the infarct, the acute pericardial reaction will by 2–3 weeks have evolved into fibrotic epicardial plaques.

Since myocardial infarcts heal by the process of fibroblastic proliferation and collagen formation, the resultant scar has less volume than the muscle it replaces. This leads to thinning of the ventricular wall. If, as occasionally occurs, the infarct scar is infiltrated with adipose tissue, the tensile strength of the scar may be reduced. Scar formation is known to be due to the process of protein (collagen) synthesis, since in experimental animals inhibition of protein synthesis results in inadequate scar formation.

The endocardial surface of a healed infarct will reveal a grayish white rindlike lining over the infarcted area. This is frequently interpreted as being part of the infarct, but in reality it is composed primarily of an organizing mural thrombus. It is important to note that immediately subjacent to the endocardial surface there is usually a zone of viable intact myocardial cells varying from 2 to 15 cells in depth. It is believed that the selective sparing of these subendocardial cells is due to diffusion of oxygen from oxygenated blood within the left ventricular cavity.

Ultrastructural Pathologic Changes

Changes in myocardial ultrastructure in the first hours following acute infarction in the human have not been defined, for obvious reasons. Moreover, the usefulness of electron microscopy to study the process of acute infarction in the postmortem state is questionable, since ultrastructural alterations produced by postmortem autolysis cannot be distinguished from those due to the infarct. Therefore all information regarding ultrastructural changes in acute myocardial ischemia has come from animal studies, in which the tissue can be fixed immediately.

Ultrastructural changes in myocardial tissue following permanent occlusion of a coronary artery have been studied in the rabbit, dog, cat, and rat. The changes described in all four species are identical, and they follow similar time courses. Thus it seems reasonable to assume that similar abnormalities occur in human tissue. Ultrastructural changes can be noted as early as 5 min following occlusion; they consist of loss of glycogen granulation and mild intracellular edema. By 15 min, changes in the muscle nuclei, particularly clumping of chromatin at the periphery of the nucleus and rarefaction of the central areas, may be noted. Between 15 min and 45 min intracellular edema increases, and prominent swelling of mitochondria, sarcoplasmic reticulum, and the Golgi complex becomes apparent. During this period the loss of glycogen continues such that by 45 min there is total depletion of intracardiac glycogen granules. At 4 hr following occlusion, a time at which there still is no histologic change noted by conventional light microscopy, the mitochondria are diffusely damaged, and focal calcium deposits are noted within the mitochondrial spaces. At this point the sarcolemma is fragmented, and intercalated disks begin to separate.

It is interesting that the myofibrils are the structures most resistant to acute occlusion, retaining normal ultrastructural patterns for many hours. At 1–2 hr following occlusion the only change noted in myofibrillar structure is a mild degree of edema separating adjacent filaments. Over a period of several hours the fibers show gradual dissolution, but changes in the nuclei and mitochondria occur well before any significant abnormality of the myofilaments can be defined.

Capillary endothelial cells of the coronary circulation are extremely susceptible to coronary occlusion and show significant edema within 20–30 min. Within hours the capillary endothelial cells are totally fragmented, and all ultrastructural architectural landmarks of these cells are abolished.

In contrast to the changes that have been described as characteristic of the central infarct area, changes in muscle cells at the periphery of the infarct are extremely variable. Between 24 and 48 hr following infarction, electron-dense material may be seen within the lumina of the T tubules at the periphery. Unusually small mitochondria may be noted, as well as mitochondria with cristae arranged in a circular pattern, cisterns with rough-surfaced endoplasmic reticulum, increased glycogen, free ribosomes, and lipid droplets. These changes are believed to be indicative of cellular regeneration. Between 4 and 7 days, dilatation of the T system, abnormal Z bands, myofilamentous lysis, and disorganization of newly formed myofilaments have been noted. Between 1 and 4 weeks the process of fibrotic replacement of necrotic material continues, and muscle cells at the periphery of the infarct that have survived show degenerative changes characterized by granularity of sarcoplasm, loss of myofibrils, and irregularity in arrangement of sarcoplasmic reticulum.

FUNCTIONAL COMPLICATIONS OF ACUTE MYOCARDIAL INFARCTION

The impairment of cardiac function that results from a single episode of myocardial infarction is variable in regard to both the degree of impairment and the temporal pattern in which the functional changes evolve.

Major factors that interact to define the degree of physiologic impairment resulting from an infarct include the following:

- the amount of muscle necrosis resulting from the acute episode
- the amount of preexisting necrosis and/or scar tissue from previous infarctions
- the anatomic site or sites of the infarction within the ventricle
- the degree of residual ischemic dysfunction persisting in myocardium that survives the acute episode but that remains partially ischemic following completion of the healing process
- the extent of atherosclerotic disease in the remainder of the coronary circulation

The impairment of cardiac function resulting from an episode of acute myocardial infarction is variable with time, evolving over the course of the illness. Characteristically and most commonly, peak dysfunction is noted in the first days after the acute episode, with gradual improvement occurring over the ensuing weeks. Traditionally, acute dysfunction (i.e., congestive heart failure, pump failure) has been ascribed to a total lack of contractile function in areas of myocardium rendered necrotic and varying degrees of contractile insufficiency in the zones of myocardium that border the necrotic center of the infarct and are marginally ischemic but viable. Similarly, the improvement in cardiac function that characterizes the healing phase of acute infarction has been ascribed to replacement of necrotic myocardium by firm scar tissue and improved perfusion of marginally ischemic areas.

Although there is no doubt that this theory is in part correct, various laboratories have recently reported alterations in metabolism in areas of myocardium remote from the infarct zone. These data suggest that a second mechanism for the depression of contractile function commonly seen in the acute phase may relate to a degree of global contractile-element failure that cannot be attributed directly to vascular insufficiency and that at this time remains unexplained. Thus the improvement in cardiac performance noted over the course of convalescence presumably relates not only to replacement of necrotic material by scar tissue and improved perfusion of ischemic areas but also to recovery of global myocardial function.

Whereas gradual improvement in ventricular function is most commonly seen following infarction, deterioration in pump function may occur, depending on the interaction of the following variables:

- the total mass of the dysfunctional yet viable ischemic tissue bordering the necrotic infarct center and the ultimate fate of this marginal tissue
- the stability of the vascular and/or hemodynamic process that initiated the acute episode, i.e., the extent of the infarct as initially defined may increase if the vascular process or hemodynamic stress (tachycardia, shock) initially responsible for the episode recurs

Extent of Necrosis

Clinicopathologic correlations have demonstrated that survival is not possible if more than 40% of the left ventricular myocardium is infarcted. Conversely, patients in whom only 5% of the left ventricular mass is infarcted have no apparent limitation in cardiac function as defined clinically, and they exhibit minimal or no abnormality of cardiac function when sophisticated catheterization and angiographic techniques are employed. The degree to which cardiac function is compromised by intermediate percentages of infarction is variable, depending in part on the site of the infarct (*vide infra*), the adequacy of the healing process, and the degree of preexisting scar.

Although pump function as determined hemodynamically in terms of cardiac output and filling pressure may show no alteration following infarction, angiographic techniques have proved to be more sensitive in defining subtle abnormalities. Gorlin and associates first noted that varying degrees of abnormal segmental wall motion can be demonstrated with ventriculography in patients with coronary disease. These investigators demonstrated that a spectrum of disorders of myocardial wall motion can be defined as to type and extent by quantitatively analyzing the patterns of wall motion of various segments of the left ventricle. Presumably the spectrum of wall motion abnormality so defined is to some degree related to the extent of ischemic dysfunction at the site. The spectrum includes hypokinesis, akinesis, dyskinesis, and ventricular aneurysm. In a hypokinetic myocardial segment, contractile activity is present, although to a significantly decreased degree. The akinetic segment is characterized by a lack of systolic contraction, but it does not bulge paradoxically during systole. A dyskinetic segment fails to contract during systole and bulges paradoxically during systole, but it does not extend beyond the border of the cardiac silhouette during diastole. In ventricular aneurysm there is thinning of the wall, and bulging of the myocardium can be noted in both systole and diastole. Clearly, if an infarct results in a hypokinetic segment, the resultant degree of cardiac dysfunction will be significantly less than if the same infarct produces a totally akinetic segment. In a similar manner a dyskinetic segment will compromise ventricular function to a greater degree than will an akinetic segment, since some of the force of ventricular contractile effort will be dissipated by the expanding dyskinetic segment. The degree of ventricular compromise caused by an aneurysm is greater than that caused by the other wall motion abnormalities; not only is the affected segment not contributing to effective ventricular systole, but it is also compromising cardiac output by functioning as an expansile reservoir into which blood may be ejected in a retrograde fashion. When function is lost in one region of the ventricular wall, compensatory hypertrophy occurs in remaining areas, and this may help sustain overall pump function.

Characteristic clinical and laboratory findings have been described in patients with ventricular aneurysm, and descriptions of these findings are available in standard textbooks. Whether aneurysm formation following infarction is related to activity, medications, or other parameters over which the physician has control is a controversial issue. At present there exist no data suggesting that aneurysm formation may be stimulated or retarded by any available therapeutic modality, and the reasons why infarction progresses to aneurysm in some patients but not in others remain obscure. Resection of ventricular aneurysm is a commonly performed cardiac surgical procedure that has gained wide acceptance in recent years. Results with this procedure are extremely encouraging, and reviews of the medical and surgical considerations relating to aneurysm resection are included in all standard textbooks on cardiology.

Discussion to this point has focused on the concept of the extent of necrosis, referring particularly to the percentage of total ventricular mass involved. An associated but distinctly separate consideration relates to the intensity of necrosis at a given site. Cardiac rupture is a rare complication of acute myocardial infarction that occurs in about 8% of fatal infarcts. The pathologic and molecular factors that determine whether the necrotic process at a given site will be so great as to result in rupture are incompletely defined, although clinically the characteristic picture is that of an elderly hypertensive patient with an extensive anterior wall infarct in whom rupture of the apex of the left ventricle occurs on the fourth or fifth day. If the site of rupture is the ventricular septum, death is not immediate as it is in the case of rupture of the free ventricular wall. Although mortality in patients with septal rupture is high, antemortem diagnosis followed by supportive therapy with cardiac assist devices and definitive surgical repair has been reported in a large number of patients. Clinically, rupture of the ventricular septum is characterized by the abrupt onset of congestive failure associated with a harsh systolic murmur. The diagnosis can be confirmed at the bedside with balloon catheterization of the right heart if an oxygen step-up at the ventricular level can be documented.

Site of Necrosis

The site at which an infarct occurs may affect the degree of functional impairment resulting from the ischemic event by numerous mechanisms.

Combined angiographic and hemodynamic evaluation of patients in either the acute or chronic stage of myocardial infarction suggests that the contribution of the anterior wall of the left ventricle to overall contractile effort of this chamber is proportionately greater than that of the inferior wall. These observations are consonant with clinical studies indicating that a more favorable prognosis is associated with infarction of the inferior wall. Thus, given the same degree and extent of infarction, less ventricular dysfunction will result from an inferior wall process than from an anterior wall process.

When either the papillary muscles or those portions of the free left ventricular wall that by geometric considerations are requisite for normal papillary muscle and mitral valve function are the sites of infarction, mitral insufficiency will result. The clinical presentation varies: on the one hand there is the asymptomatic patient who exhibits only a transient murmur associated with intermittent ischemic papillary muscle dysfunction; on the other hand there is the patient with severe mitral insufficiency and acute pulmonary edema due to infarction and/or rupture of the papillary muscle. Papillary muscle rupture is uniformly fatal; it is found at autopsy in 1% of patients dying from acute myocardial infarction. In contrast, even severe degrees of acute papillary muscle dysfunction may be compatible with life; these are amenable to treatment with vasodilator drugs, cardiac assist devices, and surgical replacement of the mitral valve. The vascular supply to the papillary muscles is identical to the vascular supply to the subendocardium, and thus this portion of the mitral apparatus is particularly susceptible to ischemia. For this reason it is not surprising that some degree of papillary muscle fibrosis is found in 80% of hearts obtained at autopsy from patients who died from or with coronary artery disease.

The clinical findings with papillary muscle dysfunction consist primarily of congestive heart failure, although the physical findings are distinctly variable and do not mimic those of classic rheumatic mitral regurgitation. Most prominently, acute failure may ensue with pulmonary edema. Sinus rhythm is generally maintained. The degree of mitral regurgitation varies with time and decreases whenever cardiac volume is reduced by whatever means.

If the site of ischemia involves the specialized conduction system, varying degrees of heart block and/or intraventricular conduction deficit may result. Classically, inferior wall infarction causes *transient* ischemic dysfunction of the atrioventricular (A-V) node but does not damage the bundle of His or the right or left bundle branches. Consequently, inferior wall infarction may be associated with Wenckebach-type second-degree heart block or complete heart block with narrow QRS complexes (i.e., pacemaker site in the bundle of His). These conduction abnormalities usually are transient and are not indicative of widespread necrosis, but rather of focal ischemia at the A-V node. In contrast, heart block resulting from an anteroseptal infarction indicates diffuse necrosis, since the block can result from a septal infarct only if the right and left bundle branches are simultaneously involved. The bundle of His is a short structure localized to the infranodal position of the interventricular septum that divides to form the right and left bundle branches. The three divisions of the conduction system radiate in different directions, so that at this junction the conduction system is transformed from a localized structure in and around the A-V node to a diffuse structure coursing through various myocardial segments. Thus when a septal infarct causes heart block, this anatomic fact indicates that the necrosis must be diffuse. The left bundle branch breaks down into a network of Purkinje fibers as it extends to more peripheral sites in the ventricle. Anatomically, the Purkinje fibers are endocardial in position, and they usually survive ischemic insult despite infarction of the overlying myocardium. As was noted previously, this is believed to be related to diffusion of oxygen from intracavitary blood. It has been postulated, but not proved, that the juxtaposition of surviving Purkinje fibers adjacent to necrotic or scarred myocardium may be of particular importance in the pathogenesis of ventricular arrhythmias associated with coronary artery disease.

It is believed that in some instances atrial arrhythmias result from atrial infarction. The present consensus is that atrial arrhythmias in the context of acute myocardial infarction may arise from at least three mechanisms: atrial infarction, atrial irritation secondary to pericarditis, or acute atrial distension due to left ventricular failure. All three mechanisms have been demonstrated, and although some atrial arrhythmias may be due to atrial infarction, a one-to-one cause-and-effect association has not been proved.

SUMMARY

Alterations of cardiac structure and function that occur consequent to acute myocardial infarction have been reviewed so as to permit correlation of structure–function relationships. Functional impairment has been shown to be variable in degree over time as the infarction process and then the healing process evolve, and it has been shown to be related to the site, extent, and intensity of myocardial necrosis. Special situations such as mitral insufficiency, heart block, etc., wherein a specific functional defect results from a particular anatomic correlation, have been reviewed. The manner in which other variables may exacerbate (hypotension, tachycardia) or ameliorate (collaterals) the evolutionary pattern of functional impairment has been considered.

REFERENCES

1. Braunwald E: *The Myocardium: Failure and Infarction.* Hospital Practice Publishing, New York, 1974
2. Fowler NO (ed): Treatment of acute myocardial infarction. In: *Cardiac Diagnosis and Treatment* (ed 2). Harper & Row, New York, 1976, p 704
3. Ferrans UJ, Roberts WC: Myocardial ultrastructure in acute and chronic hypoxia. *Cardiology* 56:144, 1971/72
4. Heggtueit HA: Morphological alterations in the ischemic heart. *Cardiology* 56:284, 1971/72
5. Titus JL: Pathology of coronary heart disease. In Ziest AN (ed): *Cardiovascular Clinics Series I, Vol 1, Coronary Heart Disease.* FA Davis, Philadelphia, 1969

3
Guidelines to Patient Management

Ezra A. Amsterdam, M.D.

Dean T. Mason, M.D.

The toll of coronary heart disease (CHD) in our society is immense. In its various presentations it is the leading cause of death and disability in this country. The annual incidence of myocardial infarction (MI) in the United States is approximately 1.4 million cases, and the mortality rate is over 50%. Many of the survivors either are incapacitated or are regarded as so and thus are lost as active, contributing members of society. Angina pectoris, another form of CHD that may occur with or without previous infarction, also significantly impairs function in a large number of patients. Sudden coronary death is the most dramatic and tragic manifestation of CHD, and is frequent, accounting for 15–20% of the total CHD mortality. Moreover, CHD strikes a large proportion of its victims in their most productive years and its occurrence under the age of 50 years is now exceedingly common.

The sequelae of MI are extensive and are consequences of the physiologic and psychologic impact of the disease. They include impairment of myocardial function with its associated signs and symptoms, general physical deconditioning, and significant psychologic symptoms. These problems can result in loss of physical working capacity, curtailment of leisure-time activities, depressed emotional outlook, and disruption of family members' roles and interpersonal relationships. Furthermore, the direct and indirect economic costs of the disease are estimated to be as high as $30 billion annually.

RATIONALE OF POST-MI REHABILITATION

Because modern methods of intensive coronary care have reduced hospital mortality resulting from acute MI, increasing attention is being directed to the

Supported in part by research program project grant HL-14780 from the National Heart and Lung Institute, National Institutes of Health, Bethesda, Maryland, and by research grants from California chapters of the American Heart Association.

29

rehabilitation of survivors of this disease in order to prevent, reverse, or diminish its long-term clinical consequences. Rehabilitation of the postinfarction patient entails a comprehensive longitudinal approach to management, with the goal of restoring and maintaining optimal physical, psychologic, occupational, social, and recreational status. It is based on the recognition that 70% or more of infarct survivors have sufficient cardiac reserve to resume their previous occupational activities and that general physical deconditioning and psychologic symptoms, including depression and impoverished self-image, are significant factors in the disability of many postinfarction patients. Rehabilitation is further predicated on the premise that adequate functional performance and amelioration of the aforementioned problems frequently can be attained by rational systematic management of the post-MI patient.

In order to achieve its broad goals the comprehensive rehabilitation effort must include complete medical evaluation and treatment, assessment of functional and work capacity, health and vocational counseling, modification of coronary risk factors, and a program of exercise. When appropriate, special procedures such as cardiac catheterization and angiography are employed, and in some cases cardiac surgery may be indicated. It should be noted that although cardiac rehabilitation programs have been used chiefly for postinfarction patients, the principles and methods are applicable to patients with angina pectoris and to patients after coronary artery bypass surgery.

Heterogeneity of MI Population

It is important to recognize that although the populations of patients with CHD and MI have in common generally similar anatomic (coronary artery disease) and pathophysiologic (myocardial ischemia and necrosis) derangements, they are heterogeneous with regard to specific qualitative and quantitative aspects of their cardiac impairment, such as type and extent of coronary and myocardial lesions (Figs. 1 and 2). These latter factors are of the utmost importance in regard to clinical course, prognosis, and the patient's potential to respond favorably to rehabilitative efforts. For example, the long-term prognosis is likely to be significantly different in two 45-year-old men who have recovered uneventfully from inferior wall MI if one has only single-vessel right coronary artery disease and the other has severe three-vessel coronary disease. The difference in outlook for the two patients is based on data that have consistently demonstrated that the number of significantly diseased coronary arteries is a major determinant of long-term survival. The heterogeneity of patients with coronary artery disease with respect to the number of coronary arteries involved is demonstrated in Figure 2. The patient's capacity to undertake the exercise training component of a rehabilitation program is limited or nil if there is persistent postinfarction cardiac failure, whereas there is much greater capacity in a patient with uncomplicated MI and no overt dysfunction (Fig. 1).

On the basis of information of the foregoing type it has been determined that a cardinal tenet in the approach to the post-MI patient must be individualization of management based on thorough evaluation. The latter will involve, in addition to history and physical examination, noninvasive techniques for cardiac evaluation that provide more sensitive and precise assessment and, in selected

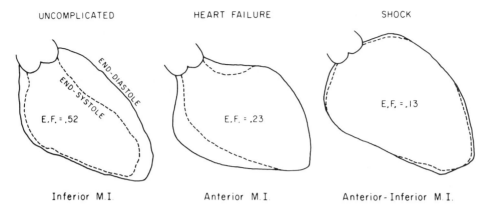

UNCOMPLICATED   HEART FAILURE   SHOCK

Inferior M.I.   Anterior M.I.   Anterior-Inferior M.I.

Figure 1. Differing degrees of left ventricular damage as indicated by diagrams of left ventricular angiograms obtained in 3 patients during acute MI (right anterior oblique position). The inferior infarction demonstrates inferior wall hypokinesis and is clinically uncomplicated. Heart failure is associated with extensive anterior wall akinesis in the anterior infarction. The anterior-inferior infarction is complicated by shock resulting from severe diffuse impairment of ventricular function. Ejection fraction (E.F.), the fraction of the left ventricular end-diastolic volume ejected during each beat, decreases with increasing involvement of left ventricular myocardium.

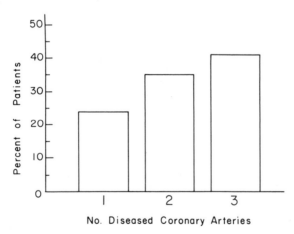

Figure 2. Extent of coronary artery disease in 382 patients with clinical ischemic heart disease evaluated by coronary angiography at the University of California, Davis, School of Medicine.

patients, definitive studies such as cardiac catheterization and coronary angiography.

CLINICAL COURSE OF MI

Complications and Management

Both short-term management and long-term management of the patient with MI are based on an understanding of the clinical course and complications of the disease, modalities of therapy, and spectrum of outcome. Complications of MI involve the heart and peripheral organs. Among the important clinical sequelae are cardiac arrhythmias, heart failure, cardiogenic shock, mitral regurgitation, ventricular aneurysm, myocardial rupture, and thromboembolism either originating as a mural thrombus in the left ventricle that embolizes to a remote artery or originating as a peripheral vein thrombus that embolizes to the pulmonary arterial bed.

Arrhythmias

The most common arrhythmias are ventricular ectopic beats. If these are frequent ($\geq$ 6 beats/min), coupled, or multiform or if they impinge on a preceding T wave, the patient should receive therapy with intravenous lidocaine. Ventricular ectopic beats occur in up to 90% of patients in the first 3–5 days in the course of MI. When they are of the primary type (i.e., unassociated with significant impairment of cardiac pump performance) they usually respond readily to lidocaine. Intravenous or oral procainamide and oral quinidine are the most commonly effective agents when lidocaine therapy fails. Sustained ventricular tachycardia and fibrillation are unusual after suppression of ventricular ectopic beats and in the absence of cardiac pump dysfunction. These are lethal arrhythmias, and they usually require immediate reversion by external direct-current countershock and institution of cardiac resuscitative efforts until resumption of normal cardiorespiratory function. In most MI patients ventricular arrhythmias are transient, and no long-term therapy is required. Opinions differ regarding the utility of long-term prophylactic antiarrhythmic therapy after recovery from cardiac arrest without subsequent ventricular ectopy.

The most important bradyarrhythmia complicating acute MI is complete heart block, which occurs in less than 10% of patients. It is most common in inferior wall infarction, in which it is usually due to reversible ischemia of the atrioventricular node; there is resumption of normal conduction in 2–7 days in all but rare instances. A temporary cardiac pacemaker is indicated during the period of heart block; it should be withdrawn after normal, stable conduction recurs. In contrast to the foregoing situation, complete heart block in anterior infarction is most commonly associated with extensive left ventricular damage that involves the two fascicles of the left bundle. This syndrome is usually fatal because of cardiogenic shock; cardiac pacing, although recommended, is usually of no avail. The uncommon survivor of this syndrome may require a permanent cardiac pacemaker.

Cardiac Failure

Cardiac failure of some degree occurs in approximately 50% of MI patients who reach the hospital, and in 15–25% it consists of severe pump dysfunction or shock. The hemodynamic consequences of acute MI are most closely related to the extent of left ventricular damage (Fig. 1). Minimal left ventricular damage is typically unassociated with significant hemodynamic consequences. Cardiac failure occurs when 20% of left ventricular myocardium is destroyed; shock is the result of damage to at least 40%, and usually more, of the left ventricle. Mild heart failure manifested only by basilar rales may require only bed rest and sodium restriction or addition of a diuretic. More severe dysfunction, including pulmonary edema, requires more intensive treatment, which may include morphine, oxygen, diuretics, digitalis, vasodilators, rotating tourniquets, and venesection. Cardiogenic shock due to MI is a dread syndrome with a mortality that approaches 100% when it is treated with conventional medical therapy (vasopressor agents). Mechanical circulatory assist devices, acute diagnostic angiography, and emergency surgery to repair the mechanical cardiac defects producing the shock syndrome in MI have resulted in some dramatic successes in the few centers where these methods are available. However, because of the massive left ventricular damage underlying shock in MI, no major reduction in its mortality rate appears likely at this time. It is important to exclude, as the basis for MI shock, nonmyocardial causes such as hypovolemia, arrhythmias, hypoxia, and severe pain, since their presence may provoke, and their correction may reverse, this syndrome when it is unassociated with extensive myocardial damage. Unfortunately, the foregoing factors are unusual causes of shock in MI.

Mitral Regurgitation
Mitral regurgitation develops in more than 50% of patients during the first 5 days of MI. However, it is of hemodynamic significance in only a minority, and it is transient in one-third, disappearing with recovery. Mitral regurgitation is usually caused by papillary muscle dysfunction due to ischemia or infarction; ventricular dilatation may also contribute to valve dysfunction. Major mitral regurgitation may be an important factor in severe cardiac failure or shock in MI.

Left Ventricular Aneurysm
Left ventricular aneurysm, or a large hypofunctioning or nonfunctioning segment of left ventricular myocardium, may occur in the area of infarction. If it is of sufficient extent, cardiac output may be decreased, with resultant left ventricular failure. Left ventricular aneurysms also may be associated with serious ventricular arrhythmias and with mural thrombi that can embolize to peripheral organs. These complications may occur acutely or in the chronic post-MI phase. Severe cardiac failure, life-threatening arrhythmias, and emboli associated with ventricular aneurysm that are unresponsive to conservative therapy are indications to consider surgical excision of the aneurysm.

Rupture of Myocardium
Rupture of the myocardium is an unusual and life-threatening complication of MI that has its highest incidence in the first week. It may involve the interventricular septum, papillary muscle, or free left ventricular wall. The latter two situations are usually rapidly fatal. Emergency repair of septal perforation during acute MI has recently been accomplished, but it is an extremely high risk procedure in this setting. Therefore treatment should be conservative if the patient can be adequately maintained thereby; surgery should be delayed, if possible, until conditions are more nearly optimal for operative intervention.

Venous Thrombi and Pulmonary Emboli
Venous thrombi and consequent pulmonary emboli may arise from several factors, including prolonged bed rest and immobility, a low-flow state due to

Table 1. Determinants of Myocardial Oxygen Consumption

Major	*Minor*
Heart rate	External work (load × shortening)
Intramyocardial tension	Activation energy
Ventricular systolic pressure	Basal energy
Ventricular volume	
Myocardial contractility	

cardiac failure, and venous disease and hypercoagulability. Measures for preventing thromboembolism include the following: early ambulation for patients with uncomplicated MI, leg exercises, supportive hose, and use of low-dose heparin for patients requiring prolonged bed rest.

Limitation of MI Size

There has recently been much interest in reducing ischemia and limiting myocardial damage in acute MI. In this regard, a rational approach to treatment of acute MI or ischemic heart disease in general is to attempt to decrease myocardial oxygen requirements to an optimal level; this favors an improved balance between myocardial oxygen supply and demand, and it is compatible with adequate cardiac pump performance to satisfy systemic circulatory requirements. Myocardial oxygen demand can be manipulated by alteration of its major determinants: heart rate, blood pressure, ventricular volume, and contractility (Table 1). Excessive elevation of any of these factors during acute MI would be a reasonable indication for its attenuation. For example, tachycardia of 120 beats/min unassociated with fever, cardiac failure, or hypovolemia would be an indication for sedation or β-adrenergic blockade in order to reduce the unnecessary myocardial oxygen cost of this disturbance, which has the potential to increase ischemia and necrosis. This approach should be employed with the utmost care, and attention must be paid to identifying and treating reversible causes of derangements such as tachycardia and hypertension before employing potent pharmacologic agents with the potential to produce cardiac failure, hypotension, and other complications. Furthermore, data are insufficient at present to advocate the use of drugs such as the nitrates for limitation of infarct size in the absence of any hemodynamic indications for their application.

BASIS FOR INDIVIDUAL PATIENT ASSESSMENT

It is important to emphasize again, in regard to the patient's potential for cardiac rehabilitation, that the effects of any of the previously mentioned complications of MI must be assessed in the individual patient. Whereas the more serious sequelae are most likely to result in major and permanent impairment of cardiac function, this is not a consistent occurrence; many of the complications of acute MI in the hospitalized patient are transient and are followed by significant recovery.

The variable recovery of function after MI can be understood from an examination of the pathophysiology of infarcted myocardium, which involves both irreversibly damaged and reversibly damaged tissue. To the extent that the early clinical consequences are related to the latter, significant structural repair, recovery of physiologic function, and subsidence of clinical abnormalities may result. Thus, as was noted previously, ventricular ectopic beats, although potentially serious, usually are readily managed and are transient. Mild cardiac failure during the acute phase of MI frequently resolves after 1–2 weeks. Furthermore, drugs such as antiarrhythmic agents, digitalis, diuretics, and anticoagulants that are necessary during the hospital phase of MI can in many cases be discontinued after function improves. On the other hand, the presence of severe cardiac failure or cardiogenic shock is usually indicative of extensive and permanent left ventricular damage. In the uncommon patient who recovers from cardiogenic shock, considerable impairment of cardiac performance would be anticipated, as well as a regimen of maintenance cardiac drugs. Similarly, a history of multiple infarctions suggests a reduction in cardiac reserve, although this factor requires assessment by both clinical evaluation and objective methods, which will be discussed later.

Contrary to prevalent belief, angina is frequent in postinfarction patients. Angina that is present prior to MI usually is not abolished after infarction; when angina is not present prior to MI, it often appears thereafter. Thus in planning for management of the post-MI patient, it should not necessarily be anticipated that angina will be absent. When angina does disappear after MI, it is frequently in association with the onset of cardiac failure related to extensive myocardial scarring and ventricular dilatation. This represents a late phase in the natural history of the patient's ischemic heart disease.

Although patients with MI differ according to the individual clinical, physiologic, and anatomic aspects of their disease, certain generalizations can be made. Thus in a population of MI patients, 75% or more will have severe multivessel coronary artery disease, and only 25% or fewer will have single-vessel disease (Fig. 2). Although a very general assessment of ventricular function can be made on the basis of clinical history and physical examination, this approach is not sufficiently precise for rational management and rehabilitation. Other aspects of the patient's status, such as functional capacity, myocardial ischemic threshold, and presence of occult ventricular ectopy, are important components of the evaluation, and they merit definitive assessment. Therefore a systematic approach involving simple and inexpensive methods as well as more complex techniques must be employed in evaluating the patient in order to determine the appropriate management. These may be applied either during or after hospitalization for MI, as indicated by the condition of the patient, the requirements of the test, the reasons for performing it, and the use to which the results will be put in management of the patient.

METHODS OF EVALUATION

Important information about the post-MI patient is gained from a variety of techniques that range from simple to very sophisticated (Table 2). Of primary

Table 2. Special Methods of Cardiac Evaluation in Assessment of the Postinfarction Patient

---

Ambulatory electrocardiographic monitoring
  Presence of arrhythmias and their relation to daily activities, including sleeping and waking

Echocardiography
  Cardiac valve function, chamber size, thickness and motion of posterior wall and septum of left ventricle, anatomy of thoracic aorta

Exercise testing
  Functional capacity, ischemic threshold, relation of arrhythmias to activity level, blood pressure response

Intracardiac electrography
  His bundle electrography for function of cardiac conduction system (including atrioventricular and intraventricular conduction), sinus node function

Nuclear cardiology
  Gated blood pool scan for determination of left and right ventricular wall motion, ejection fraction, myocardial stress perfusion scan for detection of coronary artery disease

---

importance are clinical observations of the patient, associated physical findings, electrocardiogram, and chest x-ray film. These methods can provide a rational basis for the use of several important quantitative methods: ambulatory electrocardiographic monitoring, echocardiography, and exercise testing. Specialized methods that apply in certain circumstances but are not of general application include, during the acute phase of infarction, right heart catheterization and in the hospital or posthospital phases, intracardiac electrography, nuclear cardiology techniques, cardiac catheterization, and angiography. Clinical evaluation obviously is initiated with admission of the patient to the hospital and is continuous thereafter. The choice of methods to be used subsequently must be determined by the factors enumerated in the preceding section.

Clinical Assessment

The patient's clinical course provides a reasonable basis from which to assess the severity of the MI, the patient's progress or lack thereof, the necessity for treatment and the type of treatment, and the indications for further diagnostic evaluation. The patient may be judged to have had uncomplicated MI in the absence of serious arrhythmias, symptoms and physical signs of cardiac failure, and other complications discussed previously. However, physical findings such as persistent pulmonary rales and S_3 gallop indicate cardiac decompensation, despite the absence of accompanying symptoms. These findings may clear during the hospitalization period with only short-term therapy, or they may persist despite maintenance therapy of diuretics and digitalis. The latter situation indicates a significant degree of myocardial damage and diminution of cardiac reserve. This is of importance in planning a patient's rehabilitation program in terms of activity level, work capacity, and further diagnostic studies.

Right Heart Catheterization

More precise information on cardiac functional status is provided by right heart catheterization, which can now be readily performed at the bedside by flotation catheters and is available in many institutions for selective application in acute MI patients. Right heart catheterization is applied in patients with clinical evidence of significant left ventricular dysfunction who require quantitative hemodynamic analysis as a basis for determining appropriate therapy. Right heart catheterization provides information on the two fundamental factors reflecting left ventricular function: left ventricular filling pressure, which can be indirectly measured from pulmonary artery wedge pressure or pulmonary artery diastolic pressure, and cardiac output, which can be determined by indicator dilution technique or thermodilution technique. Hemodynamic assessment provides important data about left ventricular function, and it is an accurate indicator of prognosis. Furthermore, it permits rapid bedside identification of two major complications of MI: ventricular septal perforation, which is detectable by right heart oxygen saturations and indicator dilution curves, and mitral regurgitation, which is reflected by enlarged V waves in the pulmonary artery wedge pressure curve.

Ambulatory Electrocardiographic Monitoring

As the patient progresses from intensive coronary care to regular hospital care, ambulatory electrocardiographic monitoring may be informative in regard to the presence of serious ventricular irritability and its relationship to low levels of activity, such as beginning ambulation. In many institutions telemetric monitoring is available after discharge from the coronary care unit, providing a continuous and immediately available record of cardiac rhythm in the ambulatory patient.

When a patient who is on ambulatory electrocardiographic monitoring in the late hospital phase of MI has serious ventricular arrhythmias, such as short runs of ventricular tachycardia or frequent multiform ventricular ectopic beats, there is an increased risk of subsequent sudden death. If general evaluation does not reveal a correctable cause for the arrhythmia, such as electrolyte abnormality or hypoxia, antiarrhythmic therapy should be instituted. The efficacy of therapy should be determined by periodic ambulatory monitoring, which can also provide a basis for determining the necessity of continuing antiarrhythmic therapy.

Echocardiography

Echocardiography, a noninvasive method, provides quantitative information on cardiac structure and function, thus affording evaluation of valves, chamber dimensions, thickness and motion of septal and posterior left ventricular walls, and the presence of pericardial effusion and intracardiac masses. Determination of dynamic left ventricular geometry provides a basis for estimating cardiac output, ejection fraction, and indices of contractility. Data regarding chamber volume and integrity of wall motion are of particular interest in CHD because these factors frequently reflect abnormalities resulting from ischemic myocardial damage. Thus echocardiographic evidence of left ventricular dilatation and areas of segmental asynergy in a post-MI patient can indicate significant dysfunction.

Exercise Testing (See Chapter 8)

Patients with uncomplicated MI and those who have recovered with no significant residual problem on clinical evaluation (i.e., absence of symptoms and signs of cardiac failure and myocardial ischemia at rest, adequate blood pressure at rest and during mild activity, and stable electrocardiogram) are appropriate candidates for exercise testing.

Formal exercise evaluation is usually performed 2–3 months after hospital discharge of the post-MI patient. Recently, however, it has been applied earlier, and in some institutions a low-level exercise test is performed prior to discharge from hospital. Although exercise testing can be carried out on a bicycle ergometer or treadmill, the latter is more widely used in this country. The patient's initial exercise test should be of submaximal intensity, as determined by readily available charts based on age and heart rate response. Exercise testing is an essential component of any cardiac rehabilitation program because it is the most accurate means widely available for determining cardiac reserve, cardiovascular fitness, and tolerance to physical stress. It thereby provides quantitative data regarding functional capacity, hemodynamic response to physical activity, the presence of myocardial ischemia and its activity threshold, and the occurrence of arrhythmias in relation to activity.

The exercise test is the basis for the patient's individual exercise prescription if a formal program of exercise training is to be instituted, and it can be used as a means of determining safe and appropriate levels of occupational and recreational activity. Although all "burst" activity and tasks involving heavy isometric work, such as lifting, carrying, and straining, are restricted for coronary patients because of the excessive burden they impose on the myocardium in terms of elevated peripheral vascular resistance and blood pressure, the individual approach to each post-MI patient should be emphasized in determining capacity for physical activity. Activities that are submaximal in comparison to those that can be undertaken without evidence of abnormality on a stress test would appear to be reasonable for the post-MI patient. Furthermore, the level of activity allowed should be such as to produce a heart rate 20 beats/min less than that at which an abnormality appears. Significant abnormalities on stress testing include dyspnea, chest pain, lightheadedness, exertional hypotension (a decrease of 10 mm Hg or more during exertion), ischemic ST-segment depression, serious ventricular arrhythmias, paroxysmal supraventricular tachyarrhythmias, and exertion-associated bradyarrhythmia. Exercise testing also provides a baseline against which to measure the effect of therapy, such as that for exertional angina, cardiac failure, or exercise-associated arrhythmias.

Cardiac Catheterization

Post-MI patients who manifest significant functional impairment that does not respond to conservative management are candidates for definitive evaluation by cardiac catheterization to detect surgically remediable lesions. The clinical spectrum of such problems ranges from intractable cardiac failure that precludes discharge of the patient from the hospital to angina noted on mild activity after discharge. Complications of MI and coronary artery disease amenable to surgical correction include well-defined left ventricular aneurysm, mitral regurgitation due to ischemic papillary muscle dysfunction, ventricular septal perforation, and bypassable coronary artery lesions. In general, cardiac catheterization, if elective, is not performed until at least 2 months after MI, since elective surgery is usually delayed until 2–3 months after MI in order to avoid the increased surgical risk of the early postinfarction period. However, if clinical indications necessitate intervention sooner, earlier catheterization and corrective surgery should be performed.

Intracardiac Electrography

Studies of the functional integrity of the cardiac conduction system can be performed by intracardiac electrography. This technique, which requires insertion of an electrode catheter into the right heart to record intracardiac potentials from the right ventricular septal area, provides data on the adequacy of conduction within the separate areas of the atrioventricular and the trifascicular intraventricular conduction systems. This information may be important in the evaluation of disorders such as syncope that may be related to intermittent cardiac arrhythmias. In such instances His bundle electrography may demonstrate impairment of atrioventricular or intraventricular conduction that frequently is not evident on conventional electrocardiography and that may be responsible for intermittent advanced heart block or other bradyarrhythmia. Assessment of sinoatrial node function is usually performed, if indicated, in conjunction with intracardiac electrography in order to assess the presence of sick sinus syndrome. Intracardiac electrography is also frequently combined with ambulatory electrocardiographic monitoring for investigation of the relationship between symptoms and arrythmias.

Nuclear Cardiology

Recent advances in nuclear cardiology have provided noninvasive techniques to assess ventricular function and to detect myocardial ischemia. These methods employ intravenously injected radioisotopes and a scintillation camera. Ventricular function can be measured by the gated blood pool scan method, which involves the use of an isotope that remains in the intravascular compartment and thereby permits determination of ventricular ejection fraction and wall motion. With this technique the isotope functions in a manner analogous to that of contrast medium in cardiac contrast angiography. Relative regional myocardial perfusion can be measured by detection of isotopes that are distributed throughout the myocardium in proportion to coronary blood flow. Regional hypoperfusion, as indicated by myocardial scanning, correlates well with a significant lesion in the coronary artery supplying this area. Myocardial perfusion scanning to detect ischemia must generally be performed in conjunction with maximal or angina-limited exercise stress testing in order to provoke regional ischemia.

THERAPY OF THE POST-MI PATIENT

Treatment of post-MI patients after discharge from the hospital involves certain measures common to the entire group of patients and other measures determined by the specific needs of individual patients. Therapy is directed at treatment of CHD and its complications, modification of coronary risk factors, and management of associated cardiac and noncardiac conditions. Treatment of CHD involves the therapeutic spectrum of drugs, exercise training, and surgery. In conjunction with these modalities, comprehensive rehabilitation is carried out by means of assessment of functional and work capacity, health and vocational counseling, and, when indicated, the assistance of social workers and mental health professionals.

Modification of Coronary Risk Factors

It is reasonable to attempt to decrease coronary risk factors in all patients. However, it must be recognized that in the post-MI patient coronary artery disease is well established, and the later in the course of the disease these corrective measures are undertaken, the less the degree of benefit that can be anticipated from them. Attempts to modify coronary risk factors entail little or no risk; they are employed to impede progression of coronary atherosclerosis already present and inhibit development of new lesions. The effort that is to be expended in this area will depend on a number of factors, including the patient's clinical status, attitude and cooperation, and age.

The three major coronary risk factors are hypercholesterolemia, cigarette smoking, and hypertension. Conservative measures involving diet and education may suffice for management of the first two. However, drugs may be indicated for elevated serum cholesterol, and they usually are necessary when blood pressure is persistently greater than 160/100 mm Hg. Diabetes mellitus is, of course, associated with accelerated atherosclerosis, and its control is important. Other risk factors that have been implicated in the etiology or exacerbation of CHD and that merit alteration include hypertriglyceridemia, obesity, sedentary life pattern, and emotional stress.

Treatment of CHD

The two major clinical manifestations of CHD that require ongoing management are angina pectoris and cardiac failure. Arrhythmias that produce clinical signs and symptoms or ventricular ectopic beats that pose a high risk for lethal arrhythmias and sudden death require treatment and suppression. Of course, the comprehensive rehabilitation effort is aimed directly or indirectly at reducing the risk of recurrent MI and sudden death.

Angina Pectoris
As was noted previously, angina is frequent after MI. Initial treatment of angina should consist of correction or elimination of provoking factors such as hypertension, obesity, smoking, emotional stress, anemia, and hyperthyroidism. Drugs, exercise therapy, and coronary artery bypass graft surgery are important

specific modalities of treatment, and the mechanisms of their therapeutic actions can be understood from their physiologic effects and a consideration of the pathophysiology of angina.

Angina is a manifestation of myocardial ischemia that results from disparity between cardiac oxygen supply and demand due to obstructive coronary artery disease. Treatment of angina is based on alleviation of the metabolic imbalance by increasing the myocardial oxygen supply or reducing the demand. In the treatment of angina, myocardial oxygen supply is increased by augmenting coronary blood flow through myocardial revascularization by coronary artery bypass grafting. Myocardial oxygen demand can be diminished by decreasing the hemodynamic factors that are its principal determinants: heart rate, blood pressure, ventricular volume, and contractility (Table 1). This is accomplished by drug therapy with nitrate drugs or β-adrenergic blockade or by exercise training.

Both medical therapy and surgical therapy, acting by fundamentally different mechanisms, decrease myocardial ischemia, alleviate angina, and enhance the patient's capacity for physical activity. The effects of these two approaches in angina can be elucidated on the basis of their actions on indirect indices of myocardial oxygen demand. The latter, although dependent on the four previously mentioned factors, can be closely related to heart rate and systolic blood pressure during physical activity. Thus the product heart rate × systolic blood pressure correlates closely with relative myocardial oxygen consumption during exertion, and the value of this product at which angina occurs represents an externally measurable threshold for myocardial ischemia that is reproducible for the individual patient. Medical therapy and exercise training, by reducing the exertional heart rate × blood pressure response, thus reflecting a decrease in myocardial oxygen consumption to a level more nearly compatible with the restricted flow capacity of the impaired coronary circulation, result in a more favorable balance between myocardial oxygen supply and demand and allow greater intensity and duration of work prior to attainment of the ischemic threshold. However, angina does occur when the threshold is reached (Fig. 3). By contrast, coronary bypass graft surgery is associated with elevation of the ischemic threshold or abolition of ischemia, as evidenced by the increase in heart rate × blood pressure product attainable with this therapy (Fig. 4).

The major effects of medical forms of antianginal therapy on the determinants of myocardial oxygen consumption are shown in Table 3. Myocardial oxygen demand is reduced by the nitrates by their relaxation of vascular smooth muscle. The most potent action of these agents is venodilatation, which reduces venous return and thereby decreases cardiac volume. Arterial dilatation, although less profound, is important, resulting in reduction of blood pressure.

Sublingual nitroglycerin is indicated in all patients with angina; prophylactic use is a most important and valuable application of this drug. Long-acting oral nitrates may be effective for 3 hr or more, but these agents generally must be given in doses substantially higher than those that have conventionally been recommended. Nitroglycerin ointment also has prolonged action, and it is of particular value for nocturnal angina. The chief antianginal action of β-adrenergic blockade with propranolol is reduction of heart rate; decreases in

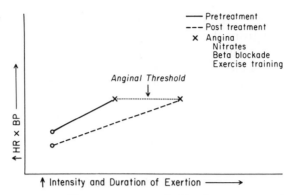

Figure 3. Typical response of heart rate × systolic blood pressure product (HR × SBP) to physical exertion in patients with angina before and after therapy with antianginal drugs (nitrates or β-adrenergic blockade) or exercise training. Duration and intensity of exertion are augmented by therapy, but angina occurs at the same HR × SBP, indicating that the major mechanism of beneficial action of these forms of treatment is reduction of myocardial oxygen demand (reflected by decreased HR × SBP) rather than increased myocardial oxygen supply.

myocardial contractility and blood pressure produced by β-adrenergic blockade also contribute to its therapeutic effectiveness. Exercise training, as applied in a prescriptive manner (see Chapter 8), is effective in angina largely because it diminishes the heart rate response to physical stress; blood pressure is also decreased, although to a lesser degree.

In addition to decreasing angina and enhancing functional capacity, the

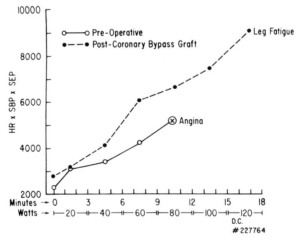

Figure 4. Exercise performance in a patient with CHD before and after coronary artery bypass graft surgery. The triple product of heart rate (HR), systolic blood pressure (SBP), and systolic ejection period (SEP) is used for indirect assessment of myocardial oxygen consumption. Surgery is associated with increased exercise capacity, abolition of exercise-induced angina, and elevated triple product (the last is consistent with increased myocardial oxygen supply) which is in contrast to the occurrence of angina with less exercise at a lower triple product before surgery.

Table 3. Major Effects of Medical Forms of Antianginal Therapy on Determinants of Myocardial Oxygen Consumption

	Nitrates	β-adrenergic blockade	Exercise training
Heart rate	↑ *	↓ ↓	↓
Blood pressure	↓	↓ (→)	↓
Myocardial contractility	↑ *	↓	?
Ventricular volume	↓ ↓	→(↑)	→(↑)

↑   Major effect.

↑   Mild to moderate effect.

*   Indirect (reflex) effect.

physiologic actions of medical and surgical antianginal therapy suggest the potential for inhibiting ischemic events such as MI and lethal arrhythmias and thereby enhancing the prognosis. This is readily apparent in the reduction or abolition of myocardial ischemia that may be achieved by surgical revascularization. However, medical therapy and exercise training, by reducing myocardial ischemia through diminution of cardiac oxygen demands, permit the myocardium to function at a level further from the ischemic threshold at rest and during activity than in the untrained or untreated state. Exercise training produces a number of additional physiologic alterations that are of further potential benefit in reducing the risk of coronary morbidity and mortality (Table 4).

Table 4. Effects of Exercise With the Potential to Inhibit Progression of Severity of Coronary Artery Disease

Exercise may increase:
  Coronary vessel caliber
  Myocardial efficiency
  Efficiency of peripheral circulation
  Fibrinolysis
  Tolerance to physical and emotional stress
  Positive emotional outlook

Exercise may decrease:
  Heart rate
  Blood pressure
  Serum lipids
  Glucose intolerance
  Obesity-adiposity
  Platelet aggregability
  Vulnerability to arrhythmias
  Sympathetic neurohumoral excess
  Psychologic stress

For treatment of mild angina, sublingual nitroglycerin and exercise training may be adequate. More severe forms of angina may necessitate the combined application of exercise and sublingual and long-acting nitrates. Addition of propranolol is necessary when daily angina persists during this regimen. Coronary bypass graft surgery is indicated when angina is unresponsive to optimal medical management and angiography reveals suitable coronary anatomy. Indications for coronary bypass surgery may be extended beyond this category in selected cases. These include the presence of left main coronary artery disease, recurrent MI in young patients, and refractory and recurrent life-threatening ventricular arrhythmias.

Cardiac Failure

The fundamental cause of cardiac failure in CHD usually is loss of contracting myocardium because of previous MI. Rarely does it occur in the coronary patient without prior MI, since contractile abnormalities in the absence of MI are usually absent or mild. Thus in the natural history of CHD that presents as angina, the initial stage is characterized by normal size and contractile function of the left ventricle, and no cardiac failure, in addition to angina. With the occurrence of MI, myocardial scarring results. Presentations of cardiac failure and angina are related to the relative quantities of myocardial fibrosis and ischemic viable myocardium, respectively. Recurrent MI produces progressively greater areas of myocardial scarring, increasing contractile deficit, and ventricular dilatation and failure. In this late stage the loss of large areas of ischemic but viable myocardium is associated with decrease or disappearance of angina.

Cardiac failure in CHD can result from several types of contractile abnormalities affecting the left ventricle. These are decreased wall motion (hypokinesis), absence of wall motion (akinesis), and paradoxic expansion or bulging during systole (dyskinesis). An aneurysm consists of a large akinetic area of the ventricle, well-differentiated from more normal tissue, frequently manifesting some dyskinesis. Aneurysms are usually associated with considerable disturbance of hemodynamic function and cardiac failure. Myocardial ischemia affecting the papillary muscles can produce mitral valve incompetence and thus contribute to cardiac dysfunction.

The major functional consequences of left ventricular failure are pulmonary congestion resulting in dyspnea and low cardiac output, the latter limiting performance of the skeletal muscles and compromising organ function. Treatment is aimed at improving cardiac function without excessively increasing myocardial oxygen requirements and inadvertently provoking ischemia. Prior to treatment of cardiac failure by specific drugs, nonmyocardial, systemic, and metabolic factors responsible for circulatory dysfunction should be identified and corrected. These include arrhythmias, pericardial effusion, poorly controlled hypertension, anemia, hypoxia, and conditions such as pulmonary emboli, hyperthyroidism, and arteriovenous shunts. Treatment of cardiac failure should also include dietary sodium restriction to reduce excessive fluid retention.

The most important drugs used in the treatment of cardiac failure are diuretics and digitalis. Vasodilator drugs have received recent attention and have been increasingly used for this condition.

Diuretics. By promoting renal loss of sodium and water, diuretics reduce elevated left ventricular end-diastolic pressure, alleviate pulmonary congestion, and enhance functional capacity without any action on the myocardium itself. Despite the decrease in left ventricular preload, cardiac output usually is unaltered or falls only a small amount after diuretic therapy. Functional capacity is improved without major alteration in cardiac output because of diminution of both pulmonary congestion and the limiting symptom, dyspnea. These relationships can be represented by cardiac performance and ventricular function curves, as shown in Figure 5. As indicated, the relationship between left ventricular performance and filling pressure (preload) in the normal heart is represented by a steep curve. As myocardial contractility decreases, there is less augmentation of performance in response to increases in preload, and the function curve is depressed. Clinical cardiac failure due to CHD usually is associated with considerable depression of the left ventricular function curve. The low cardiac output and elevated left ventricular filling pressure in this condition are represented by a point relatively far to the right on the depressed function curve. Therefore, in this state, preload can be reduced considerably with little reduction of cardiac output. These relationships provide the basis for enhancement of clinical status by diuretic therapy in cardiac failure. Diuretic therapy also produces its bene-

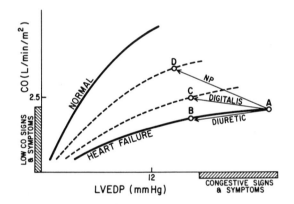

Figure 5. Relationship between ventricular performance, represented by cardiac output (CO), and left ventricular preload, represented by left ventricular end-diastolic pressure (LVEDP), in a normal individual and in a patient with congestive heart failure. Point A is the point at which the failing left ventricle operates before treatment. B represents the shift in ventricular performance on the original function curve after diuretic therapy, involving a reduction in LVEDP to a point no longer associated with congestive signs and symptoms. C indicates alteration in ventricular function after digitalis, producing a curve reflecting increased myocardial contractility, which results in an improved relationship between CO and LVEDP. In this example both low cardiac output and circulatory congestion are alleviated by the enhanced cardiac function. D represents the augmented ventricular function resulting from vasodilator therapy by nitroprusside (NP). It is emphasized that the ventricular function curve in the latter instance does not reflect increased myocardial contractility; rather, the improved relationship between CO and LVEDP results from reduced afterload to left ventricular ejection produced by the vasodilator.

ficial actions without increasing myocardial oxygen demands. Overzealous use of the diuretics can produce excessive fluid loss, significant reduction of cardiac output, and hypotension. Precautions against the electrolyte abnormalities that can result from these agents should also be taken.

Digitalis. Digitalis is a positive inotropic agent that augments myocardial contractility, resulting in improved cardiac output. As a result of enhanced left ventricular ejection, end-diastolic volume and pressure are decreased, and pulmonary congestion is alleviated. Improved cardiac performance also results in reduction of the compensatory tachycardia that may be associated with cardiac failure, further augmenting cardiac output by improved diastolic filling due to the increased diastolic filling time resulting from reduced cardiac rate. Digitalis is particularly useful in cardiac failure associated with atrial fibrillation and a rapid ventricular response. The glycoside decreases the excessive ventricular rate by its action of increasing the refractory period of the atrioventricular node, with consequent reduction of the frequency of impulse conduction to the ventricles, thereby augmenting left ventricular filling and cardiac output. Digitalis and diuretics are frequently used together in treating cardiac failure.

The effect of digitalis on cardiac performance in heart failure is depicted in Figure 5. In contrast to the diuretics, digitalis results in an improved function curve, reflecting increased myocardial contractility, and performance is shifted up and to the left. Because the increase in myocardial contractility raises myocardial oxygen demand, digitalis has the potential to augment myocardial ischemia in CHD. However, its net effect in the ischemic failing heart is more likely to result in reduced myocardial oxygen demand and decreased ischemia. By reduction of elevated ventricular volume and rate, the drug decreases cardiac oxygen requirements, actions that tend to override its augmenting effect on oxygen consumption due to increased contractility. However, inappropriate use of digitalis in CHD in the absence of cardiac failure or atrial fibrillation could result in unopposed elevation of myocardial oxygen consumption and increased ischemia.

Vasodilators. There has been considerable interest in the use of vasodilator drugs to treat cardiac failure. These agents, which have no direct myocardial actions, alleviate circulatory failure, increasing cardiac output and reducing pulmonary congestion, by their favorable effects on cardiac loading conditions. The use of vasodilators to treat cardiac failure represents an extension of previous physiologic approaches to this problem. Stroke volume is determined by three fundamental factors (Table 5): myocardial contractility, preload, and afterload, or resistance to left ventricular ejection. The first factor may be stimulated with digitalis. Increasing the preload is clinically applicable only in hypovolemia, since preload is usually excessive in cardiac failure. Reduction of afterload has the potential for improving stroke volume and cardiac output and, through enhanced ventricular emptying, also diminishing elevated preload. As was noted previously in regard to the physiologic actions of the nitrates, the most commonly used vasodilators in cardiac failure, these drugs reduce elevated left ventricular volume and pressure and decrease resistance to left ventricular

Table 5. Determinants of Stroke Volume

Determinant		Effect on stroke volume
Myocardial contractility	↑	↑
Preload	↑	↑
Afterload	↓	↑

ejection. Whereas preload is consistently reduced by the nitrates, their influence on cardiac output will be determined by the interaction of their separate effects on preload and resistance to left ventricular ejection, as represented by peripheral arterial resistance. If adequate preload is maintained after nitrate therapy (filling pressure ≥ 12 mm Hg), the reduction in peripheral resistance usually results in increased stroke volume and cardiac output. However, if preload is reduced excessively, cardiac output will fall despite the decrease in peripheral resistance. These therapeutic mechanisms are ideal in CHD because cardiac pump performance is enhanced without a rise in myocardial oxygen requirements. Indeed, by reducing resistance to left ventricular outflow and thereby allowing the ventricle to expend more of its contractile energy in shortening than in developing isovolumic pressure, the vasodilators have the potential to augment ventricular function while reducing myocardial oxygen needs. The effects of a vasodilator on ventricular function in cardiac failure are shown in Figure 5. Although ventricular performance is elevated to a higher function curve, this does not represent increased myocardial contractility, since the improved relationship between cardiac performance and preload is the result of reduced afterload. Thus ventricular function curves represent comparative contractility only if afterload is constant.

Vasodilators employed in clinical practice exert dilating actions on both arteries and veins, although the relative effects on the two systems differ with the individual agents. The increase in cardiac output by the nitrates is less than the reduction they produce in left ventricular volume and pressure, since their venodilating action predominates over their arterial dilating effect.

The nitrates are used when conventional therapy of cardiac failure is unsuccessful. The long-acting oral agents are employed as in the treatment of angina. Other oral vasodilator agents used in cardiac failure are hydralazine and prazosin. In initial trials the latter agent has shown considerable promise in increasing depressed cardiac output. The major hazards associated with the vasodilator drugs are hypotension and decreased cardiac output, the latter being related to excessive reduction of preload.

Cardiac Surgery. Corrective surgery is indicated when cardiac failure is related to one of the aforementioned mechanical defects and conservative management is unsuccessful. Coronary bypass graft surgery is rarely performed alone for cardiac failure; it is more commonly employed in conjunction with one of the other major surgical corrective procedures.

PERSPECTIVE ON PHYSICAL ACTIVITY
IN THE POST-MI PATIENT

Recent recognition of the potential therapeutic and prophylactic roles of physical activity in CHD has stimulated increased interest in practical application, and this aspect of treatment merits special consideration here. As was noted previously, a systematic approach to physical activity is an important component of comprehensive cardiac rehabilitation after MI. It begins in the coronary care unit and continues through convalescence and recovery in progressive stages, as described in Chapters 4 and 8.

Early institution of physical activity for MI patients is a departure from the traditional practice of prolonged bed rest and severe activity restriction; its rationale is based on demonstrated safety, proven advantages, and potential for further benefits, as well as on the deleterious effects of inactivity. Early ambulation in patients with uncomplicated MI has resulted in shortened hospitalization; many patients now are discharged after 2 weeks, affording major economic and personal advantages. Systematic physical activity after MI has been shown to be associated with fewer complications related to bed rest, psychologic gains, enhanced cardiac function, and earlier and higher frequency of return to work. As was discussed previously, exercise training can also improve exertional capacity and alleviate symptoms of myocardial ischemia. Current evidence supports the rationale and safety of early activity after MI and exercise training after recovery. However, to gain the benefits and maintain the safety of an activity program in the hospital and during the posthospital course after MI, emphasis must be placed on proper patient selection, individualization of prescribed activity, and careful attention to potential hazards. It is stressed that an activity program should be initiated *only* in the stable patient with uncomplicated MI (absence of cardiac failure, shock, arrhythmias, continuing pain, and noncardiac complications).

Phases of Physical Activity After MI
(See Also Chapters 4 and 8)

Physical activity after MI involves several progressive stages that begin in the coronary care unit and continue through the remainder of the hospitalization, convalescence, and recovery phases. The physician is responsible for prescription of activity, although he may work closely with a nurse, physical therapist, physical educator, and others.

Coronary Care Unit

Activity is initiated on day 2 or day 3 of the coronary care unit phase of MI. Consisting initially of low-energy functions such as self-care and progressing to the use of a chair, if tolerated, it prevents the deleterious influence of immobilization. Activity is evaluated by subjective response, electrocardiographic monitoring, and blood pressure measurement. The occurrence of untoward effects indicates that the activity is excessive, necessitating its discontinuance and reevaluation of clinical status.

Remainder of Hospitalization

In patients who progress satisfactorily from intensive coronary care, activities are increased during this phase. In the uncomplicated patient these include increased time in a chair, rhythmic exercises of extremities and trunk, and progressive ambulation in the room and then the hospital corridor. Before being discharged the patient should be able to walk in the corridor without difficulty at least three times daily for 3 days. The patient totally free of complications may be ready for discharge within 2 weeks.

During the latter phase of hospitalization, the patient and family should be educated regarding appropriate activities after returning home. Topics that should be covered include avoidance of isometric exertion and "burst" activity, the use of stairs, travel, activity in relation to alteration of environmental temperature, and sexual activity. Instruction in the use of nitroglycerin is essential; the drug should always be carried and should be taken at the onset of angina.

In order to provide the patient intelligent guidance in the sensitive area of sexual relations, it is important that the physician be well informed on the emotional and physiologic implications of sexual activity. The physician should deal with this topic directly and openly, since the patient may be reluctant to discuss it, and clarification can obviate much of the apprehension and disability associated with misunderstanding. Sexual activity in middle-aged post-MI patients has been found to produce a peak heart rate of 90–144 beats/min (average 117) for 10–15 sec, which is equivalent to the energy expenditure in climbing one flight of stairs. Resumption of sexual activity at reduced intensity is thus well within the capacity of the asymptomatic convalescing post-MI patient, especially if the patient has progressed satisfactorily on the type of activity plan described here. If angina is provoked by sexual activity, modification of intensity and use of prophylactic nitroglycerin may eliminate this problem.

A rational prescription for early posthospital activity is based on assessment of the patient's functional capacity before discharge. This can be determined by evaluating the response to hospital activity in terms of cardiac rate, blood pressure, and electrocardiogram. If indicated by the patient's specific needs, exertional capacity can be measured by a low-level treadmill test (e.g., to 70% predicted maximum heart rate).

Convalescent Phase

The objectives of physical activity during the convalescent phase are continued augmentation of physical capacity to attain a level consistent with return to the patient's employment or, if the latter is precluded by its excessive demands, complete self-care and safe pursuit of certain social and recreational activities. Limited sexual activity also is resumed during this period. Most light household and personal-care activities, except those involving vigorous effort, can be undertaken safely. In asymptomatic patients, walking constitutes an important aspect of physical rehabilitation. This activity can be increased in duration and rate to an individual optimum—a level that provides the benefits of exercise without symptoms or other untoward effects. Careful physician consultation and supervision are essential during the convalescent period in order to reevaluate clinical status, including recent history with regard to the effects of activity, physical examination, and resting electrocardiogram. Patients who progress without symptoms will generally be capable of returning to most forms of work within 8–12 weeks following MI.

The convalescent activity program may be pursued in a supervised group, if one is available, or by the patient alone. Physician guidance is mandatory in either circumstance, since objective assessment of physical capacity (for determination of the individual activity program) and periodic reevaluation are important aspects of the program. Supervised exercise permits patients to strive for higher levels of activity with increased physiologic benefits. In an unsupervised setting, such activity might exceed prudent levels. Furthermore, the motivation and support provided by the group contribute to increased adherence. Activities of relatively high intensity, such as jogging, are proscribed at this stage for unsupervised coronary patients. However, walking is an excellent form of exercise from which considerable benefit can be derived. A progressive increase to a peak of walking 4 mph for 30 min reflects a relatively high capacity for activity that is more than that required by most forms of work, including bricklaying, for example. In order to obtain benefit from exercise, this type of activity should be carried out on at least 3 days per week. (See Chap. 8.)

Maintenance

The aim of the maintenance phase, beginning 10–12 weeks after MI, is further enhancement and maintenance of function at an optimum level to allow desired and appropriate occupational and leisure activities. Activity can be continued in an organized program or on an individual basis, with increasing levels of exertion, consistent with capacity, rational goals, and safety. In order to obtain a "training effect" (increase in physical working capacity and maximal oxygen consumption) from exercise, it is necessary to maintain 65–75% maximal capacity for 20–30 min at least 3 times each week. For these higher levels of exertion, formal exercise testing and prescription are indicated. Furthermore, higher levels, 70–80% of maximal capacity, should not be undertaken in the coronary patient without on-site supervision. When a higher-intensity exercise program has been followed successfully for 6 months to 1 year, unsupervised activity should be considered in selected patients. In this group, treadmill exercise testing to a level of 10–12 mets should be tolerated without adverse effects in terms of symptoms, signs, and electrocardiogram. In patients not engaged in a formal exercise program, exercise testing may be used as a guide to physical activities and maximum permissible heart rate (20 beats/min below the rate associated with signs or symptoms, thereby providing a safe margin from adverse effects).

SUMMARY

Comprehensive cardiac rehabilitation after acute MI is aimed at restoration of optimal functional status. It is based on residual cardiovascular capacity, which is, in the majority of postinfarction patients, sufficient for most moderate occupational, recreational, and personal functions. Rehabilitation seeks to prevent functional impairment related to physical deconditioning by promoting appropriate activity; it includes application of medical and surgical therapy when indicated. Individualization in evaluation and management of postinfarction patients is necessary because the nature and extent of underlying cardiac abnormalities vary, and therefore therapeutic indications and prognoses can differ widely. Results of rehabilitation efforts are most satisfactory when a program is pursued in a systematic manner on a long-term basis. The program must include patient education and selection of rational therapy, as indicated by continuing evaluation.

ACKNOWLEDGMENTS

The authors gratefully acknowledge the skilled assistance of Ms. Kristen Cowan and Mrs. Carol Loscutoff.

REFERENCES

1. Amsterdam EA, Hughes JL III, Miller RR, et al: Physiologic approach to the medical and surgical treatment of angina pectoris. In Naughton JP, Hellerstein HK (eds): *Exercise Testing and Exercise Training in Coronary Heart Disease*. Academic Press, New York, 1973, Chap 8

2. Wenger NK, Gilbert CA: Rehabilitation of the myocardial infarction patient. In Hurst JW, Logue RB, Schlant RC, Wenger NK (eds): *The Heart*. McGraw-Hill, New York, 4th ed, 1978, Chap 62G

3. Kellermann JJ: Rehabilitation of patients with coronary heart disease. *Prog Cardiovasc Dis* 17:303, 1975

4. James W, Amsterdam EA (eds): *Coronary Heart Disease, Exercise Testing and Cardiac Rehabilitation*. Symposia Specialists, Miami, 1977, p 183

5. Amsterdam EA, Wilmore JH, DeMaria AN (eds): *Exercise in Cardiovascular Health and Disease*. Yorke Medical Books, New York, 1977

4

Early Ambulation After Myocardial Infarction: Rationale, Program Components, and Results

Nanette Kass Wenger, M.D.

The changing pattern of care for the patient with myocardial infarction in the 1970s is characterized by an increase in early resumption of physical activity and a consequent decrease in imposed invalidism and by earlier discharge from the hospital for appropriately selected patients.

HISTORICAL PERSPECTIVE

Over 200 years ago Heberden advocated physical activity for patients with angina pectoris and described its beneficial effect, but this wisdom was forgotten following the clinical description of myocardial infarction by Herrick in 1912 (1). In the early 1900s patients were almost completely immobilized at bed rest for a minimum of 6–8 weeks; protracted bed rest and hospitalization were the mainstays of treatment. It was believed that any physical exertion would markedly increase the occurrence of ventricular aneurysm and ventricular rupture and that the worsening of arterial hypoxemia with activity would increase the risk of arrhythmia, recurrent myocardial infarction, and sudden cardiac death. Activities as strenuous as climbing stairs were deferred for at least a year, and a return to productive work or to normal living was unusual.

Pathologic studies of the healing process following myocardial infarction reported by Mallory et al. (2) reinforced this empiric custom of the 1920s and

Program and materials developed in part under grants from the Vocational Rehabilitation Services, State of Georgia Health Services; and the Division of Vocational Rehabilitation, U.S. Department of Health, Education and Welfare.

53

1930s of prolonged bed rest after myocardial infarction; they demonstrated that at least 6 weeks were required for transformation of necrotic myocardium into firm scar tissue: "To advise less than three weeks in bed is unwise, even for patients with the smallest myocardial infarcts." Lewis (3) also recommended a minimum of 6–8 weeks of bed rest for patients with coronary occlusion: "during the whole of this period the patient is to be guarded by day and night nursing and helped in every way to avoid voluntary movement or effort." Patients were cautioned to lie as still as possible for fear of arrhythmia, asystole, or myocardial aneurysm formation or rupture.

Jetter and White (4) detected a higher incidence of myocardial rupture among postinfarction patients in mental hospitals than among patients in private hospitals; they postulated that this was attributable to the increased activity of mentally deranged patients, as compared with the enforced bed rest of patients hospitalized for routine private medical care.

The Levine (5, 6) "chair treatment of acute coronary thrombosis" in Boston in the 1940s began "the present trend in coronary care . . . liberalization of the rigid restrictions of activity hitherto practiced." Levine is credited with emphasizing that "long continued bed rest saps morale, provokes desperation, unleashes anxiety and ushers in hopelessness of the capacity of resuming a normal life." His regimen allowed the patient to sit in a chair for 1–2 hr, beginning the first day after myocardial infarction. Although no control series was ever done, no complications attributable to this management appeared among the 81 patients initially reported. The sitting position was believed to be beneficial because it increased peripheral venous pooling, decreased venous return, and reduced cardiac work. Levine further theorized that this therapeutic approach would diminish thromboembolic and respiratory complications, a thesis that subsequently has been well documented and accepted. An enhanced sense of well-being and easier activity resumption were also described (6).

Dock (7) also emphasized the excessive risk of thromboembolism and vasomotor instability with immobilization; he favored the use of a bedside commode (rather than a bedpan) as a means of avoiding or lessening the Valsalva maneuver.

Harrison (8) cited the "abuse" of bed rest as a therapeutic measure for patients with cardiovascular disease and warned that excessive physician caution would result in incapacitating cardiac neurosis in postinfarction patients. He emphasized that both John Hunter and Sir William McKenzie had lived active lives after apparent myocardial infarctions that had not been treated by bed rest.

As early as the 1940s the cardiac catheterization studies of Stead et al. (9) demonstrated that fear and anxiety markedly increased cardiac output. It was therefore suggested that enforced bed rest might exert a paradoxic effect, with the patient's fear of impending death or disability or concern about prolonged invalidism resulting in increased cardiac work as a response to emotional stress.

In 1950 Irvin and Burgess (10) further criticized the customary lengthy immobilization at bed rest; they noted that there were few data to support advocacy of prolonged immobilization, and there was mounting evidence of its deleterious effects. They emphasized that bed rest could be "advantageously and safely shortened."

Even as recently as the early 1970s clinical practice in the United States varied considerably, with the duration of bed rest varying from 1 day to 4 weeks after uncomplicated myocardial infarction and the duration of hospitalization varying from 2 to 6 weeks or more (11–13). Many physicians continued to perpetuate the misconception that the optimal pattern of care for the patient with uncomplicated myocardial infarction was prolonged bed rest and hospitalization. Recent data have increasingly confirmed that most of the serious complications of myocardial infarction occur during the first few days of hospitalization and that the overwhelming majority of patients with uncomplicated completed myocardial infarction have little or no in-hospital mortality and very few significant late complications (14). These data and information concerning the risks of needlessly prolonged activity restriction have encouraged early mobilization and early discharge from the hospital for appropriately selected patients after myocardial infarction. Indeed, Rose (15) has suggested that the burden of proof now lies with the physician who advocates extensive activity restriction as being beneficial for the patient with uncomplicated acute myocardial infarction.

PHYSIOLOGIC BASIS

Information about the deleterious effects of prolonged immobilization at bed rest provided the impetus for early ambulation or early mobilization programs for patients with acute myocardial infarction (16, 17). Comparable regimens are equally appropriate, and necessary, for patients who have undergone coronary bypass surgery.

The most marked alteration after immobilization at bed rest is a decrease in physical work capacity. In a study (16) of healthy young college students placed at strict bed rest for 21 days (formerly the traditional management for the myocardial infarction patient) it was found that physical work capacity decreased by 20–25%, and at least 3 weeks of physical activity training were required to restore pre-bed-rest status. The higher the degree of physical fitness prior to bed rest, the longer the training required to return to the prior functional level after resumption of activity. Therefore one must question whether the post-illness fatigue, weakness, and tiredness of the patient who has been at prolonged bed rest for myocardial infarction (or indeed for any other medical problem) are due to the disease process or to the therapy that has been imposed for the illness.

Furthermore, when the patient is first mobilized after a period of bed rest, there often occurs significant tachycardia and orthostatic hypotension, neither of which is desirable for the postinfarction patient (18). Although loss of normal postural vasomotor reflexes plays a role, these responses are due in large part to the hypovolemia that occurs with bed rest; patients may sustain a decrease of 700–800 cc in circulating blood volume after a week to 10 days of strict bed rest (19). It is interesting that patients with congestive heart failure, who obviously do not have decreased circulating blood volume, do not manifest this tachycardia and postural hypotension when mobilized after a period at bed rest (18). To further compound the problem in the patient who experiences hypovolemia as a response to immobilization at bed rest, plasma volume decreases to a greater extent than does red blood cell mass (20), thus increasing blood viscosity and thereby predisposing to thromboembolism; this occurs in a setting of bed rest, which precludes use of the leg muscle pump, adding the thromboembolic risk of venous circulatory stasis to that of increased blood viscosity (21).

There is a modest decrease in pulmonary ventilation due to depression of lung volume and vital capacity at bed rest (5), which perhaps is of major significance only in the patient with associated chronic pulmonary disease; negative nitrogen and protein balances occur (22, 23). Our surgical colleagues find this of concern in the postoperative patient in regard to wound healing; perhaps internists and cardiologists should be equally concerned in the setting in which we hope to optimize healing of a necrotic area of myocardium.

Finally, there are decreases in skeletal muscle mass and muscular contractile strength and efficiency; contractile strength may diminish by 10–15% within the first week at bed rest (24). This means that inefficiently contracting muscle demands more oxygen for the same amount of work to be performed, and this increased demand is imposed on an impaired oxygen transport system and myocardium.

Early ambulation efforts are therefore designed to avert or lessen these deleterious or deconditioning effects of prolonged immobilization at bed rest, a limited but important goal. Additionally, these programs have been shown to lessen the varying degrees of anxiety and depression that are concomitants of acute myocardial infarction (25–27). The gradual progressive increases in activity that are allowed each day provide tangible reinforcement of the physician's statement that the patient is improving and can expect to return to a normal or near-normal life-style.

PATIENT SELECTION AND PROGRAM COMPONENTS

Appropriate selection of patients for early ambulation is crucial, as is surveillance of their activity. Early ambulation may begin as early as the first days in the coronary care unit for the patient with uncomplicated myocardial infarction— the patient without significant dysrhythmia, heart failure, shock, or persistent or recurrent chest pain. Patients with these complications require appropriate care at bed rest, and ambulation should be initiated only when these complications have been controlled; these patients often require more prolonged hospitalization. Although physicians tend to remember more clearly their patients with life-threatening complications, patients with uncomplicated myocardial infarction comprise over half of all patients admitted to coronary care units in the United States (28, 29); in general, they tend to be younger patients and those with first episodes of myocardial infarction.

Activities in the coronary care unit should be isotonic and of low intensity, 1–2 mets, i.e., one to two times the resting metabolic rate (1 met = approximately 3.5 cc O_2/kg body weight per minute). Such activities include self-care, eating, active and passive arm and leg movements, use of a bedside commode, and sitting in bed or in a bedside chair. Indeed, some of these activities do not entail augmented physical activity; for example, less energy is required to use a bedside commode than to use a bedpan (30, 31), and cardiac output and myocardial work are less in the sitting position than in the recumbent position (32). DeBusk and associates (33) demonstrated no significant increase in cardiac work (rate-pressure product) with postural change or with selected passive and active exercise performed by patients in the coronary care unit.

At Grady Memorial Hospital and Emory University School of Medicine in Atlanta, Georgia, a prototype early ambulation program has been operative for over a decade (34) (Table 1). Their suggested guidelines for monitoring appropriate responses to early ambulation and the safety of early ambulation activities in the coronary care unit include the following: a heart rate response no greater than 120 beats/min; no chest pain, dyspnea, or excessive fatigue; no occurrence of dysrhythmias; no change in ST-segment displacement on the electrocardiogram or monitor as evidence of ischemia; no decrease in systolic blood pressure greater than 15–20 mm Hg. The usual response to exercise is a slight increase in systolic blood pressure; in this clinical setting, a fall in systolic blood pressure usually indicates that cardiac output is inadequate to meet demands.

An inappropriate physiologic response to any level of activity signifies that the work load is excessive and requires that the patient's activity plan be revised, that the patient be returned to a less demanding stage, and that the clinical status be reevaluated. When the response is appropriate, the patient may be allowed to progress to the next activity level.

After the patient leaves the coronary care unit and is in a progressive care unit or in a general medical area, the goal of the physical activity program is to continue to prevent the deleterious physiologic and psychologic effects of bed rest and to increase cardiovascular function to a level that will enable the patient to perform a reasonable degree of self-care and usual household activities by the time of discharge from the hospital. Currently this discharge is often as early as the 10th to the 14th day for the patient with uncomplicated myocardial infarction (14). A variety of physical activities may be employed (34–36), but the basic requirements are that they be of low intensity (2–3 mets) and be supervised by a trained individual who can monitor the physiologic response parameters previously cited. In general, low-intensity dynamic (not isometric) rhythmic calisthenics are used to maintain muscle tone and joint mobility, but an important part of the prescribed activity is a walking program that gradually increases the distance walked and the speed of walking. Isometric activities should be avoided because they do not elicit (as do dynamic exercises) a heart rate response proportional to the intensity of the activity; instead, they are associated with a sudden and significant increase in blood pressure (37). A sudden increase in blood pressure is poorly tolerated by an ischemic left ventricle, and places the patient at increased risk of life-threatening arrhythmias. Ideally, activities should be performed several times each day, interspersed with rest periods.

Increments in the intensity of in-hospital daily activities should parallel the serial progression of prescribed exercise, and recreational and diversional activities of a comparable work level should be offered. It is desirable for patients who will have to climb stairs at home to practice doing so before dismissal from the hospital; accomplishing this safely under supervision in the hospital will decrease the anxiety of the patient and family faced with the problem of stair climbing at home.

Formal low-intensity exercise testing prior to hospital discharge after myocardial infarction is currently used mainly as a research procedure, but it also has several potential clinical benefits (28). It allows more precise definition of safely

Table 1. Fourteen-Step Myocardial Infarction Rehabilitation Program[a]

1	Passive ROM[b] to all extremities (5× ea): patient to do *active* plantar and dorsiflexion of ankles several times/day.	Feeding self, sitting with bed rolled up to 45°, trunk and arms supported by over-bed table.	Initial interview and brief orientation to program.
2	Repeat exercises of Step 1.	1. Feed self. 2. Partial A.M. care (wash hands, face, brush teeth) in bed. 3. Dangle legs on side of bed (1×).	Light recreational activity, such as reading.
3	Active assistive exercise in shoulder flexion; elbow flexion and extension; hip flexion, extension, and rotation: knee flexion and extension: rotation of feet (4× ea).	1. Begin sitting in chair for short periods as tolerated, 2×/day. 2. Bathing whole body. 3. Use of bedside commode.	More detailed explanation of program. Continue light recreation.
4	Minimal resistance, lying in bed in above ROM, 5× ea. Stiffen all muscles to the count of 2 (3×).	1. Increase sitting 3×/day. 2. Change gown.	Begin explanation of what is an MI[b]. Give patient pamphlets to read. Begin craft activity: 1. Leather lacing. 2. Link belt. 3. Hand sewing, embroidery. 4. Copper tooling.
5	Moderate resistance in bed at 45° above ROM exercises; hands on shoulder, elbow circling (5× ea arm).	1. Sitting ad lib. 2. Sitting in chair at bedside for meals. 3. Dressing, shaving, combing hair—*sitting down*. 4. Walking in room, 2×/day.	Continue education about healing of heart, reasons for early restrictions in activity.
6	1. Further resistive exercises sitting on side of bed, manual resistance of knee extension and flexion (7× ea). 2. Walk to bathroom and back (note if patient needs help).	1. Walk to bathroom, ad lib if patient can tolerate. 2. Stand at sink to shave.	Continue craft activity or supply patient with another one. Patient may attend group meetings in a wheelchair for no more than 1 h.

Table 1. (Continued)

7	1. Standing warm-up exercises: a. Arms in extension and shoulder abduction, rotate arms together in circles (circumduction), 5× ea arm. b. Stand on toes, 10×. c. May substitute abduction, 5× ea leg. 2. Walk length of hall (50 ft) and back at average pace.	1. Bathe in tub. 2. Walk to telephone or sit in waiting room (1×/day).	May walk to group meetings on the same floor.
8	1. Warm-up exercises: a. Lateral side bending 5× ea side. b. Trunk twisting. 5× ea side. 2. Walk 1½ lengths of hall, down 1 fl stairs, elevator up.	1. Walk to waiting room, 2×/day. 2. Stay sitting up most of the day.	Continue all previous craft and educational activities.
9	1. Warm-up exercises: a. Lateral side bending, 10× ea side. b. Slight knee bends, 10× with hands on hips. 2. Increase walking distance, walk down one flight of stairs.	Continue above activities.	Discussion of work simplification techniques and pacing of activities.
10	1. Warm-up exercises: a. Lateral side bending with 1-lb weight (10×). b. Standing—leg raising leaning against wall, 5× ea. 2. Walk two lengths of hall and downstairs, take elevator up.	Continue all previous ward activities.	1. Patient may walk to OT[b] clinic and work on craft proj. for ½ h. a. Copper tooling; b. woodworking; c. ceramics; d. small weaving proj. e. metal hammering; f. mosaic tile. 2. Discussion of patient's home exercises.
11	1. Warm-up exercises: a. Lateral side bending with 1-lb weight, leaning against wall, 10× ea side. b. Standing, leg raising, 5× ea. c. Trunk twisting with 1-lb weight, 5× ea. side. 2. Repeat part 2 of Step 10.	Continue all previous ward activities.	Increase time in OT clinic to 1 h.

Table 1. (Continued)

12	1. Warm-up exercises: a. Lateral side bending with 2-lb weight, 10×. b. Standing—leg raising, leaning against wall, 10× ea. c. Trunk twisting with 2-lb weight, 10×. 2. Walk down two flights of stairs.	Continue all previous ward activities.	Continue craft activity with increased resistance.
13	Repeat all exercises of Step 12.	Continue all previous ward activities.	Complete all projects.
14	1. Warm-up exercises: a. Lateral side bending with 2-lb weight, 10× ea. side. b. Trunk twisting with 2-lb weight, 10× ea. side. c. Touch toes from sitting position, 10×. 2. Walk up flight of 10 stairs and down.	Continue all previous ward activities.	Final instructions about home procedures and activities.

[a] Reprinted with permission from JW Hurst (ed), *The Heart* (ed 4), McGraw-Hill, New York, 1978, p. 1305.

[b] ROM = range of motion, MI = myocardial infarction, OT = occupational therapy.

tolerated activity levels, and it may permit identification of treatable mechanisms of impairment. The less severely impaired patient may be allowed to progress more rapidly to normal activity levels, and the more severely incapacitated patient who requires more gradual and supervised increases in activity level can also be distinguished. Finally, actual performance of a low-intensity exercise test may decrease the common fear among patients who have sustained myocardial infarction—that physical activity will result in recurrent myocardial infarction or in sudden cardiac death. (See Chap. 8.)

Although they are not in the strictest sense components of early ambulation, recommendations for physical activity during the early weeks of convalescence at home deserve mention. Most patients who have not become deconditioned during the course of uncomplicated myocardial infarction can and do return to work by 8–12 weeks after infarction, typically returning to their former jobs (12). Therefore the posthospital program should be designed to effect a gradual increase in endurance. A walking program that progressively increases the speed of walking and the distance walked is recommended. Prescription of the heart rate that is to be attained and self-monitoring of pulse rate assure an appropriate level of activity. A patient who can walk at a speed of 3.5 mph without difficulty is performing at a level of 4–5 mets. Such patients can be expected to return to most relatively sedentary occupations in today's society, which generally require an energy expenditure of 3–4 mets. Patients whose occupations require high levels of physical activity may require more intense and more prolonged exercise training before resuming their occupations.

RESULTS

Experience with nonrandomized in-hospital early mobilization programs (38–40) uniformly suggests favorable results in terms of self-care, improved patient's outlook and emotional status, earlier discharge from the hospital, and earlier and more complete return to work (41). The 10-year follow-up data of Brummer et al. (42) showed no significant differences in outcome as bed rest was progressively decreased from 16.2 to 10.3 days and hospitalization was decreased from 22.6 to 18.9 days. No apparent detrimental effects of early mobilization and hospital discharge for patients with uncomplicated myocardial infarction were found in other studies (43, 44) where hospital discharge was as early as 3–18 days.

McNeer and associates (45) at the Duke University Medical Center studied 522 consecutive patients with myocardial infarction; 51% of patients had uncomplicated clinical courses through day 4, with no subsequent hospital mortality or late complications. They advocated a controlled trial of early mobilization and discharge from hospital at 7 days, citing major economic benefits if the safety of such an approach could be documented. The feasibility of this approach has been repeatedly demonstrated, as has its cost-effectiveness; and McNeer and associates (45a) subsequently documented its safety in a small selected subgroup of patients with uncomplicated infarction.

More recently, several well-designed controlled studies have documented the safety of early ambulation for appropriately selected patients after myocardial infarction. There was no increase in morbidity or mortality and no increase in complications; indeed, some studies suggested that a more favorable outcome was associated with early mobilization. Early mobilization and earlier discharge from hospital commonly go hand in hand, the former facilitating the latter.

Groden and Brown (46) in Glasgow compared the effects of early and late mobilization after myocardial infarction on psychologic tests administered at discharge from the hospital and 1 year later. Eighteen patients were mobilized on day 14 and were discharged from the hospital on day 21; 27 patients were mobilized on day 25 and were discharged from the hospital after 35 days. The group that was mobilized earlier had lower neuroticism scores at discharge, but these scores did not persist at 1 year, which suggests that the initial advantages of early mobilization may be lost when patients return to the home environment.

In a subsequent study Groden (47) compared 50 male patients mobilized on day 15 and discharged by day 22 with 55 male patients who remained at bed rest for 25 days and were hospitalized for a total of 36 days. There were no adverse effects of early mobilization; benefits included reduction in psychologic complications and earlier return to work.

A British study of early ambulation coordinated by Harpur (48) mobilized 95 patients on day 8, had them walking by day 11, and had them home by day 15.

They were compared with a randomized population of 104 patients who were mobilized on day 21, allowed to walk by day 24, and discharged on day 28. Patients with complications of myocardial infarction (asystole, ventricular fibrillation, ventricular tachycardia, left ventricular failure, and hypotension) were not included in the study. No medical disadvantages (increased morbidity or mortality) were associated with early ambulation. The outcomes were comparable after 8 months of follow-up, with no differences in incidences of coronary deaths, recurrent myocardial infarction, congestive heart failure, significant arrhythmias, or ventricular aneurysm. However, earlier return to work was documented in the early mobilization group.

Lamers et al. (49) described a controlled study of early mobilization after uncomplicated myocardial infarction conducted in The Netherlands. No differences were observed in clinical outcomes or laboratory data between 102 patients mobilized on day 10 and 100 patients mobilized on day 20; no differences were evident at 18 months post infarction. The authors concluded that mobilization after 9 days and discharge after 3 weeks were safe for patients with uncomplicated myocardial infarction.

In a study at the Massachusetts General Hospital in Boston (50), 69 patients with uncomplicated myocardial infarction were discharged from the hospital at 2 weeks and 69 patients were discharged at 3 weeks post infarction. No differences were observed during the 6 months of follow-up in terms of angina, heart failure, ventricular aneurysm, recurrent infarction, coronary death, or in anxiety and depression, or return to work. The authors emphasized that the additional week of hospitalization did not appear to benefit patients with uncomplicated myocardial infarction and that the shorter hospital stay yielded substantial savings in costs of medical care and more optimum use of hospital beds.

In 1973 Boyle and Lorimer (51) reported a randomized trial of 538 patients with uncomplicated acute myocardial infarction; half were mobilized at 7 days after admission and discharged on day 21; the other half were mobilized on day 21 and discharged on day 28. Review at day 28, at 3 months, and at 1 year showed no differences in mortality or morbidity; early mobilization permitted improved utilization of hospital beds.

Hayes et al. (52) in Britain compared a total of 189 patients, uncomplicated at 48 hr, who were randomized into a group mobilized immediately and discharged after a total of 9 days in the hospital and a second group mobilized at 9 days and discharged at 16 days. No differences were observed in mortality or morbidity as reflected by the incidence of recurrent chest pain or myocardial infarction, heart failure, dysrhythmia, or venous thromboembolism detected either clinically or by ^{125}I-labeled fibrinogen scanning; the incidences of clinical deep vein thrombosis and pulmonary embolism were low in both groups and did not contribute to mortality in either group.

The Geneva study of Bloch et al. (53) randomized 154 patients with uncomplicated myocardial infarction at day 2 into an early mobilization group (beginning physical activity at day 2–3 and hospitalized for a mean duration of 21.3 days) and a traditional hospital regimen group (at strict bed rest for 3 weeks or more and hospitalized for a mean duration of 32.8 days). No differences in mortality or morbidity or in the results of an exercise test were evident between the two groups at 1 year; however, the early mobilization group had resumed work earlier and had a significantly lower incidence of disability (psychologic factors were the primary contributors to the disability).

Early mobilization trials have been characterized by progressively earlier ambulation in recent years. Indeed, the early mobilization groups of the earlier studies are comparable to the late mobilization groups in the later reports. Additionally, some earlier reports did not characterize myocardial infarction patients as complicated or uncomplicated; even when this was done the time after infarction at which this decision was made varied considerably.

Nevertheless numerous controlled studies throughout the world have confirmed the safety of supervised early mobilization regimens for appropriately selected patients. There have been no increases in hospital complications or follow-up complications of myocardial infarction (angina pectoris, recurrent myocardial infarction, dysrhythmias, congestive heart failure, ventricular aneurysm, cardiac rupture, sudden cardiac death, etc.) (51, 52); indeed, some studies have suggested a more favorable outcome. The complications of prolonged immobilization at bed rest (thromboembolism, pulmonary atelectasis, cardiovascular deconditioning, anxiety and depression) have been effectively reduced. Significantly greater disability has been demonstrated at follow-up examination in the traditional hospital regimen groups than in the early ambulation groups (53).

SUMMARY

Early ambulation for appropriately selected patients after uncomplicated myocardial infarction is no longer controversial. The benefits of early ambulation programs appear to be prevention of deconditioning and the other complications of prolonged bed rest, prevention or amelioration of anxiety and depression, greater physical capability and improved patient self-image at time of hospital discharge, and the economic advantages inherent in shorter hospitalization, more nearly optimal use of hospital beds, and an earlier and more complete return to work. This approach has proved desirable, feasible, cost-effective, and safe.

REFERENCES

1. Herrick JB: Clinical features of sudden obstruction of the coronary arteries. *JAMA* 59:2015, 1912

2. Mallory GK, White PD, Salcedo-Salgar J: The speed of healing of myocardial infarction: A study of the pathologic anatomy in seventy-two cases. *Am Heart J* 18:647, 1939

3. Lewis T: *Diseases of the Heart*. Macmillan, New York, 1933, p 49

4. Jetter WW, White PD: Rupture of the heart in patients in mental institutions. *Ann Intern Med* 21:783, 1944

5. Levine SA: Some harmful effects of recumbency in the treatment of heart disease. *JAMA* 126:80, 1944

6. Levine SA, Lown B: The "chair" treatment of acute coronary thrombosis. *Trans Assoc Am Physicians* 64:316, 1951

7. Dock W: The evil sequelae of complete bed rest. *JAMA* 125:1083, 1944

8. Harrison TR: Abuse of rest as a therapeutic measure for patients with cardiovascular disease. *JAMA* 125:1075, 1944

9. Stead EA Jr, Warren JV, Merrill AJ, et al: The cardiac output in male subjects as measured by the technique of right atrial catheterization. Normal values with observations on the effect of anxiety and tilting. *J Clin Invest* 24:326, 1944

10. Irvin CW Jr, Burgess AM Jr: The abuse of bed rest in the treatment of myocardial infarction. *N Engl J Med* 243:486, 1950

11. *Modern Medicine* July 23, 1973, pp 67–70

12. Wenger NK, Hellerstein HK, Blackburn H, et al: Uncomplicated myocardial infarction. Current physician practice in patient management. *JAMA* 224:511, 1973

13. Duke M: Bed rest in acute myocardial infarction. A study of physician practices. *Am Heart J* 82:486, 1971

14. Swan HJC, Blackburn HW, DeSanctis R, et al: Duration of hospitalization in "uncomplicated completed acute myocardial infarction." An ad hoc committee review. *Am J Cardiol* 37:413, 1976

15. Rose G: Early mobilization and discharge after myocardial infarction. *Mod Concepts Cardiovasc Dis* 41:59, 1972

16. Saltin B, Blomqvist G, Mitchell JH, et al: Response to exercise after bed rest and training. *Circulation* 37–38(Suppl 7):1, 1968

17. Chobanian AV, Lille RD, Tercyak A, et al: The metabolic and hemodynamic effects of prolonged bed rest in normal subjects. *Circulation* 49:551, 1974

18. Fareeduddin K, Abelmann WH: Impaired orthostatic tolerance after bed rest in patients with myocardial infarction. *N Engl J Med* 280:345, 1969

19. Hyatt KH, Kamenetsky LG, Smith WM: Extravascular dehydration as an etiologic factor in post-recumbency orthostatism. *Aerosp Med* 40:644, 1969

20. Miller PB, Johnson RL, Lamb LE: Effects of moderate physical exercise during four weeks of bed rest on circulatory functions in man. *Aerosp Med* 36:1077, 1965

21. Broustet JP, Dubecq M, Bouloumie J, et al: Rehabilitation of the coronary patients: Mobilization program in the acute phase. *Schweiz Med Wochenschr* 103:57, 1973

22. Lynch TN, Jensen RL, Stevens PM, et al: Metabolic effects of prolonged bed rest: Their modification by simulated altitude. *Aerosp Med* 38:10, 1967

23. Deitrick JE, Whedon GD, Shorr E: Effects of immobilization upon various metabolic and physiologic functions of normal men. *Am J Med* 4:3, 1948

24. Bonner CD: Rehabilitation instead of bed rest? *Geriatrics* 24:109, 1969

25. McPherson BD, Paivio A, Yuhasz MS, et al: Psychological effects of an exercise program for post-infarct and normal adult men. *J Sports Med Phys Fitness* 7:95, 1967

26. Cassem NH, Hackett TP: Psychiatric consultation in a coronary care unit. *Ann Intern Med* 75:9, 1971

27. Hackett TP, Cassem NH: Psychological adaptation to convalescence in myocardial infarction patients. In Naughton JP, Hellerstein HK (eds): *Exercise Testing and Exercise Training in Coronary Heart Disease*. Academic Press, New York, 1973

28. Report of the Task Force on Cardiovascular Rehabilitation, National Heart and Lung Institute: Needs and Opportunities for Rehabilitating the Coronary Heart Disease Patient, December 15, 1974. Washington, DC, US Department of Health, Education, and Welfare publication (NIH) 75-750

29. Report of the Joint Working Party of Royal College of Physicians of London and the British Cardiac Society on Rehabilitation after Cardiac Illness: Cardiac rehabilitation 1975. *JR Coll Physicians Lond* 9:281, 1975

30. Benton JG, Brown H, Rusk HA: Energy expended by patients on the bedpan and bedside commode. *JAMA* 144:1443, 1950

31. Wanka J: Bedpan vs. commode in patients with myocardial infarction. *Cardiac Rehabil* 1:7, 1970

32. Coe WS: Cardiac work and the chair treatment of acute coronary thrombosis. *Ann Intern Med* 40:42, 1954

33. DeBusk RF, Spivack AP, van Kessel A, et al: The coronary care unit activities program: Its role in post-infarction rehabilitation. *J Chronic Dis* 24:373, 1971

34. Wenger NK: Coronary Care—Rehabilitation after Myocardial Infarction, prepared for the Coronary Care Committee, Council on Clinical Cardiology and the Committee on Medical Education, American Heart Association, Dallas, Texas, EM609, November 1973

35. Acker J: Early ambulation of post-myocardial infarction patients. In Naughton JP, Hellerstein HK (eds): *Exercise Testing and Exercise Training in Heart Disease*. Academic Press, New York, 1973, p 311

36. Zohman LR: Early ambulation of post-myocardial infarction patients. In Naughton JP, Hellerstein HK (eds): *Exercise Testing and Exercise Training in Heart Disease.* Academic Press, New York, 1973, p 329

37. Nutter DO, Schlant RC, Hurst JW: Isometric exercise and the cardiovascular system. *Mod Concepts Cardiovasc Dis* 41:11, 1972

38. Royston GR: Short stay hospital treatment and rapid rehabilitation of cases of myocardial infarction in a district hospital. *Br Heart J* 34:526, 1972

39. Tucker HH, Carson PHM, Bass NM, et al: Results of early mobilization and discharge after myocardial infarction. *Br Med J* 1:10, 1973

40. Takkunen J, Huhti E, Oilinki O, et al: Early ambulation in myocardial infarction. *Acta Med Scand* 188:103, 1970

41. Mulcahy R, Hickey N: The rehabilitation of patients with coronary heart disease: A comparison of the return to work experience of national health insurance patients with coronary heart disease and of a group of coronary patients subjected to a specific rehabilitation programme. *J Ir Med Assoc* 64:541, 1971

42. Brummer P, Kallio V, Tala E: Early ambulation in the treatment of myocardial infarction. *Acta Med Scand* 180:231, 1966

43. Chaturvedi NC, Walsh MJ, Evans A, et al: Selection of patients for early discharge after acute myocardial infarction. *Br Heart J* 36:533, 1974

44. Adgey AAJ: Prognosis after early discharge from hospital of patients with acute myocardial infarction. *Br Heart J* 31:730, 1969

45. McNeer JF, Wallace AG, Wagner GS, et al: The course of acute myocardial infarction. Feasibility of early discharge of the uncomplicated patient. *Circulation* 51:410, 1975

45a. McNeer JF, Wagner GS, Ginsburg PB, et al: Hospital discharge one week after acute myocardial infarction. *N Engl J Med* 298:229, 1978

46. Groden BM, Brown RIF: Differential psychological effects of early and late mobilisation after myocardial infarction. *Scand J Rehabil Med* 2:60, 1970

47. Groden BM: The management of myocardial infarction. A controlled study of the effects of early mobilization. *Cardiac Rehabil* 1:13, 1971

48. Harpur JE, Kellett RJ, Conner WT, et al: Controlled trial of early mobilization and discharge from hospital in uncomplicated myocardial infarction. *Lancet* 2:1331, 1971

49. Lamers HJ, Drost WSJ, Kroon BJM, et al: Early mobilization after myocardial infarction: A controlled study. *Br Med J* 1:257, 1973

50. Hutter AM Jr, Sidel VW, Shine KI, et al: Early hospital discharge after myocardial infarction. *N Engl J Med* 288:1141, 1973

51. Boyle JA, Lorimer AR: Early mobilisation after uncomplicated myocardial infarction. Prospective study of 538 patients. *Lancet* 2:346, 1973

52. Hayes MJ, Morris GK, Hamptom JR: Comparison of mobilization after two and nine days in uncomplicated myocardial infarction. *Br Med J* 3:10, 1974

53. Bloch A, Maeder J-P, Haissly J-C, et al: Early mobilization after myocardial infarction. A controlled study. *Am J Cardiol* 34:152, 1974

5
The Potential for Preventing Reinfarction

Henry Blackburn, M.D.

In French medicine cardiac rehabilitation is called cardiac readaptation, a term that is consistent with French realism and the ability to adapt to circumstances. In contrast, the American ideal is ambitiously optimistic: to *prevent* reinfarction and to *prolong* life and *improve* its quality—never to accept the coronary event as end-stage vascular disease. This preventive ideal is pursued aggressively with an advanced technology by which we seek to reconstruct vessels and revascularize muscle surgically, reduce cardiac work and infarct size and suppress electrical instability pharmacologically, support ventricular function mechanically, and eventually replace the worn-out and failing heart with a partial and temporary prosthesis or even a complete and permanent prosthesis. But this volume is concerned primarily with physiologic ways of improving the efficiency of the oxygen delivery system, and this chapter will deal with simple approaches to the classification of risk after myocardial infarction, as well as safe and hygienic preventive management against reinfarction.

Prognosis for coronary patients has been improved and is now quantifiable. Risk assessment provides a rational basis for the practice of preventive cardiology, pointing out where observation and therapy may best be applied. The viewpoint taken here emphasizes the desirability of preventive efforts at the earliest possible stage of coronary heart disease (CHD), but disparages no reasonable or promising intervention at *any* stage.

Part of the information on diagnosis of high risk in coronary patients described in this chapter derives from the Coronary Drug Project, a collaborative trial fully supported by the National Heart, Lung, and Blood Institute (NHLBI) (USPHS grant HL-11898). Other findings derive from the experience in the Seven Countries Study, supported by the NHLBI (USPHS grant HL-94697) and by the American Heart Association, the National Diet-Heart Study (USPHS grant HE-07381), the Cooperative Study on Physical Activity and Prevention of Coronary Heart Disease, supported by the USPHS, Heart Disease Control Division (USPHS grant HE-03088), and the Heart Attack Risk Reduction Trial (HARRT), sponsored by the Minnesota Heart Association and by the Preventive Cardiology Award of Mutual Service Insurance Companies, St. Paul, Minnesota.

PERSPECTIVE

Cardiac symptoms and signs have traditionally provided clues to prognosis and therapy for the perceptive physician. Promotion of health, *hygieia* in the classic sense of a healthy mind in a healthy body, is also in the best medical tradition. But how many have fully heeded the fathers of modern cardiology, such as Sir James Mackenzie and Paul Dudley White, who proposed that medical prognosis is a fine art of medicine, and prevention the highest aim of the profession? Many cardiologists have heard, and some have acted—in their personal lives and in their practice. Hear Sir James (1) in 1916:

> I would ask you to realize for a moment what is the highest object at which the profession should aim, and then to consider how the object should be obtained. The highest duty, undoubtedly, is the prevention of disease. We are, however, far from obtaining this object in most instances for the simple reason that the danger is upon us before we are aware of it. Clinical research at the present date deals with disease at an advanced stage. To acquire knowledge of the life history of chronic diseases, it is necessary to be able to follow individual cases from the start to the finish. It must at once be apparent to you that this necessary knowledge cannot be acquired in a laboratory. The great field of investigation, the hospital ward, cannot afford sufficient opportunities, although the world has been taught to look in that direction for the advancement of medical science. Investigation of prognosis can only be carried out by those who have the opportunity of watching individuals during the whole course of the disease. You will best realize that what is called "prognosis" is a coping-stone which completes the edifice of your education.

In the more than 60 years since that time, technology applied to the diagnosis and therapy of cardiovascular diseases has made up the mainstream of cardiological training, investigative effort, and practice. Now, however, prediction, rehabilitation, and prevention of cardiovascular diseases are emerging in a vigorous response to the challenge laid down by Sir James at the beginnings of modern cardiology.

CLASSIFICATION OF RISK AFTER INFARCTION

Multiple Risk Indicators

Simple, practical, and objective office assessment of coronary risk is now possible among survivors of uncomplicated infarction. Data from the Coronary Drug Project (CDP) (Table 1) are highly relevant because the patients were ambulatory and largely uncomplicated, typical of patients likely to be encountered in office and clinical practice concerned with prevention (2,3).

The CDP experience provided the 16 prognostically important indicators listed in Table 1. They are statistically significant and additively predictive of sudden death or reinfarction and are listed in decreasing order of their independent contributions to risk prediction. The patients who contributed to the data base were men 35–64 years of age who survived one or more infarctions. Because the mortality rate for women is comparable to that for men, post infarction, it is reasonable to extrapolate these predictive findings to women.

Table 1. Coronary Drug Project: 16 Entry Prognostic
Factors for Death in 3 Years Among Myocardial Infarction
Survivors (2789 Placebo-treated Men, Ages 35–64)[a]

ST-segment depression (rest electrocardiogram)
Cardiomegaly (chest x-ray)
NYHA functional class
Ventricular conduction defect (rest electrocardiogram)
Diuretic therapy
Intermittent claudication
Serum total cholesterol
Frequent ventricular premature beats ($\geq$ 10% beats, rest elec-
    trocardiogram)
Physical inactivity
Q-QS waves (rest electrocardiogram)
Heart rate (rest electrocardiogram)
Number of prior infarctions
Systolic blood pressure
Diastolic blood pressure
Oral hypoglycemic therapy
Number of cigarettes smoked

[a]From CDP Research Group (3), with permission.

The findings derive from common elements of medical history, physical examination, chest x-ray, clinical laboratory tests, and conventional electrocardiogram.

Five of the top 16 predictors of 3-year mortality in CDP men are electrocardiographic, 7 come from medical history, 2 come from physical examination,
and 2 come from laboratory tests. Overall, the strongest predictors are the extent
of electrocardiographic residuals after infarction and the indicators of myocardial dysfunction. The top 16 factors have significantly positive relationships to
risk, above and beyond their intercorrelation with other risk characteristics.

An analytic procedure using 10 risk factors (Fig. 1) successfully discriminates
ambulatory infarction survivors in the CDP having reinfarction rates differing
by a factor of 12 for men in the highest and lowest deciles of estimated risk. The
index predicts over one-third of eventual cases from the upper 10% of risk
scores and over half of cases from the upper 20%. Application of the risk
equation to independent populations within the CDP (e.g., university versus
nonuniversity clinics) reveals that the profile remains efficiently predictive. A
simple, universal, objective, and powerful means is available to identify risk
among infarction survivors, and it uses common noninvasive medical procedures. The adjusted regression coefficients to compute risk are contained in the
original source (3). Of great practical importance are those risk indicators that
are directly causal and those among the possible causal influences that potentially
are modifiable.

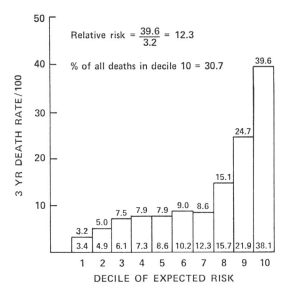

Figure 1. Expected and observed 3-year mortality for each decile of estimated risk; multiple logistic regression analysis with 10 variables, placebo group, 2789 men, CDP as of Nov. 1, 1972 (numbers inside bars show expected 3-year death rate per 100). [Reproduced by permission from CDP Research Group (3).]

Modifiable Risk Factors

The important risk influences for a first coronary event (blood lipid levels, diet, blood pressure, and cigarette smoking) appear also to influence subsequent risk among infarction survivors (3) (Table 1). It seems remarkable that prognostic relationships persist post infarction for these measures, which presumably affect underlying and precipitating mechanisms of the primary coronary event. Their significant and independent contributions to risk estimates, within categories of similar disease severity, suggest that these factors are also involved in mechanisms that alter the recurrence rate, or the survival from reinfarction. This, in turn, gives promise that a multiple-factor approach to risk reduction is a rational approach for preventive cardiology in postinfarction patients, as well as in high-risk persons before infarction.

Nonmodifiable Risk Indicators

The electrocardiogram was long considered to be so unrelated to ventricular structure or function as to have little serious interest for prognosis. The CDP found otherwise (2). The contribution of conventional 12-lead electrocardiographic items to 3-year prognosis in the CDP is given in Table 2. An electrocardiogram that reverts to "normal" following infarction is associated with an extremely favorable prognostic status, about 1% mortality per year (at the average age of 53 years) as compared to over 4% per year in those with any electrocardiographic residuals. Significant numbers of the infarction "community" (5–10%) may so revert and apparently are at low risk.

Table 2. Coronary Drug Project: Resting Electrocardiographic Risk Indicators Among Myocardial Infarction Survivors (Placebo-treated Men, Ages 30–64)[a]

ST-segment depression
T-wave amplitude in lead V_5
Any major electrocardiographic code (Minnesota code)
Negative T waves
Q-QS waves
Frequent ventricular premature beats
Ventricular conduction defects
Atrial fibrillation

[a]From CDP Research Group (2), with permission.

On the other hand, the electrocardiographic patterns "nonspecific ST and T wave findings" and "left hypertrophy or strain" so commonly considered innocuous in clinical practice are highly unfavorable in prognosis. They need to be recognized among the more powerful independent indicators (albeit unmodifiable?) of future mortality risk among infarction survivors.

Similarly, patients with intraventricular block or complete left bundle branch block have an increased risk of death, as compared to infarction survivors having tracings without these findings. In contrast, a stable pattern of complete right bundle branch block, even when associated with left anterior or posterior hemiblock, is not prognostically unfavorable among recovered ambulatory survivors of myocardial infarction. Atrial fibrillation and frequent or complex ventricular premature beats (VPB) are important predictors of excess risk.

The items in Table 2 contribute additively and significantly to risk prediction. Using the top five electrocardiographic predictors and ignoring clinical findings, 34.4% of deaths observed were in the upper decile of risk scores, as compared to 4.6% in the lower decile, a risk ratio of 7.5; 42.7% of deaths were concentrated in the upper two deciles (20%) of risk estimates, based on resting electrocardiogram alone, at entry into the CDP.

These data provide evidence that, other things being equal, electrocardiographic depolarization and repolarization findings, conduction defects, and arrhythmias, and their "severity," are prognostically important. Obviously the prognosis also depends on the clinical state in which the electrocardiographic findings are observed, whether in the acute phase, in late hospital or early posthospital convalescence, or, as in the CDP, in late convalescence.

Psychosocial Risk Indicators

The positive relationships between the following psychosocial variables and CHD have been summarized by Jenkins, among others:

· social and demographic variables, including incongruity between past or expected status and present or attained status (prospective study)
· mobility, both in jobs and geographically, and changes in occupation between generations (case–control study)

· anxiety and neuroticism precede coronary disease, particularly angina pectoris (prospective study), whereas excessive denial and repression are widely reported in CHD patients
· life dissatisfactions and environmental stress are more prevalent among CHD patients (case–control studies)
· a syndrome of "coronary-prone behavior" (prospective study)
· psychologic and social factors relate differently to particular CHD end points such as myocardial infarction and angina pectoris

Despite these interesting suggestions, there is little evidence concerning the influences of behavior, personality, and life stress on recurrence or mortality rates after myocardial infarction (5,6) and the effectiveness of modifying these characteristics in an attempt to reduce the risk of reinfarction: "Our present knowledge of social and psychologic factors of coronary disease . . . is still too rudimentary to permit comments on the implications of these findings for control programs" (4). However, if the same logic is used as in multiple physiologic risk factor reduction, the thoughtful practitioner concerned with prevention might try to reduce the stress of life, now complicated and threatened by the coronary event, and give support to the patient in finding ways to live well with the disease.

Other Prognostic Indices

Numerous indices have been developed for predicting in-hospital mortality based on data compiled early in the course of myocardial infarction. Because these indices are not strongly related to later survival, the equations, which take into consideration acute-phase arrhythmias, shock, heart failure, dyspnea, and serum enzyme elevation, are omitted from this discussion (7–9).

A number of prognostic indices measured at the end of hospitalization or in early convalescence and variably followed thereafter have also been computed for CHD. In general, the extent of myocardial dysfunction is the major prognosticator, whether expressed as left ventricular ejection fraction, ventriculographic pattern, end-diastolic volume, or functional aerobic impairment (7,10–12). Other strong indicators are the extent and distribution of coronary artery stenosis defined angiographically (13,14). These more specific measures tend to confirm the noninvasive indicators from later-stage measurements (2,3,15–17). Of the simple noninvasive measures, continued cigarette smoking was the factor that in one study best discriminated future nonfatal from fatal reinfarctions (18).

SUMMARY OF THE SIMPLE NONINVASIVE
POSTINFARCTION RISK PROFILE

Among infarction survivors, the factors that predict excessive risk of future reinfarction, coronary sudden death, and death from all causes include the following: cardiac size on posteroanterior chest x-ray; the presence or absence on the electrocardiogram of nonspecific ST-T findings, major conduction defects, specific arrhythmias, and size of residual Q-QS waves; the simple NYHA

(New York Heart Association) functional class; diuretic or digitalis therapy; history of intermittent claudication. By contrast, reversion to "normal" in the electrocardiogram post infarction is a very favorable indicator. The value of the coronary risk profile (Table 1) derives from its power to classify risk, its simplicity, its noninvasiveness, and its broad applicability to coronary patients with an uncomplicated clinical course. Other newer noninvasive procedures, including echocardiography and scintillography, may permit more precise definition of excess risk in coronary patients who do not require angiography and ventriculography.

Modifiable factors that contribute significantly to risk post infarction include level of total serum cholesterol, arterial pressure, and number of cigarettes smoked. Habitual sedentary activity and behavioral patterns may influence risk and may be modifiable.

POTENTIAL FOR PREVENTION OF REINFARCTION: THE EVIDENCE

Multifactor Risk Reduction

Unequivocal evidence is not yet at hand that cardiac reinfarction can be prevented, life prolonged, or death delayed by any means, including multifactor hygienic risk reduction, pharmacologic, or surgical. This is due in part to the vagaries of the disease and in part to the problems of design, operation, and cost of adequately controlled trials, the weakness of any intervention based solely on single characteristics of risk, and the equivocal results of the trials (generally of less than ideal design) that have been carried out thus far.

A definitive clinical trial to resolve this question would involve the following: aggressive and effective intervention on the multiple risk factors of blood pressure, smoking, and blood lipid levels in one group of patients; identical multiple risk factor intervention plus systematic physical conditioning in another group; conventional laissez-faire "best medical care" and advice in another group. Such a design would determine the contributions of specific preventive programs as compared to usual care and should delineate any added contribution of physical conditioning to the multiple risk factor approach. Such trials have been proposed, and a few, with limited sample sizes, are under way (19–21). It will be costly to determine a definite answer to the simple question whether or not reinfarction or CHD death can be delayed, but it will probably be more costly not to answer it.

Single-Factor Risk Reduction

Rehabilitation Physical Activity Programs—Uncontrolled
Results from convalescent cardiac rehabilitation programs, none of which has been adequately controlled, indicate that gradually progressive physical activity prevention programs have generally low mortality when administered by careful, competent, and devoted investigators to groups of select, highly motivated, volunteer coronary patients without severe functional impairment. They rarely appear to be harmful and possibly are beneficial. Much has been learned about

technique and safety in such pilot programs (22–24). However, some patients so treated receive no benefit, some deteriorate during such programs, and the optimal exercise prescription remains to be determined (22–28).

Rehabilitation Physical Activity Trials—Controlled

Results of adequately controlled and randomized trials of physical activity rehabilitation after myocardial infarction suggest a possible but not overwhelming beneficial effect of cardiovascular conditioning on reinfarction and survival. The Gothenburg trial data are as follows: Follow-up averaged over 4 years in men below 55 years of age; there were 30 deaths among 158 trained patients, as compared to 37 deaths among 157 controls, and 28 as compared to 30 nonfatal reinfarctions. The study had inadequate statistical power and sample size to give great confidence that this is a truly negative result (27,28). Preliminary data from a Helsinki trial in progress are comparable, i.e., insufficient power to demonstrate any but gross differences, perhaps of a magnitude it would be unrealistic to expect for any therapy after infarction (29).

However, symptomatic effects are more certain. The threshold for angina pectoris (possibly for arrhythmias and other electrocardiographic manifestations of ischemia during graduated exercise) can be significantly raised and cardiovascular function improved in ideally supervised intensive conditioning programs. But it must be questioned how much benefit might be obtained through less intensive and less formal, but longer or more frequent, exercise programs.

The evidence is not conclusive regarding whether programs of intensive supervised exercise for rehabilitation among patients with angina and/or patients recovered from myocardial infarction are effective in prolonging life or are widely indicated and advisable. Results of current collaborative trials are needed before mass adoption of therapeutic efforts using intensive exercise in CHD patients. Moreover, better information is required about optimal exercise prescriptions and about the costs of such programs (19,20). Finally, such intensive multifactor interventions would provide the ideal control groups for bypass surgery trials.

Risk Factor Reduction Programs

Evidence is also limited in regard to how reductions in the levels of primary coronary risk factors (serum lipids, blood pressure, and cigarette smoking) affect reinfarction rates in CHD patients. The potential for reducing other risk factors (relative weight, uric acid levels, behavior pattern, etc.) that have significant, if lesser, relationships to primary development of atherosclerosis, sudden cardiac death, and myocardial infarction has likewise not been systematically explored in postinfarction patients. Their relatively weak influences in primary event prediction and the difficulties inherent in assessing and modifying behavior or life stresses suggest that their preventive potential will remain untested in the near future.

Lipid-lowering Trials

The CDP results (30) are applicable to patients who have survived with good functional recovery for several months to years after an initial myocardial infarction. The lipid-lowering drugs studied (estrogen, dextrothyroxine, clofi-brate, and niacin) did not improve long-term survival after infarction. On the contrary, unfavorable side effects and toxicity, particularly with estrogen and dextrothyroxine, resulted in more harm than good. The United Kingdom studies on clofibrate demonstrated a beneficial effect on mortality in patients with angina; however, the effect was not related to the lipid-lowering property of the drug (31,32). Lipid-lowering drugs and ileal bypass surgery currently are being tested experimentally among infarction survivors and those at high coronary risk.

Diet trials, in contrast to drug trials, have shown no harmful effect. In Oslo the Leren study (33) of survivors of myocardial infarction followed for over a decade showed that dietary modification of serum lipids had a positive effect on the rate of nonfatal reinfarction but had no significant effect on sudden coronary death rate or total coronary death rate. Because effects were not demonstrated for all manifestations of coronary disease and because of other problems inherent in trials that involve health behavior (such as sufficient numbers of subjects and events and effective blinding of subjects and investigators to the results), the Oslo study must be considered suggestive but not definitive.

Aspirin Trials

Preliminary results of studies on the use of aspirin are encouraging in terms of preventing reinfarction among infarction survivors (34–36); full-scale trials of aspirin and Persantine-aspirin are currently in progress.

Blood Pressure-lowering Trials

Adequately controlled studies of the effect of blood pressure reduction on recurrence rates in ambulatory patients recovered from infarction have not been performed. The results of a trial among stroke patients were negative (37). There is also a lack of evidence regarding the effects of proper management of elevated blood pressure on the initial coronary attack rate, although controlled trials are approaching completion. The collaborative Veterans Administration hypertension trials, which established the overall efficacy of blood pressure lowering, were inadequate in terms of sample size to answer the question about reduced CHD incidence. Thus their "negative" results for coronary events were essentially "no results." However, in those same VA trials, differences among the treatment groups suggested that similarly favorable results over a long period, or in a sample several times larger, would have demonstrated a significant effect of blood pressure lowering for the end points of sudden death and coronary death in hypertensive middle-aged veterans. However, no attempt at positive or nega-tive extrapolation of these results is appropriate (38,39).

Thus the trials reported to date among CHD patients regarding lipid lowering or blood pressure control by diet or drugs or combinations thereof have pre-sented no definitive evidence that nonfatal reinfarction rate or coronary death rate is significantly modified by such therapy. However, the results of a recent drug trial with β-adrenergic blockade were encouraging in terms of improved survival after myocardial infarction (10). These results require confirmation, which are being sought in a collaborative NHLBI propranolol trial.

Observations on Cessation of Smoking

The evidence concerning the effects of cessation of cigarette smoking on death rate and reinfarction among coronary patients is based on observed experience; no controlled experiment has been made. CDP data indicated an improved prognosis for those men who stopped smoking cigarettes "spontaneously" after entry in the study, but this finding was not statistically significant after differences in the severity of clinical disease were taken into account. In the Gothenburg multiple risk factor intervention trial the rate of reinfarction among those who continued to smoke after infarction was twice as high as the rate among those who stopped; there were also higher cardiovascular and total mortality. The favorable rate in smokers who stopped smoking was not related to less severe infarction clinically; on the contrary, those who stopped smoking had larger infarctions and more severe clinical disease. On the basis of multivariate analysis of clinical characteristics it was estimated that the group that stopped smoking after myocardial infarction had a higher expected risk of dying than the group that continued to smoke. Despite the fact that the study was not a controlled experiment, the results suggest that altering smoking habits after infarction is effective (18,21). A randomized controlled trial concerning cessation of smoking in high-risk patients is in progress in the United Kingdom, but several years will be required to determine the outcome (40).

Behavior Change

Study of systematic efforts to modify risk-related health behavior is just beginning. These efforts range from behavior modification approaches based on learning theory to eating behavior (amount and composition of diet), smoking, and life-style. Further development and comparative testing of various change strategies are believed to be essential to risk factor reduction for individuals, groups, and entire communities (41). These strategies have been well reviewed in respect to eating, smoking, and aggressive behavior patterns (11,42–45). There are indications that information, motivation, and skills for change can be more effectively and practically imparted than they have been in our traditional, authoritative, prescription-oriented medical practices.

SUMMARY OF EVIDENCE ON RISK FACTOR REDUCTION

Our ability to measure and diagnose differences in risks of reinfarction and sudden death among coronary patients has been vastly improved in the last decade by means of simple clinical findings and common measurements as well as more sophisticated measurements of cardiac anatomy and function. Modifiable primary coronary risk characteristics appear to retain an influence on risk after infarction. Experimental interventions on primary risk factors and on exercise habits have produced suggestive evidence that a systematic, positive multifactor approach to preventing reinfarction may be effective.

Most of the scientific and practicing community agree that it is good medical practice to treat not only cardiac manifestations but also single and combined coronary risk factors, post infarction and in patients with angina. It is increasingly being accepted that although there is not yet full experimental evidence of the beneficial effect of such an approach, it is harmless to intervene, always by hygienic means and, were indicated, by the least toxic of the lipid-lowering and blood pressure-reducing drugs. It is also being accepted that moderate levels of unsupervised physical activity and more intensive appropriately supervised exercise programs are effective ways of improving cardiac function. They also have the potential to reduce the risk of reinfarction.

A RATIONALE FOR PREVENTIVE PRACTICE

In coronary disease, as in most chronic diseases, the more advanced the disease process the poorer the prognosis and probably the less the potential for important intervention. But CHD is probably more amenable than most chronic diseases to characterization of risk and prognosis. CHD is perhaps more strongly related to risk elements that can be modified in rational, hygienic, self-determined, safe, and effective ways. Consequently it seems inappropriate and inconsistent to reject safe and reasonable interventions on health habits such as overeating, cigarette smoking, and sedentary life-style. Strong associations and logical mechanisms exist to justify attempts at risk factor reduction. Experiments in man and animals have suggested a powerful potential for the arrest of progress, or actual regression, of "mobile" fatty portions of atherosclerotic plaques. Similarly, mechanisms exist whereby risk factor reduction may have effects on thrombogenesis and platelet function, cardiac workload and myocardial oxygen requirement, catecholamine activity, myocardial excitability, and ventricular fibrillation threshold. All these mechanisms could be affected favorably by safe, palatable, moderate, hygienic, and at times pharmacologic approaches to the reduction of primary coronary risk factors. Let us now consider how to implement the potential for preventing reinfarction in coronary patients.

TECHNIQUES FOR PREVENTING REINFARCTION

How to Measure Serum Lipids

A casually drawn sample for determination of serum cholesterol level is the best method for rapid office risk screening. The effect of a meal is not much greater than the laboratory measurement error. In office management of coronary patients, measurement of total serum cholesterol and fasting triglycerides is first indicated. Good laboratories perform these analyses, refrigerate the plasma specimen at 4°C, and inspect it the next day to report any chylomicron layer.

Phenotyping provides increased understanding for management but little more precision in risk estimation than does evaluation of total cholesterol, triglycerides, and chylomicrons. But high-density lipoprotein (HDL) cholesterol appears to provide added information for estimating risk. Because HDL cholesterol contributes independently to risk, and because it does not vary with total cholesterol level, it is usefully obtained as part of a complete risk assessment.

However, because HDL cholesterol is rather insensitive to dietary change, it figures little in nutritional prescriptions. It is interesting that only vigorous habitual conditioning exercise, weight reduction, and perhaps moderate alcohol consumption tend to elevate the HDL cholesterol level. This is now believed to be a desirable change, independent of low-density lipoprotein (LDL) and total cholesterol lowering, which is the main need and the focus of the eating patterns recommended here; however, research is needed in this area.

A baseline cholesterol determination is essential to understanding and handling an individual patient's lipid levels over a period of time. One determination gives only a rough estimate of "true" cholesterol level; a more precise value is obtained by averaging multiple determinations over a relatively short time—before starting intervention. The relative merits of two, three, four, or more baseline laboratory determinations are depicted in Figure 2. This curve illustrates the decreasing width of the range (confidence interval) around the "true" level obtainable by averaging two or more determinations and using these to estimate individual variations. A considerable increase in precision is achieved by the third or fourth determination because of the greater information about the individual's cholesterol variability (46). Three baseline determinations in a short period may be reasonable and practical, whereas 10 determinations clearly are not.

Guidelines are needed to inform patients about cholesterol values and their changes during intervention. These must take into consideration individual variations as well as measurement error. In the absence of specific knowledge about an individual's past serum cholesterol level, we have employed an arbitrary

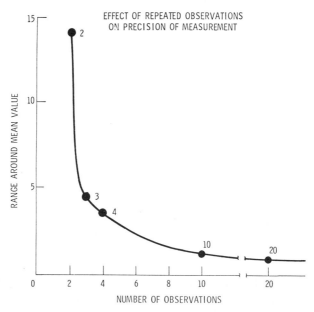

Figure 2. The "range around the mean value" decreases, and precision increases, with the frequency of observations made. A considerable increase in precision occurs by the third or fourth measurement. The range is the average number of true intraindividual standard deviations in an interval that has 95% probability of containing the true mean. [Reproduced by permission from Blackburn (46).]

unit of variation based on the variations found in relatively stable experimental populations: ± 15 mg/dl. Under these circumstances a change of 22 mg/dl, based on one follow-up cholesterol value and one baseline value, is probably a real change; 42 mg/dl is almost surely so. These are substantial changes that are not easily attained, and therefore they leave most cholesterol-lowering results uncertain.

A practical approach to this problem is necessary because emotional swings, which are tied to the very uncertain swings in individual blood lipid values, are devastating to effective intervention. Our approach is as follows:

· explain to the patient at the outset that the phenomena of biologic and technical variability exist in all risk measurement
· explain that we will from the beginning focus on actual changes in eating behavior and food choices, rather than on each blood test result
· explain that after a few months we will show averaged levels and a graph of blood cholesterol and pressure trends over time in order to assess progress

Under these conditions a slope can be drawn through points indicating the general direction of change. Averaging will be more sensitive to detecting real change. For example, a change of 12 mg/dl in serum cholesterol level is likely a real change—when a mean of three follow-up determinations is compared with a mean baseline value from three determinations.

How to Measure Dietary Patterns

Effective intervention on the affluent American way of eating requires some basic information on the patient's eating habits. As in taking a medical history, important or deviant phenomena are often exposed by a systematic diet history. Otherwise, one can miss vital information on the patient. A patient recently encountered ate a gallon of ice cream weekly, i.e., over 300 g or about 3000 calories of butterfat per week; otherwise, the patient ate quite unremarkably.

Two types of dietary information are useful, one acquired with a food diary and the other with a food pattern questionnaire (see Appendices 2.1 and 2.2). For practical reasons the diary is confined to 3 days and is best kept on different sets of 3 days, involving one nonworking day. It is completed near the time of a counseling visit. Although the patient may be "showing off" during the recorded days, the diary provides information, education, and motivation. The simple recording of eating behavior appears to influence that behavior. The food pattern questionnaire is more likely than is the diary to show the overall patterns and peculiarities in eating. Both are of value in assessing a patient's progress in understanding and adherence, as well as in providing a basis from which to relate reported diet changes to measured serum lipid changes.

Dietary Intervention

Modification of the habitual way of eating to achieve weight control and reduction in serum lipid levels is central to effective preventive care in patients recovered from myocardial infarction. The physician may inform himself about the simple principles of a prudent diet and gather information and materials about lipid-reducing and weight-reducing ways of eating as outlined here, or patients may be referred to other professionals (dietitians) for these matters, but the needed facts and procedures are easily available without the physician having to become a full-time student of nutrition.

Beyond the components of the prudent diet necessary for successful intervention on eating habits are a clear plan, patient self-testing of knowledge, some "change skills," and supportive involvement of the family. Such a plan is within the scope of the physician and staff in office or clinical practice (47). Regular nutritional counseling may best be handled by a member of an office or clinic staff who has been specially trained by a physician and nutritionist for such a function. Occasionally a hospital dietitian may be recruited. Emphasis should be on the long-term preventive approach rather than on short-term disease-oriented teaching. The desirable modifications are established among the five basic food groups, setting simple goals for change in each, and following up by periodic review and discussions with the patient and family. Actual shopping choices and eating changes are reviewed, the food pattern and diet diary are evaluated, lipid levels are measured at intervals of 6–12 weeks until new habits are established (46).

Nutrition Program

The dietary goals for most patients are similar to those recommended by all the major deliberative bodies that have thoughtfully considered the diet–heart issue. The goals include establishing an energy balance, reducing consumption of saturated fat, partially replacing saturated fat with polyunsaturated fat, reducing dietary cholesterol, and reducing simple sugars and salt. These recommendations are fully reviewed and summarized elsewhere (38,48,49).

Food Groups

Over 90% of all fat intake is contained in three food groups:

· meat, fish, and poultry
· dairy products and eggs
· cooking fats and oils

The other two major food groups are low in fat and "neutral" in serum lipid effect (when there is caloric balance):

· cereals and starches
· fruits and vegetables

Treatment begins with the staff's diet evaluation (food diary and questionnaire), followed by an introductory presentation from the physician or other staff person to provide:

· opportunity for a deliberate commitment by the patient to the prevention program (preferably written)
· simple repeated facts about the effects of specific types of foods, and amounts, on levels of blood lipids
· specific short-term goals for change in eating pattern

a program for achieving and maintaining an appropriate long-term pattern of food choices, food preparation, and eating habits

Generally, at least three sessions are required to provide the minimal basic information about the prudent way of eating. These meetings must include the person who prepares most of the home meals. Special sessions are useful for reviewing individual questions on menu choices for those who eat out much of the time, on shopping and brand-name guides, etc. Patients should be involved in monitoring the local availability and price of approved products and collecting this information for others.

The simplest goals and messages are sought for each of the food groups:

Meat, Fish, and Poultry. Reduce the frequency of eating meats to average one serving daily. Reduce the size of the meat serving, and remove visible fat. Select lean cuts and types of beef (veal, ground lean round, tenderloin, chuck roast) and lean pork chops. Increase fish and fowl. Avoid sausage, bacon, cold cuts, frankfurters, bologna, ordinary hamburger, and organ meats.

Dairy Products and Eggs. Decrease the use of butter and spreads, whole milk, ice cream, cream, cheese, and egg yolks. This does not mean that they are totally prohibited. Milk is a rich food, not to be used as a thirst-quenching beverage. Emphasize low-fat skim milk products, yogurt, sherbets, cottage cheese, egg substitutes, egg whites, and cheese in small portions or as seasoning. For food preparation, replacement of butter with soft margarines is suggested.

Fruits and Vegetables. Emphasis is on "unlimited" intake of vegetables. Legumes are also recommended in all forms: beans or peas or as ingredients in casseroles and salads.

Cereals and Starches. Free use of cereal grains or starches should be encouraged within the limits set for weight control. Sweet baked goods are to be avoided unless made at home under prudent recipes. Reduced consumption of simple sugar and alcohol calories is often desirable as a part of effective intervention on elevated weight, serum lipids, and blood pressure.

Cooking Fats and Oils. Reduce total fat consumption. Liquid oils and soft margarines should be used for only partial replacement of fats needed in food preparation; a surfeit of polyunsaturated fats is not desirable. With a little practice, oils and margarines are generally as successful in food preparation and baking as are hard fats.

Salt. Salty foods should be avoided; no salt should be added at the table, and lesser amounts of Lite Salt (half potassium) should be employed in cooking.

Eating Out
Physicians and patients alike bemoan the problems of adhering to a prudent diet when eating in restaurants. On eating out there may be an atmosphere of celebration, which can lead to an orgy of overdrinking and overeating. It is customary to get, and to feel, stuffed. Rarely, however, is there a total absence of

good food choices. To document this contention, the following list of food choices was culled by Laboratory of Physiological Hygiene nutritionists from menus taken from "greasy spoons," cafeterias, and leading restaurants in the Twin Cities, Minnesota. The foods listed usually are acceptable in terms of low fat or relatively low saturated fat and cholesterol constituents:

· soups and appetizers: onion soup, consommé, tomato juice, gazpacho, pickled herring, shrimp or crabmeat cocktail, salad tray
· entrées (avoid sauces and gravies): broiled fish, such as salmon, pike, haddock, snapper, and trout; chicken, baked or broiled (not Chicken Kiev); turkey; broiled tenderloin or sirloin (the leanest of beef cuts); roast leg of lamb or lamb chops; baked ham; teriyaki; chicken almond; pepper steak; sukiyaki or tempura; beef and snow pea pods; chow mein with steamed rice
· vegetables and potatoes: any and all vegetables, without added butter or cream sauce
· salads: any vegetable or fruit salad with dressing, except whipped cream or cheese-based dressings; also chef salad (without eggs), cabbage salad, tossed salad, potato salad (without eggs), fruit salad
· desserts: ices, sherbets, fruit, melon, angel food cakes, baked apples
· drinks: wines, any cocktail or after-dinner drink except those made with ice cream or cream
· sandwiches: chicken, turkey, tuna salad, chicken salad, peanut butter, broiled lean ground beef, fish patties
· beverages: beer, carbonated beverages, skim milk, buttermilk, coffee, tea, consommé, fruit juices

Lobster, shrimp, and shellfish are relatively high in cholesterol and low in saturated fat, but when eaten occasionally they are advantageous in comparison with many cuts of meat. Newer analyses of shellfish, adjusting for water content, indicate that they are not as high in cholesterol as older analyses indicated.

Many restaurants will serve margarine instead of butter if requested. In addition, in many restaurants the waiter will tell the customer who inquires what fat is used in deep frying. If a liquid vegetable fat is used it is likely to be cottonseed oil or peanut oil and is thus relatively "neutral" in terms of serum lipid effects. There is a trend toward the use of other relatively neutral, partially saturated deep-fry fats in commercial food preparation, but there is not yet any widespread commercial use of the polyunsaturated liquid vegetable oils for frying.

In the long run, market availability of leaner cuts of meat and low-fat dairy products, as well as more varied international foods, and restaurant use of liquid fats rather than hard fats in food preparation depend on customer interest and demand. Therefore it may be useful to encourage patients to make intelligent requests when eating out and shopping.

Public Myths and Professional Misconceptions About Diet and Blood Lipids

Carbohydrate-induced Hyperlipidemia. The clinical matter of carbohydrate-induced hyperlipidemia remains a confused subject. There have been many valid reports about the short-term elevations in serum triglycerides that occur on shifting to low-fat diets. Other reports have described patients especially sensitive to the lipid-raising effects of alcohol. There is much to learn about the control of very low density lipoproteins and serum triglycerides and their independent importances in atherosclerosis, if any. However, some specific facts should be kept in mind:

Well-designed long-term experiments have shown that the prudent diet (low fat, low saturated fat, high carbohydrate), combined with weight reduction where indicated, results in a lowering of elevated serum cholesterol and serum triglyceride levels in the majority of hyperlipidemias encountered in clinical practice (50,51).

The loosely used term low-carbohydrate diet really means a high-fat diet, because protein intake is not readily variable. Such a diet is rarely indicated or required for lipid lowering. In countries where serum lipid levels are generally very low (and where, incidentally, CHD is uncommon), high-carbohydrate (low-fat) diets have been habitually consumed for centuries. This does not negate the idea that restriction in total calories and in simple sugar and alcohol calories is, on the whole, usually desirable in patients. Moreover, serum lipid levels usually rise during periods of weight gain, irrespective of the composition of the diet. But the carbohydrate sensitivity question, as with the question of specific lipid phenotype and HDL/LDL ratio, should not obscure the central issue: mass hyperlipidemia in affluent populations is related primarily to widespread habitual overeating of saturated fat, cholesterol, and total calories (38,52).

Low-Carbohydrate and High-Protein Diets. Needless to say, the Stillman-Atkins types of low-carbohydrate (very high fat, ketosis-inducing weight reduction) diets are totally wrong in their claims that fat "calories don't count." When they are effective in weight reduction, it is probably primarily because of appetite suppression. Such reduction diets are highly suspect in terms of their poorly documented claims that they lower serum lipid values, although this may happen temporarily during an active period of negative caloric balance. Such high-fat diets are totally incongruous with any reasonable and healthful long-term eating pattern.

Similarly misleading are other so-called high-protein diets prevalent in the United States: the drinking man's diet, the "Mayo diet," and various protein-supplement diets. Large proportions of the calories in the commonly regarded high-protein foods of such diets (especially steak and eggs) are fat calories rather than protein calories. The dangers of rapid weight reduction on poor-quality liquid protein preparations are becoming evident.

Every physician's office would do well to keep, perhaps next to the *Physicians' Desk Reference*, a copy of U.S. Department of Agriculture handbook number 8 on the composition, in protein, fat, and carbohydrate calories, of all common foods (see Appendix, p. 104).

Dietary Cholesterol. The relative importance of dietary cholesterol versus dietary fat remains controversial. The effect of dietary cholesterol in "natural" diets may best be characterized by the formula of a Minnesota group (53) based on numerous experiments in man in caloric balance:

$$\Delta C = 1.35(2\Delta S - \Delta P) + 1.5\Delta Z$$

where ΔC indicates change in serum cholesterol, ΔS indicates change in saturated fat calories, ΔP indicates change in polyunsaturated fat calories, and ΔZ is the square root of change in dietary cholesterol intake. This means that saturated fats raise serum cholesterol (monounsaturated fats are neutral) and polyunsaturated fats lower serum cholesterol. Thus the saturated fats are twice as powerful and efficient at raising cholesterol as the polyunsaturated fats are at lowering cholesterol. Dietary cholesterol within the usual range of United States intake raises serum cholesterol by a factor equal to the square root of the amount of cholesterol added. The effect of eating cholesterol is strongest at the low end of the range of cholesterol consumption. But even in a culture heavily dependent on meat and dairy products the dietary cholesterol effect on average serum cholesterol level is important in terms of population risk.

The Minnesota $2S-P$ formula clearly shows that the most efficient way to reduce serum lipid levels among men in caloric balance is to reduce total consumption of saturated fat, reduce dietary cholesterol, and add polyunsaturated fat. In actual practice, and in natural diets around the world, the first two measures generally go together automatically, and increasing the polyunsaturated fat is not necessary for a significant cholesterol-lowering effect in those partaking of our common affluent high-fat eating pattern.

Polyunsaturated Fats. The Minnesota group believes that significant additions of polyunsaturated fats to the United States diet or other affluent diets (i.e., total replacement of saturated-fat calories by polyunsaturated) are neither necessary nor desirable, despite the fact that a somewhat greater serum-cholesterol-lowering effect might be anticipated therefrom in Americans. Why? Figure 3

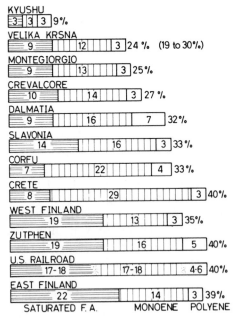

Figure 3. Average percentages of total calories in diets provided by saturated, monoene, and polyunsaturated fatty acids. [Reproduced by permission from Keys (54).]

shows that the primary difference in the fat composition of natural diets among working populations lies in the proportion of saturated fat calories consumed. There is no correlation of polyunsaturated-fat intake with serum cholesterol levels or with CHD incidence in these populations; no natural diet studied contained more than 8–10% of calories as polyunsaturated fat (54).

Reduced consumption of saturated fat is the natural experiment thoroughly proven by centuries of use to be safe, effective, and salubrious. Consequently there appears to be no indication for great increases in polyunsaturated-fat consumption in American or other Western diets. However, partial replacement of the common saturated fats by polyunsaturated fats is reasonable in some circumstances: for purposes of palatability; when fat is necessary in food preparation; when many calories are needed, as for the young or for very active persons. The American Heart Association prudent diet includes 30–35% fat calories, made up one-third each of saturated, monounsaturated, and polyunsaturated fatty acids.

Medical-Surgical Lipid Lowering

Lipid-lowering drug therapy is part of the traditional medical armamentarium. Its techniques are well described in the general medical literature. The negative CDP results provide a balancing caution against long-term use of many lipid-lowering preparations. Ileal bypass surgery is still very much an investigative procedure for coronary patients with elevated LDL cholesterol levels, but its lipid-lowering effect is impressive and sustained.

Obesity

Consideration of obesity is an integral part of evaluation and management of all coronary patients, particularly patients with hypertension. Significant improvement in blood pressure control can be achieved by the loss of fat tissue and sodium involved in simple weight reduction. Added benefits are obvious: lipid lowering, improved glucose tolerance, greater mobility, enhanced and healthy self-image. It is even likely that early intervention to prevent obesity in coronary patients and in those persons who stop smoking (for that matter, in the general population) would result in mass reductions in frequency and severity of hypertension, hyperlipidemia, and glucose intolerance.

The seven-countries study conducted by Keys and the Minnesota group (54) in many rural and small-town populations tends to confirm Dr. Jean Mayer's theory that the mass phenomenon of obesity and caloric imbalance is probably more closely related to a mass decrease in physical activity than to "excess" caloric intake. The greater the mean daily caloric intake, the thinner the population. Caloric intake in such "natural" populations is a good measure of habitual physical activity. The conclusion is that long-term sedentary lifestyle is essential to mass adiposity in a population. If we were more active as a population, we would be less likely to eat our way to being fat. As with the dietary fat/serum lipid/CHD relationship, we must separate the question of an individual's high risk (which may be due primarily to a particular personal or hereditary factor) from the question of high risk of an entire population. In the latter situation it is likely that cultural and environmental factors overwhelmingly influence the mass phenomenon. Systematic revision of daily life to include regular activity probably is necessary to any successful individual or mass program of weight control.

In the United States and in other cultures where there are strong social pressures for high-fat high-caloric eating, and where food intake also functions as an escape or substitute pleasure, it is possible that eating habits play a greater role in energy balance than in the hard-working rural cultures of the seven-countries study. But long-term caloric balance or weight control clearly requires an increase in habitual physical activity among most persons and coronary patients engaged in sedentary occupations.

Measurement

The use of standard height–weight tables to determine weight excess over the "ideal," followed by nude inspection of the amount and distribution of adipose deposits, is sufficient for most purposes of evaluation before and during intervention. A frequency of weighing for the individual is not established; for those making little progress in weight reduction, more frequent weighing is indicated.

This discussion does not address gross obesity, which is a special physiologic, metabolic, and psychologic challenge. In "garden-variety" positive caloric balance there is a cyclic but slowly "losing" curve of excess caloric intake over output—from school days into advanced middle-age.

Intervention for Weight Reduction

Computation of the exercise required to lose 1 lb (3600 kcal, or 10 hr of walking-jogging) can cause confusion—and inaction! The important point about physical activity and body weight is the very small amount of long-term frequent caloric excess that eventuates in moderate obesity. Often this amounts to only 50–150 calories average daily excess intake over expenditure. Such a small but frequent excess intake can be balanced by only 10–30 minutes of brisk walking daily. In contrast to the frustrating problem of weight reduction, this provides a much happier perspective, that is, the long-term potential for correction, maintenance, and prevention of obesity by moderate regular exercise.

Large numbers of middle-aged American men and women would find little problem with energy balance if they simply eliminated one cocktail, switched to skimmed milk products, and walked briskly for 15–30 min daily. Most would have no long-term weight problem if they also adopted the prudent diet with its reduced frequency of meat eating, reduced portion sizes, and reduced butterfat and baked-goods consumption.

Changing Eating Behavior and Reducing Weight

The principles of modifying behavior, which will be described later in this chapter, must be applied systematically (43,44,55). First, it must be determined that the patient is ready to make a commitment to long-term change. Self-recording of the 3-day food record is carried out, and the eating-pattern questionnaire is completed. Three meals per day are prescribed, with low-calorie between-meal snacks—no skipped meals, no fasting, no formula diets! Portion sizes are reduced, as are alcoholic drinks, where indicated. Exercise is recommended in the form of brisk walking daily or a more vigorous activity prescription based on functional testing. A continuing educational and demonstration program is carried out concerning the amount and composition of foods, as described herein. Weekly visits to the staff at the outset can be used to deal with emotional responses and stresses that deregulate appetite (56) and to provide regular feedback on progress (43,44).

Evaluation and Intervention for Hypertension

Methods for baseline evaluation of blood pressure, as well as a progressive stepped-care program for hypertension, are part of the traditional knowledge and armamentarium of physicians; they require only implementation. The staff of an office or clinic should be trained to take blood pressures of all patients on all visits in standard fashion, to average the results of several determinations, and to forward those results with the patient's chart to the physician at each visit. The number of pressure determinations is dictated by the same factors discussed in regard to the number of lipid measurements; three readings per visit seem optimal. In addition to the stepped-care therapeutic program and the program for weight reduction and salt restriction, which are essential factors in hypertension control, there must be a regular systematic follow-up procedure in which patients are called back at regular intervals to have their intake of medications checked by pill counts (and sometimes chemical determinations of the urine) and their blood pressure levels followed. The degree of awareness of the importance of this systematic approach to hypertension is now so high among the profession, and the sources of information are so general among the physician and patient populations, that no detailed consideration of this very important aspect of prevention will be presented here.

An important new complication of diuretic therapy has recently been described in the Laboratory of Physiological Hygiene and elsewhere (57). The average cholesterol-lowering effect of the prudent diet is largely cancelled in high-risk men by the usual doses of either of the more commonly used diuretics (hydrochlorothiazide and chlorthalidone). This finding should be kept in mind, not necessarily for the choice of antihypertension therapy, but for interpretation of results of combined intervention on diet and hypertension. Similarly, the hypertensive and thrombogenic complications of synthetic estrogens or birth control pills must be kept prominently in mind when giving preventive advice to women patients post infarction.

Finally, stress management and relaxation therapy in hypertension are still in an early experimental stage (58).

Evaluation and Modification of Smoking Habits

Assessment of smoking habits is indicated for all patients (see example form in Appendix 4). Such assessment consists of information on current amounts of each type of tobacco smoked, the degree of inhalation, the duration of the habit, and previous experience with cessation of smoking, as well as an attempt at determination of the reasons for smoking.

Clinical measurements may aid motivation and maintenance of smoking cessation by indicating progress. Lung function tests are the least likely to show changes, but when the values are diminished at the outset they provide a powerful indication of the serious risk from continued smoking and, presumably, a motivation to stop. Inexpensive equipment for simple measurement of CO in expired air is available and has been used effectively for immediate feedback regarding the physiologic effects of smoking cessation. Plasma thiocyanate levels also show "improvement" on cessation of smoking and serve as unobtrusive objective measures of success. The half-life of expired CO is $\pm$ 4 hr, and that of plasma thiocyanate is $\pm$ 7 days, which permits a range of evaluations.

A physical examination emphasizing the nose, throat, chest, and vascular state of the lower extremities is a basic part of effective evaluation of the patient who smokes, and it can help to establish a credible basis for intervention on smoking.

Intervention on Smoking

The fact that there exist so many antismoking approaches and gimmicks is probably good evidence that none is superior. The theoretical bases of current antismoking research are not strong, the controlled trials are few, and long-term maintenance is ignored in most cessation programs. The physician may therefore choose and polish the available approaches with which he is most comfortable, or he may devise his own (59–61).

As with most therapy, individual tailoring is desirable. Unfortunately there is no certain way of assessing beforehand which patient will respond best to a particular approach. Nevertheless, the physician should use a simple and forceful recommendation about the important health matter of smoking on completion of the baseline workup. For example: "I think you must stop smoking. Would you like to set a target date now?"

A simple and direct approach used by practitioners is to ask, when examining the throat: "What do you smoke?" On examining the chest: "How much are you smoking these days?" When finished with the examination, outline the findings by system, explaining the effect of smoking, and add: "The first thing to do is to stop smoking. We'll give you all the help we can. If you can't quit cold now, we'll outline a reduction program leading up to a quitting date in a few weeks. Let's set the date now."

Results with this direct and authoritative approach are far from 100% effective over the long term. They may average about 20% sustained effect, certainly a worthwhile result of preventive practice.

Rationalizations to avoid intervention on habits and life-style are numerous: it is an invasion of privacy; self-determination, including self-destruction, is an individual's right; it is basically unfruitful to try to change people's habits; physicians are poorly trained to handle behavior change; etc. Generations of physicians have thus avoided entering the "privacy" of their patients' health behavior. Fortunately, these attitudes are changing in the profession, and the need for skills and facilities to change smoking behavior is recognized.

On the other hand, if the physician approaches his smoker patients ferociously about stopping, or if he appears self-righteous and fanatic, or if he attempts to bully or charm patients into stopping before they have thought out their decisions, the rate of recidivism may be higher. The physician's role is to initiate such thinking, offer support and give a reasonable time for the patient to prepare for change, guide the patient to a personal decision to stop, and, finally, never reject the failing patient. The thoughtless professional attitude "Do as I say or get another doctor" has never been good medical practice; neither is it so for preventive practice. Patience and persistence will enhance therapeutic success (60).

Although cessation of smoking is the goal, reduction of the amount smoked and change in the type of smoking are held out to those who cannot, for the time being, stop absolutely. They are not satisfactory alternatives.

Education about the noxious nature of tobacco smoke and its effects on the body may contribute to the success rate and should be provided by the physician. Audiovisual aids and brochures for use in individual or group counseling are listed in the Appendix. These appear useful adjuncts to start people thinking seriously about stopping smoking. They illustrate the frequent rationalizations for smoking, and they provide a platform for preventive action (61,62).

Most larger communities in the United States have several varieties of group antismoking clinics. They are usually of two types, the 5-day approach of the Seventh Day Adventists or the longer-term behavior modification approach. Although there is no established way of choosing between them, the behavior modification approach may be best for people who are more organized and meticulous or who have more time; perhaps the 'hard sell' works for more impulsive or hurried types.

One of the strongest of human protective mechanisms is the revulsion produced by an overwhelmingly unpleasant encounter. Aversive techniques are used in research studies to reduce smoking; however, most physicians are not prepared to acquire these techniques, which employ electrical shocks, ammonia fumes, emetics, and a host of unpleasant stimuli. Rapid puffing, however, is a different aversive therapy that has been used with variable long-term results. Many physicians are averse to aversive conditioning, as well as to trance states, etc., but these may be justified when simple counseling and self-determination have failed. They are certainly more acceptable techniques when divorced from pecuniary motives and philosophical proselytizing.

Relaxation and breathing exercises encourage active participatory behavior for the tense smoker and may be useful as a substitute or as a way to cope with stress without reaching for a cigarette.

Evaluation of Behavior, Stress, and Personality

Often infarction survivors spontaneously modify the frenetic aspects of their behavior and become more serene, with a regularly paced life. Others return to their original aggressive, urgent style. Others develop crippling neuroses, obsessions, or depression. Still others, perhaps most patients, change little in their behavior, which may or may not have been healthy. Characterizing behavior helps the physician to deal with it, and this is perhaps not inherently more difficult than characterizing diet. However, it requires a habitual and systematic approach. A few guidelines (63) may be helpful:

· Try to separate aspects of behavior and stress reactions from basic personality.
· Evaluate the patient's behavior during a pleasant nondirected conversation, making observations on voice, mood, gestures, and vitality. Try to elicit an

organized account of the patient's behavior at work before the infarction and currently. Note deadline behavior, which involves hostility when delayed, overtime work, work taken home, responsibilities and organizational activities in and outside work. Use the Jenkins Activity Survey or the Rosenman-Friedman Interview to aid in characterizing the range of aggressive and nonaggressive behavior (5,63).

· Evaluate personality during a nondirected conversation. Explore life dissatisfactions regarding work, income, education, living conditions, family life, and goals by means of questionnaires such as Cattell's 16 personality factors or the MMPI (4).

· Evaluate stress by directed questions about patterns of work, responsibility, play, meals, sleep, child development, marital situation, travel, and alcohol and drug consumption. Assess current and recent stress by means of questionnaires on life events and life change (4,64).

Modifying Psychosocial Factors

While there is a lack of evidence regarding modifiability of behavior, it remains possible to proceed with prudent approaches that encourage behavior pattern change and modification of psychosocial traits and exposures. Behaviors such as obsessive eating, drinking, and smoking or avoidance of physical activity are of particular concern in preventive practice. Moreover, catecholamine "rages," flight-or-fight "storms," and constant states of anxiety, insecurity, hostility, and arousal are hardly healthy ways of living for coronary patients or anyone else. The approaches of a few thoughtful people who are attempting to deal with these problems merit our attention. The elements of universal good sense in their recommendations should be incorporated into a prudent program of preventing reinfarction (11,63,65–68).

The steps recommended by Friedman and Rosenman for altering frantic, unwise behavior include the following:

· a thoroughgoing self-examination and self-evaluation in regard to intelligence, creativity, humor, adaptability, leadership, professional and leisure activities, credos, and essential values

· specific advice for "hurry sickness," including orderliness of the work environment, listening rather than talking, periods of quiet solitude, and periods of moderate physical activity

· "drills" against hurry sickness, against hostility, and toward changing values

More complete reviews of behavioral techniques in risk factor modification provide excellent introductions to this topic (11,42,44,65,66,69), in particular a new self-help book on skills for behavior change by Farquhar (42).

A systematic evaluation of the coronary patient's behavior and psychosocial status is possible in present-day medical practice and is clearly warranted in understanding and helping patients. Human behavior and values can be modified, and that accomplishment is possible in a proportion of cases comparable to those in many other medical interventions. But there is little support for the strongly negative tone of this advice to patients (63) from Rosenman and Friedman: "Remember that if you can't succeed at altering your behavior pattern, you aren't being protected against heart disease, no matter how little cholesterol you now eat, how little cigarette smoke you now inhale, or how many miles you run each day!" The very fact that behavior pattern characterization is independent of these other risk factors in predictive equations is good evidence that healthful modification of any or all of them has preventive potential.

Physical Activity Evaluation and Intervention

Much of this volume is concerned with functional testing and appropriate activity prescription for the postinfarction patient. The metabolic and circulatory advantages of regular activity for the coronary patient are effectively outlined in other chapters and elsewhere (23,25,26,70). Moreover, exercise is a superb outlet for aggression, a tranquilizer for anxiety, and a tonic for depression. Intelligently used, it is an important adjunct to all preventive strategies for the coronary patient.

A PRACTICAL SYSTEM OF INTERVENTION

Numerous formal disciplines and informal intervention procedures are available to the physician. The steps outlined below are useful in attempts to modify behavior and to get patients involved in their long-term self-management. Classic behaviorism as explicated in practical guides for self-management is adaptable to office practice for most patients.

How can the practitioner intervene more effectively for prevention among CHD patients? Simple steps for evaluation and intervention on patients' health habits and behavior are compatible with individual or group treatment programs in either solo or group practice. They can be carried out by office staff with training, support, and direction from the physician abetted by self-help guides and materials (11,42,44,46). Following are 10 important steps of preventive practice.

Do a Traditional Medical Workup

A medical workup is required to establish baseline values for the risk factors used in assessing risk (diagnosis), to guide the prevention plan (treatment), to provide better understanding of any related medical problems, and to give credibility and authority to the preventive program (prescription). In addition to the traditional workup, there should be systematic coverage of health behavior: eating and drinking patterns, diet diary, smoking, physical activity, and psychosocial questionnaires, which will be described later.

Make Clear Recommendations for Change

One of the obvious mistakes in preventive practice has been the ambivalence with which physicians have recommended that patients stop smoking or otherwise change health behavior. An unambiguous, positive, authoritative (but kind) recommendation for a course of action should follow promptly after medical history, physical, and laboratory evaluation. When prescribing an explicit preventive program, the physician should emphasize that it is just as important as any prescription given for medication or surgery.

Set a Personal Example

The physician's continuing credibility and authority with patients and community alike require that he make an effort to live by what he recommends.

Seek a Firm Commitment

The patient must make a commitment to adhere to the preventive program. A commitment ensures that the patient confronts and accepts the importance of the matter of prevention and behavior change. A simply written and signed contractual agreement may reinforce the commitment to specific goals of the preventive prescription.

Provide the Basic Information

It is essential to intervention that the patient know what factors need to be changed, as well as why and how. Instructions and audiovisual aids are increasingly available in the areas of concern, i.e., smoking, eating, drinking, physical activity, stress management, and pill-taking.

Set Distinct and Realistic Goals

Specific short-term goals lead to successive achievements and are preferable to vague, distant, or unrealistic targets.

Offer Alternatives

Once the specific goals are set, the various ways of reaching them should be spelled out for the patient to choose. To this extent the treatment is tailored to the individual patient and is self-determined.

Encourage Participation in Decisions for Change

The greater the extent to which the patient understands his problem, seeks information, sets his own goals, makes choices, explores alternatives, and generally participates in and takes responsibility for change in his own health behavior, rather than depending on the physician or others, the more propitious the long-term results.

Provide Skills and a Framework for Change

The information about change is vital, but a framework for change must also be provided by the physician when announcing the plan of preventive care. It is a substantial part of the motivation required for the patient to change. Assuming that the information and the motivation are provided, there are also many behavioral skills involved in unlearning such overlearned habits as smoking, sloth, and overeating. These will be discussed shortly.

Establish Systematic Follow-up

Evaluation, treatment, new knowledge, and support must be kept up to date by frequent and systematic office appointments. A very short visit for measurement of risk characteristics should be followed by a return visit for more complete discussion and preventive treatment, based on the patient's progress. Greater emphasis is placed on changing the patient's risk-related behavior than on changing any risk factor levels.

These are some essentials for effective prevention in the area of health habits and reduction of coronary risk characteristics. Involvement of the physician is central. Any practitioner can easily master the information, methods, and organizational aspects of such a practice. Results will depend on the degree of warmth, enthusiasm, and curiosity brought to the task and on the self-help skills the patient can acquire.

SELF-HELP SKILLS

Modifying Risk-related Behavior: Self-determined Change

Advances in learning theory have greatly expanded the possibilities for helping patients change ingrained behavior (11,42,44,69,71). Learning theory ignores the underlying psychodynamic causes of behaviors such as smoking or compulsive eating and deals with the behaviors themselves. The theory is that risk-related behavior is learned in the same way that other things are learned and thus can be unlearned. Thus the result of successful behavior modification is reduction of symptoms and improved function, quite irrespective of any underlying cause of the disturbance. Specific techniques applicable to risk factor reduction and change of risk-related behavior are outlined in Table 3 and will be summarized here.

Identifying the Problem. Behavioral aspects related to given risk factor elevations are identified. The problem is stated with and for the patient; e.g., habitually

Table 3. Techniques of Behavior Change Practice[a]

Self-observation and record keeping: to confront self and give
   feedback on progress
Stimulus control: to reduce temptation by removing it
Modeling: to demonstrate the behavior
Guided practice: to train in skills
Shaping: to introduce new preferences
Reinforcement: to give social reinforcement and
   self-reinforcement

[a]From Stunkard (71), with permission.

high fat intake; evening drinking and gorging; heavy salting of foods; dependence on cigarettes.

Self-observation. Regular recording of the problem activity involves the patient in the problem. It identifies problem areas and increases the patient's awareness of these areas and of the frequency of the behavior. It permits specific instructions to be given and is of assistance in monitoring progress during the process of change. Often it has some effect, albeit temporary, on the actual behavior being recorded. Self-observation involves the patient in learning to discriminate between behaviors, to count and chart, to evaluate, and to set goals; its techniques have been well described, and forms are available for the charting of eating and smoking behavior (11,44).

Environmental (Stimulus) Control. Patients should be taught to remove cigarettes from their usual places and to make undesirable foods less readily available and desirable foods more accessible, i.e., to reduce temptation by removing it.

Demonstration and Guided Practice. It is believed that the best way of teaching new behavior is by careful demonstration of the behavior—followed promptly by guiding the patient through a practice of the desired act. This is particularly useful in nutritional counseling. Games may be used to demonstrate and implement knowledge of food composition; shopping instructions may be followed by food choice drills; menu reading may be followed by eating out. There are many varieties of food preparation demonstrations and exercises that can be used.

Self-control (Shaping) of Preferences. It is important to make an active effort to develop new tastes by continually trying new things: "The eating causes the liking as much as the liking causes the eating." Changes that are small and progressive are easier to achieve without discomfort. Such a protracted and graduated shaping of eating pattern change is described in detail by Farquhar for reducing fat, salt, and sugar in the habitual diet (42).

Reinforcement. Praise, rewards, and prompt feedback on progress are well-known inducements to learning and to change in behavior. They can easily be built into the office practice of prevention. There probably are as many forms of self-reward and reinforcement as there are individual tastes. The greater the extent to which this system of self-support and social support can be built into the family for mutual help in stopping smoking or in exercising together, the better the chance for permanent change.

Contracting and Cueing. Recording each goal in a written contract is a useful incentive, as is providing oneself with cues to aid behavior, such as placing a bathing suit or athletic gear in one's car.

    These kinds of processes have been particularly well formulated in a self-help manual by Farquhar (42), an experienced medical practitioner of behavior change; the techniques of self-directed change may be arranged in steps applicable to each risk behavior:

- problem identification
- commitment
- problem awareness
- action plan
- self-observation
- goal-setting
- self-reward
- urge suppression
- social support

Maintenance of Intervention

If the steps of preventive practice as outlined are followed, if the patients' goals in intervention are compatible with the physician's goals, and if the patients have assumed major responsibility for their interventions, then a significant proportion of patients with long-term good results is to be expected. In addition, the preventive approach must include systematic checks on status. It is useful during maintenance visits to collect a minimum of information regarding dietary recall and work and life patterns, following a sampling of risk factor status. These data should be reviewed with the patient in a direct interview by the physician to match the reported behavior with the recorded risk factor levels. There is no ideal frequency for such visits; the intervals can be lengthened as the individual requires less support. Emphasis is placed on improved risk behavior. Objective risk factor change is provided only when clear trends of success, or its lack, are established by serial observations.

Dealing With Failure of Intervention

The varying degrees of failure of intervention on risk factors for CHD are comparable to other ups and downs in physician–patient relationships. Learning to deal with failures involves recognition and awareness and the need for occasional confrontation about lack of progress. The patient should be given an indication that the physician knows that behavior is being indulged in that is blocking effective risk factor reduction. During the periodic interview and evaluation the mechanisms for change, as well as the characteristics of life-style and work and home behavior, are considered in building a fresh contract and commitment to a particular behavior change, with new short-term and long-term prevention goals. It is to be preferred that the methods and targets agreed to in a renewed contract be those the patient suggests. The contract should then be signed and given to the patient, with a copy being kept on file. A calendar of targets, dates, and revisits should also be filled out and given to the patient.

The gist of this approach is to acknowledge reality, avoiding false appearances of compliance that can eventually alienate the patient and that are clearly ineffective in reducing risk factors. When the truth is faced, the real issues may be tackled and a new agreement reached (72).

CONCLUSION

The persistence of significant relationships between primary risk factors and recurrence rate in coronary patients is evidence that these factors affect long-term atherogenesis and that their influences remain active after the first event. These relationships provide the rationale for the preventive interventions described here. On the other hand, the weaknesses of these relationships after infarction, relative to functional status, indicate other considerations:

· we probably have to achieve maximal risk factor reduction to be effective in CHD patients after infarction
· we probably have to achieve multiple risk factor reduction to have any significant impact on the rate of reinfarction

For example, the preventive practitioner should not remain complacent about the patient who stops smoking but puts on weight and has associated increases in blood pressure and serum lipid values. We must attempt to market the entire preventive package (e.g., it is always much easier to prevent the increment in weight on cessation of smoking than it is to correct it).

There are important lessons to be learned from negative results of well-designed clinical trials; e.g., drug-induced single-factor lipid lowering is inadequate in itself to modify subsequent life course for the majority of recovered myocardial infarction survivors. Such results lead not to therapeutic nihilism but rather to therapeutic realism. From that viewpoint, therapy must be tailored to the level of risk, and it must be effective and multiple, coming from a variety of portals into the preventive process.

Finally, we must ask honestly to what extent therapy can be expected to prolong life when certain processes have gone on insidiously for years and when the first clinical manifestation occurs only after vascular and organ damage is far advanced. We should not be content with improving the quality of life by interventions that only reduce symptoms or that have short-term salubrious influences; we must be equally concerned about the quantity of life. It is difficult to be impressed with the argument that the quality of life in the coronary patient is more important than the quantity; the quality of life means little if one is not alive to appreciate it.

Thus the ultimate therapeutic and public health goal is to reduce excessive and premature morbidity and mortality. Clearly the program is more promising if preventive efforts are applied early.

SUMMARY

The potential for coronary risk factor reduction is believed to be great within the setting of medical practice. Identification of risk factors for reinfarction, as well as problem-oriented diagnosis and therapy to modify them, can become routine and effective. The framework of an announced preventive practice is in itself a powerful influence for change. A prevention-oriented approach involving history, physical examination, laboratory diagnostic workup, and treatment regimen can lead to problem identification and strategies for change in health behavior. The authority of the physician can give patients the motivation to initiate change in risk-related behavior. Information and skills for self-help can be provided by office staff. Systematic follow-up is conducive to maintenance of behavior change. The physician should emphasize the benefit that the entire family of the coronary patient will derive from such improvements as a smoke-free home, a low-fat diet, a loving environment, and physical activities that promote health. Skills can be learned that can be used to cope with situations that interfere with the patient's new behavior pattern at work, at home, and with friends. Professional guidelines and self-help materials are outlined, and their sources are cited.

REFERENCES

1. Mackenzie J: *The Principles of Diagnoses and Treatment in Heart Affections* (ed 2). Oxford University Press, London, 1916

2. Coronary Drug Project Research Group: The prognostic importance of the electrocardiogram after myocardial infarction. *Ann Intern Med* 77:677, 1972

3. Coronary Drug Project Research Group: Factors influencing long-term prognosis after recovery from myocardial infarction. *J Chronic Dis* 27:267, 1974

4. Jenkins CD: Psychologic and social precursors of coronary disease. *N Engl J Med* 284:244, 1971

5. Jenkins CD, Zyzanski SJ, Rosenman RH, et al: Association of coronary-prone behavior scores with recurrence of coronary heart disease. *J Chronic Dis* 24:601, 1971

6. Jenkins CD, Zyzanski SJ, Rosenman RH: Risk of new myocardial infarction in middle-aged men with manifest coronary heart disease. *Circulation* 53:342, 1976

7. Helmers C: Short and long-term prognostic indices in acute myocardial infarction. *Acta Med Scand Suppl* 55, 1973

8. Norris RM, Caushey DE, Deening LW, et al: Coronary prognostic index for predicting survival after recovery from acute myocardial infarction. *Lancet* 2:485, 1970

9. Peel AAF, Semple T, Wang I, et al: A coronary prognostic index for grading the severity of infarction. *Br Heart J* 24:745, 1962

10. Bruce RA: The benefits of physical training for patients with CHD. In Ingelfinger FJ, Ebert R, Finland M, Relman A (eds): *Controversy in Internal Medicine*. WB Saunders, Philadelphia, 1974

11. McAlister A, Farquhar J, Thoresen CE, et al: Behavioral science applied to cardiovascular health. A survey of progress in the modification of risk-taking habits in adult populations. Health education monograph 4, CB Slack, Thoroughfare, NJ, 1976

12. Murray J: Personal communication regarding coronary prognostic indices after myocardial infarction. University of Washington

13. Bruschke AVG, Proudfit WL, Sones FM Jr: Clinical course of patients with normal, and slightly or moderately abnormal coronary arteriograms. *Circulation* 47:935, 1973

14. Oberman A, Jones WB, Riley CP, et al: Natural history of coronary artery disease. *Bull NY Acad Med* 48:1109, 1972

15. Juergens JL, Edwards JE, Achor RWP, et al: Prognosis of patients surviving first clinically diagnosed myocardial infarction. *Arch Intern Med* 105:444, 1960

16. Oxman HA, Connolly DC, Nobrega FT, et al: Factors influencing the subsequent prognosis of patients surviving their first myocardial infarction. *Circulation* 45:(Suppl II):200, 1972 (abstract)

17. Weinblatt E, Shapiro S, Frank CW, et al: Prognosis of men after myocardial infarction: Mortality and first recurrence in relation to selected parameters. *Am J Public Health* 58:1329, 1968

18. Wilhelmsson C, Vedin JA, Elmfeldt D, et al: Smoking and myocardial infarction. *Lancet* 1:415, 1975

19. Report of Task Force on Cardiovascular Rehabilitation. National Heart and Lung Institute, December, 1974

20. WHO Working Group on Rehabilitation Programs for Patients with Myocardial Infarction, Prague, October 4–7, 1971. EURO 8206(6), WHO Regional Office for Europe, Copenhagen

21. Sanne H, Elmfeldt D, Wilhelmsen L: Preventive effect of physical training after myocardial infarction. In Tibblin G, Keys A, Werkö L (eds): *Preventive Cardiology*. Almqvist and Wiksell, Stockholm, 1972, p. 154

22. Hellerstein HK: Exercise therapy in coronary disease. *Bull NY Acad Med* 44:1028, 1968

23. Wenger NK: Benefits of a rehabilitation program following myocardial infarction. *Geriatrics* 28:64, 1973

24. Zohman LR: Cardiac rehabilitation: Its role in evaluation and management of the patient with coronary heart disease. *Am Heart J* 85:706, 1973

25. Blackburn H: Disadvantages of intensive exercise therapy after myocardial infarction. In Ingelfinger FJ, Ebert R, Finland M, Relman A (eds): *Controversy in Internal Medicine II*. WB Saunders, Philadelphia, 1974, pp 162–173

26. Leon AS, Conrad J, Hunninghake D, et al: Exercise effects on body composition, work capacity and carbohydrate and lipid metabolism of young obese men. *Med Sci Sports* 9:60, 1977

27. Sanne H: Exercise tolerance and physical training of non-selected patients after myocardial infarction. *Acta Med Scand* Suppl 551, 194:124, 1973

28. Wilhelmsen L, Sanne H, Elmfeldt D, et al: A controlled trial of physical exercise on risk factors, non-fatal myocardial infarction and death. *Prev Med* 4:491, 1975

29. Kentala M: Physical fitness and feasibility of physical rehabilitation after myocardial infarction in men of working age. *Ann Clin Res* 4(Suppl 9):1, 1972

30. Coronary Drug Project Research Group: Clofibrate and niacin in coronary heart disease. *JAMA* 231:360, 1975

31. Physicians of the Newcastle-upon-Tyne region: Trial of clofibrate, in the treatment of ischaemic heart disease. *Br Med J* 4:767, 1971

32. Report by Research Committee, Scottish Society of Physicians: Ischemic heart disease. A secondary prevention trial using clofibrate. *Br Med J* 4:755, 1971

33. Leren P: The Oslo diet-heart study: Eleven year report. *Circulation* 42:935, 1970

34. Boston Collaborative Drug Surveillance Group: Regular aspirin intake and acute myocardial infarction. *Br Med J* 1:440, 1974

35. Coronary Drug Project Research Group: Aspirin in coronary heart disease. *J Chronic Dis* 29:625, 1976

36. Elwood PC, Cochrane AL, Burr ML, et al: A randomized controlled trial of acetyl salicylic acid in the secondary prevention of mortality from myocardial infarction. *Br Med J* 1:436, 1974

37. Hypertension-Stroke Cooperative Study Group: Effect of antihypertensive treatment on stroke recurrence. *JAMA* 229:409, 1974

38. Blackburn H: Progress in epidemiology and prevention of coronary heart disease. In Yu P, Goodwin J (eds): *Progress in Cardiology*. Lea & Febiger, Philadelphia, 1974, pp 1–36

39. Veterans Administration Cooperative Study Group on Antihypertensive Agents: Effects of treatment on morbidity in hypertension. *JAMA* 213:1143, 1970

40. Rose GA: Personal communication

41. Farquhar J, Maccoby N, Alexander JK, et al: Community education for cardiovascular health. *Lancet* 1:1192, 1977

42. Farquhar J: *The American Way of Life May Be Hazardous to Your Health*. WW Norton, New York, 1978

43. Leon GR: A behavioral approach to obesity. *Am J Clin Nutr* 30:785, 1977

44. Leon GR: Behavior modification in reducing risk factors for ischemic heart disease. In Long C (ed): *Prevention and Rehabilitation in Ischemic Heart Disease*. Williams & Wilkins, Baltimore (in press)

45. Lichtenstein E, Danaher BG: Modification of smoking behavior: A critical analysis of theory, research and practice. In Heisen M, Eisler RM, Miller PM (eds): *Prognosis in Behavior Modification*. Academic Press, New York, 1976

46. Blackburn H: Coronary risk factors. How to evaluate and manage them. *Eur J Cardiol* 2:249, 1975

47. Grimm R, Blackburn H: Heart Attack Prevention Workshop. Practical Guides to Preventive Practice. Laboratory of Physiological Hygiene, School of Public Health and Center for Continuing Medical Education, University of Minnesota, Minneapolis

48. Levy R, Rifkin B, Ernst N, et al (eds): *Nutrition in Heart Disease*. Raven Press, New York, 1978

49. Report of the Intersociety Commission on Heart Disease Resources: The primary prevention of atherosclerosis. *Circulation* 42:A-55, 1970

50. Hall Y, Stamler J, Cohen DB, et al: Effectiveness of the low saturated fat, low cholesterol, weight-reducing diet for the control of hypertriglyceridemia. *Atherosclerosis* 16:389, 1972

51. Hulley SB, Wilson WS, Burrows M, Nichaman MZ: Lipid and lipoprotein responses of hypertriglyceridemic outpatients to a low-carbohydrate modification of the A.H.A. fat-controlled diet. *Lancet* 2:551, 1972

52. Blackburn H: Diet and mass hyperlipidemia. A public health approach. In Levy R, Rifkin B, Ernst N, Dennis B (eds): *Nutrition in Heart Disease*. Raven Press, New York, 1978

53. Keys A, Parlin RW: Serum cholesterol response to changes in dietary lipids. *Am J Clin Nutr* 19:175, 1966

54. Keys A (ed): Coronary heart disease in seven countries. *Circulation* 41(Suppl 1): 211, 1970

55. Stuart RB: *Slim Chance in a Fat World. Behavioral Control of Obesity*. Research Press, Champaign, Ill, 1972

56. Hickey N, Mulcahy R: Effect of cessation of smoking on body weight after myocardial infarction. *Am J Clin Nutr* 26:385, 1973

57. Grimm RH, Leon AS, Hunninghake D, Blackburn H: Diuretic effects on plasma lipids and lipoproteins. American Federation for Clinical Research, 1978 (abstract)

58. Shapiro AP, Schwartz GE, Ferguson DCE, et al: Behavioral methods in the treatment of hypertension. *Ann Intern Med* 86:626, 1977

59. Jarvik M (ed): Research on Smoking Behavior. Research monograph 17. US Government Printing Office, Washington, DC, 1977

60. Lichtenstein E, Danaher BG: What can the physician do to assist the patient to stop smoking? In Brashear RE, Rhodes ML (eds): *Chronic Obstructive Lung Disease: Clinical Treatment and Management*. CV Mosby, St Louis, 1978, p. 227

61. Pechacek TF, McAlister A: Strategies for the modification of smoking behavior: Treatment and prevention. In Ferguson J, Taylor B (eds): *Advances in Behavioral Medicine*. Spectrum Press, New York, 1978

62. Department of Health, Education, and Welfare: The Smoking Digest. Office of Cancer Communications. National Cancer Institute, National Institutes of Health, Bethesda, Oct. 1977

63. Friedman M, Rosenman RH: *Type A Behavior and Your Heart*. Alfred A Knopf, New York, 1978

64. Romo M, Siltanen P, Theorell T, et al: Work behavior, time urgency and life dissatisfactions in subjects with myocardial infarction. *J Psychosom Res* 18:1, 1974

65. Enelow AJ (ed): Applying Behavioral Science to Cardiovascular Risk. Report of a working conference of the American Heart Association, 1975

66. Pomerleau O, Bass F, Crown V: Role of behavior modification in preventive medicine. *N Engl J Med* 292:1277, 1975

67. Stocksmeier U (ed): *Psychological Approach to the Rehabilitation of Coronary Patients*. International Society of Cardiology Scientific Council on Rehabilitation. Springer-Verlag, Berlin, 1976

68. Williams RL, Long JD: *Toward a Self-managed Life Style*. Houghton Mifflin, Boston, 1975

69. Bandura A: *Principles of Behavior Modification*. Holt, Rinehart & Winston, New York, 1969

70. Fletcher GF, Cantwell JD: *Exercise and Coronary Heart Disease. Role in Prevention, Diagnosis and Treatment*. Charles C Thomas, Springfield, Ill, 1973

71. Stunkard AJ: Presidential address, 1974: From explanation to action in psychosomatic medicine: A case of obesity. *Psychosom Med* 37:195, 1975

72. Lewis H: How Intervention Fails. MRFIT project, Boston University, 1975

73. Moss AJ, DeCamilla J, Davis H, et al: The early posthospital phase of myocardial infarction. *Prognostic Stratification* 54:58, 1976

74. Pomerleau OF, Pomerleau CS: *Break the Smoking Habit*. Research Press, Champaign, Ill, 1977

75. Shapiro S, Weinblatt E, Frank CW, et al: The H.I.P. study of incidence and prognosis of

coronary heart disease. Preliminary findings on incidence of myocardial infarction and angina. *J Chronic Dis* 18:527, 1965

76. Taylor HL, Jacobs D, Schucker B, et al: A questionnaire for the assessment of leisure time physical activities. *J Chronic Dis* (in press)

77. Wilhelmsson C, Vedin JA, Wilhelmsen L, et al: Reduction of sudden death after myocardial infarction by treatment with alprenolol. Preliminary results. *Lancet* 2:1157, 1974

APPENDIX 1.1: MODEL WORKSHOP ON HEART ATTACK PREVENTION, PRACTICAL APPROACHES TO RISK FACTOR REDUCTION*

Workshop Objectives

To provide knowledge, skills, and practical procedures needed by busy medical practitioners and allied personnel to reduce patients' risk factors for cardiovascular diseases. Practical methods for modifying eating patterns, blood lipid levels, blood pressure levels, smoking habits, body weight, and physical activity levels will be demonstrated and practiced. A kit of risk management materials is provided for use by practitioners and their office aides. The kit and process are a realistic incorporation of risk reduction into a prevention-oriented practice setting.

Prior Evening

Check-in and measurement of participant risk factors (blood pressure, blood lipids, smoking habits, and medical questionnaire); distribution of risk kit and pretest questionnaire.

First Day

7:00– 8:30   Nature Walk
             Breakfast
8:30–10:00   *General Session*
             Purpose and Goals of the Preventive Cardiology Workshop, R. Grimm, Jr., M.D.
             Introduction to Cardiovascular Disease Prevention: Need, Potential, and Strategies, H. Blackburn, M.D.
             Current Status of Risk Factors
             Habitual Diet, H. Blackburn, M.D. (10 minutes)
             Elevated Blood Lipids, R. Luepker, M.D. (10 minutes)
             Smoking Habits, R. Grimm, Jr., M.D. (10 minutes)
             Elevated Blood Pressure, R. Prineas, M.B.B.S., Ph.D. (10 minutes)
10:00–10:15 Activity Break

*Developed by the Center for Continuing Medical Education, The Medical School, The School of Public Health, The Laboratory of Physiological Hygiene, University of Minnesota, Minneapolis, Minnesota.

10:15–11:00   Physical Activity, R. Crow, M.D. (10 minutes)
              Diabetes, A. Leon, M.D. (10 minutes)
              Obesity, D. Halvorsen (10 minutes)
              Behavior Pattern, M. Mittelmark, Ph.D. (10 minutes)
11:00–11:50   Panel Discussion and Questions, H. Blackburn, M.D.
11:50–12:00   Summary and Announcements, R. Grimm, M.D.
12:00– 1:30   Lunch and Rest Period
 1:30   *Practical Aspects of Risk Assessment and Management*
 1:30– 2:00   *Risk Assessment* (physicians and allied personnel)
              1. Individual vs. Group Risk, D. Jacobs, Ph.D.
              2. Risk Computation Demonstration, R. Thorsen, M.D.
 2:00– 3:00   Small Group Risk Computation Exercises, R. Grimm, M.D., R. Thorsen, MD., D. Jacobs, Ph.D., and G. Fraser, M.D.
 3:00– 3:15   Activity Break
 3:15– 5:00   *Practical Risk Management* (physicians and allied personnel), R. Grimm, M.D., M. Mittelmark, Ph.D., B. Cox, R.N., and K. Lenz, R.D.
              1. Problem Identification
              2. Commitment and Contracting
              3. Self-monitoring Records
              4. Environmental Stimulus Modification
              5. Demonstrations
              6. Guided Practice
              7. Creating New Preferences
              8. Reinforcement
              9. Evaluation and Follow-up
 5:00– 6:30   Activity Break
 6:30– 7:00   Social Time
 7:00– 8:00   Group Dinner
 8:00–10:00   Audiovisual Exhibits (attendance optional for all)
              1. Brochure and Book Ordering
              2. Slide-Tape Projections
              3. Film Projections

Second Day

 7:00– 8:00   Nature Walk (Use of Pedometers)
 8:00– 8:30   Breakfast
 8:30–10:00   *Eating Pattern Assessment and Management* (allied-personnel-oriented, but all are welcome), T. Ashman, W. Thorpe, D. West, K. Lenz, and N. Foster
              1. Food Recall Records, Eating Pattern Questionnaire, Food Scores, Food Models
              2. Counseling Techniques

　　　　　3. Eating Behavior Change Techniques
　　　　　　　a. Problem Identification
　　　　　　　b. Commitment and Contracting
　　　　　　　c. Self-monitoring Records
　　　　　　　d. Environmental Stimulus Modification
　　　　　　　e. Demonstrations
　　　　　　　f. Guided Practice
　　　　　　　g. Creating New Preferences
　　　　　　　h. Reinforcement
　　　　　　　i. Evaluation and Follow-up

8:30–10:00　*Hypertension Assessment and Management* (physician-oriented, but all are welcome), R. Grimm, M.D., A. Leon, M.D., R. Prineas, M.B.B.S., Ph.D., and R. Gillum, M.D.
　　　　　1. Blood Pressure Measurement, Variability, Record Keeping, Target Pressures, Pill Counts
　　　　　2. Step-up Drug Therapy
　　　　　3. Step-down Drug Therapy
　　　　　4. Side Effects and Adherence
　　　　　5. Nondrug Adjuncts to Therapy

10:00–10:15　Activity Break

10:15–12:00　*Weight Control and Physical Activity* (physicians and allied personnel), R. Crow, M.D., A. Leon, M.D., Dan Halvorsen (Ph.D. candidate), and K. Lenz, R.D.
　　　　　1. Activity–Weight Relationship
　　　　　2. Weight, Build, Obesity Measurement
　　　　　3. Activity Assessment
　　　　　4. Obesity Management
　　　　　　　a. Problem Identification
　　　　　　　b. Commitment and Contracting
　　　　　　　c. Self-monitoring Records
　　　　　　　d. Environmental Stimulus Modification
　　　　　　　e. Demonstrations
　　　　　　　f. Guided Practice
　　　　　　　g. Creating New Preferences
　　　　　　　h. Reinforcement
　　　　　　　i. Evaluation and Follow-up

12:00– 1:30　Lunch and Rest Period

1:30– 3:00　*Smoking Assessment and Management,* M. Mittelmark, Ph.D., T. Pechacek, Ph.D., E. Rotman, M.S., and R. Grimm, M.D.
　　　　　1. Smoking Questionnaire, Self-recording Smoking Behavior, Carbon Monoxide and Thiocyanate Monitoring
　　　　　2. Smoking Cessation Counseling
　　　　　3. Self-help Techniques for Smokers
　　　　　　　a. Problem Identification
　　　　　　　b. Commitment and Contracting
　　　　　　　c. Self-monitoring Records
　　　　　　　d. Environmental Stimulus Modification

              e. Demonstrations
              f. Guided Practice
              g. Creating New Preferences
              h. Reinforcement
              i. Evaluation and Follow-up

3:00– 3:15   Activity Break

3:15– 4:30   Small Group Practice Exercises (Eating and Smoking Intervention)

4:30– 5:00   Use of Risk Reduction Kit (physicians and allied personnel), R. Grimm, M.D.
              1. Kit Explanation
              2. Prevention Visit Protocols
              3. Handling Variability
              4. Handling Failures
              5. Family Involvement

5:00   Workshop Closure, H. Blackburn, M.D.

APPENDIX 1.2: CHD RISK FACTOR REDUCTION MATERIALS

Risk Factors and Risk Appraisal

Brochures

1.1 Smoking and Heart Disease. American Heart Association, No. EM393 PHE ($1.40/100)

1.2 Smoker's Self-testing Kit (CDC). National Clearing House for Smoking and Health, No. HSM 74-8716

1.3 Facts: Smoking and Health. National Clearing House for Smoking and Health, No. HSM 73-8717

1.4 Poison Gases in Your Cigarettes. Reader's Digest Reprint Office, Pleasantville, New York 10570

1.5 Heart Quiz. American Heart Association, No. 51-012-A, EM4 PHE ($1.45/125)

1.6 L.P.H. Quiz Slide Rule. Laboratory of Physiological Hygiene, University of Minnesota

1.7 American Heart Association Coronary Risk Factor Handbook

Books

1.8 Farquhar J: *The American Way of Life May Be Hazardous to Your Health*. WW Norton, New York, 1978

Films

1.9 *What Goes Up*. Hypertension—answers questions about blood pressure. American Heart Association, available through local branch (16 mm, $85, available for loan)

Reducing Risk Factors

Book

2.1 Farquhar J: *The American Way of Life May Be Hazardous to Your Health*. WW Norton, New York, 1978

Brochures

2.2 Reduce Your Risk of Heart Attack. American Heart Association, No. EM392 ($4.95/100)

2.3 Why Risk Heart Attack? American Heart Association, No. M414 PHE ($1.90/100)

Eating Pattern Change

Cookbooks

3.1 Agriculture Handbook 8, U.S. Department of Agriculture, Superintendent of Documents, U.S. Government Printing Office

3.2 *The American Heart Association Cookbook.* David McKay, New York ($7.95)

3.3 Zane P: *The Jack Sprat Cookbook.* Harper & Row, New York ($10.95)

3.4 Lamb LE: *Food and Cooking for Health.* Viking Press, New York ($10.00)

3.5 Keys A, Keys M: *Eat Well and Stay Well.* Doubleday, New York ($5.95)

3.6 Keys A, Keys M: *The Benevolent Bean.* Doubleday, New York ($5.95)

3.7 Keys A, Keys M: *The Mediterranean Way to Eat Well and Stay Well.* Doubleday, New York

Brochures

3.9 A Diet for Today. Best Foods Division, CPC International, Department X, P.O. Box 307, Coventry, Connecticut 06238

4.1 The Way to a Man's Heart. American Heart Association, No. EM455 PHE ($3.30/100)

4.2 Recipes for Fat-controlled, Low Cholesterol Meals. American Heart Association, No. 50-020A, EM455A PHE ($4.35/100)

4.3 Heart Saver Handbook. Chicago Heart Association, Chicago, Illinois

4.4 Beef Chart—Retail Cuts of Beef. Where They Come From and How to Cook Them. National Live Stock and Meat Board, 444 North Michigan Avenue, Chicago, Illinois 60611

4.5 Sensible Eating Can Be Delicious. Fleischmann's, Box 1180, Elm City, North Carolina 27822

4.6 Cooking With Egg Beaters. Fleischmann's, Box 1180, Elm City, North Carolina 27822

4.7 Questions and Answers About Fats and Oils in Our Diet (Best Foods Publication No. 3576-73-3B). CPC International, International Plaza, Englewood Cliffs, New Jersey 07632

4.8 Cooking with Corn Oil—Mazola. Best Foods Division, CPC International, International Plaza, Englewood Cliffs, New Jersey 07632

4.9 Let's Cook Fish. U.S. Department of Commerce, Booklet No. I49.49/2:8 ($0.60, $45/100)

5.0 The Prevention of Heart Disease Begins in Childhood. Fleischmann's, Box 1180, Elm City, North Carolina 27822

5.1 Healthy Eating for Teenagers. American Heart Association, No. 42-002a EM 484 PHE ($5.90/100)

Slide-Tape

5.4 Heart Saver Slide-Tape Show, Units I–VI. Chicago Heart Association, Chicago, Illinois

Films

5.5 *Three Times a Day.* General introduction and discussion of the food pattern to lower serum cholesterol, with a tour of the grocery store. Medcom, 2 Hammarskjöld Plaza, New York, New York 10017 (16 mm, cost on request)

5.6 *Our Way of Life.* General description of the poor nutritional food pattern that accompanies the fast pace of American lives. American Heart Association, available through local branch. (16 mm, cost $100, also available for loan)

5.7 *Eat Right to Your Heart's Delight.* Low-fat meat preparation. International Producers Services, 3518 Cahuenga Boulevard, West Hollywood, California (16 mm, cost on request)

5.8 *Eat to Your Heart's Content.* American Heart Association, available through local branch. (16 mm, cost $100, also available for loan)

5.9 *Food, Energy and You.* Wexler Film Productions, Los Angeles, California 90038 (16 mm, cost on request)

Smoking Cessation

Books

6.1 *The Smoking Digest.* DHEW Office of Cancer Communications. National Cancer Institute, National Institutes of Health, Bethesda, Maryland 20014

6.2 Pomerleau OF, Pomerleau CS: *Break the Smoking Habit.* Research Press, Champaign, Illinois, 1977

6.3 Brengelmann JC: *Manual on Smoking Cessation Therapy* (for staff of Federal Center for Health Education, Cologne, West Germany). SA Studer, Geneva, 1975

Brochures

7.1 How to Stop Smoking. American Heart Association, No. 51-013A EM487 PHE ($4.35/100)

7.2 If You Want to Give Up Cigarettes. American Cancer Society, No. 2666LE.

7.3 When a Woman Smokes. American Cancer Society, No. 2051LE.

7.4 Unless You Decide to Quit. National Clearing House for Smoking and Health. Superintendent of Documents, U.S. Government Printing Office, No. HSM 72-7522

7.5 Yes, There Are a Lot of Good Reasons for Women to Quit Smoking. DHEW Publication No. HSM 73-8713

7.6 Staying Alive. DHEW Publication No. HSM 73-8705

Slide-Tapes

8.1 A Physician Talks About Smoking. Health and economic costs of smoking; 30 color slides and booklet. National Audiovisual Center, Sales Branch, Washington, D.C. 20409

Films

9.1 *Quit, Quit Again.* Relates the necessity of multiple attempts to quit; 4 case studies. National Clearing House for Smoking and Health. U.S. Public Health Service, Health Services and Mental Health Administration, Rockville, Maryland 20852 (Super-8 cassette, cost on request)

9.2 *Ashes to Ashes.* Describes the smoking problem in America today with well-documented clinical evidence and research; true case history of a surgeon who tries to stop smoking. Searle Educational Systems, G.D. Searle Co., Box 5110, Chicago, Illinois 60680 (16 mm, cost $250)

9.3 *Bill Talman.* Straightforward pitch on the consequences of smoking and lung cancer. Trigger Films, American Cancer Society, available through local branch (16 mm, loan only)

9.4 *The Embattled Cell.* Actual time-lapse motion picture of living cancer tissue and division of living cancer cells. Deals with the impact of cigarette smoking. American Cancer Society, available through local branch (16 mm, loan only)

Physical Activity

Books

10.1 *Exercise Your Way to Fitness and Heart Health.* No. 5724-75-38A Best Foods Division, CPC International, International Plaza, Englewood Cliffs, New Jersey 07632

10.2 *The Royal Canadian Air Force Exercise Book.* Available through most bookstores ($1.95)

Hypertension

Brochures

11.1 Watch Your Blood Pressure! The High Blood Pressure Information Center, 120/80 National Institutes of Health, Bethesda, Maryland 20014

11.2 Hypertension: High Blood Pressure. DHEW Publication No. NIH 1714 ($0.50, $37.50/100)

11.3 High Blood Pressure and How to Control It. American Heart Association, No. EM32 PHE ($6.00/100)

Weight Control

Brochures

12.1 A Guide for Weight Reduction. American Heart Association, No. 50-034-A ($6.75/100)

12.2 Fleischmann's Margarine Calorie Subtractor. Publication No. MF10997. Fleischmann's, Box 1180, Elm City, North Carolina 27822

12.3 Calories and Weight: The USDA Pocket Guide. Home and Garden Bulletin No. 153. Superintendent of Documents, U.S. Government Printing Office, Washington, D.C. 20402 ($0.30, $22.50/100)

12.4 Planning Fat Controlled Meals for 1200 and 1800 Calories. American Heart Association, No. EM288A PHE ($12.52/100)

12.5 Planning Fat Controlled Meals for 2000-2600 Calories. American Heart Association, No. EM288A PHE ($12.00/100)

12.6 Are You Really Serious About Losing Weight? Pennwalt Prescription Products, PO Box 1710, Rochester, New York 14603 (free of charge to physicians)

Books

12.7 Stuart RB: *Slim Chance in a Fat World. Behavioral Control of Obesity.* Research Press, Champaign, Illinois, 1972

12.8 Jeffrey DB, Kats RC: *Take It Off and Keep It Off. A Behavioral Program for Weight Loss and Healthy Living.* Prentice-Hall, Englewood Cliffs, New Jersey 07632

To Order Materials

American Cancer Society
219 East 42nd Street
New York, New York 10017

Superintendent of Documents
U.S. Government Printing Office
Washington, D.C. 20402

Laboratory of Physiological Hygiene
School of Public Health
Stadium Gate 27
Minneapolis, Minnesota 55455

American Heart Association
7320 Greenville Avenue
Dallas, Texas 75231

National Clearing House for Smoking and Health
5401 Westlund Avenue
Bethesda, Maryland 20016

APPENDIX 2.1: FOOD SELECTION RECORD

List below the amount of each food and how often you eat it. This includes all meals and snacks. Example:

Food	Amount	Frequency
Butter	2 pats	Every day
Beef	4–5 ounces	Six times a week
Pie, cake	2 servings	Every day
Milk	2 cups	Every day

Food	Amount	Frequency
Milk: Whole		
Skim or buttermilk		
Low fat (2%)		
Butter		
Cream, sweet or sour		
Ice cream		
Cheese (except cottage)		
Beef		
Lamb, pork, ham		
Bacon		
Frankfurters, cold cuts		
Pie, cake (commercial baked goods)		
Danish, donuts, sweet rolls		
Cookies, crackers		
Eggs		
Liver, kidney, brains		
Oysters, shrimp, clams		
Fish		
Chicken		
Margarine		
Vegetables (raw or cooked)		
Citrus fruit		
Bread, cereal		
Vegetable oil (in salads or cooking)		

APPENDIX 2.2: THREE-DAY FOOD RECORD

Name: _____

From _____ to _____

Directions for Recording Your Food Intake

Each day list all foods and beverages that you ate at meals, coffee breaks, and for snacks. Write down what you ate immediately after each meal to be sure you remember everything you ate and how much.

Do not forget to record:

Alcoholic beverages	Cream
Soft drinks	Nuts
Butter	Jams
Margarine	Jellies
Chips	Preserves
Popcorn	Sugar
Gravies	Candy
Sauces	Milk
Dressings	

Instead of writing out the measure, you may use these shorter abbreviations:

Tablespoon = Tbsp. or T.
Teaspoon   = tsp. or t.
Ounce   = oz.
Cup   = c.
Slice   = sl.
Piece   = pc.

Note: You can measure the size of the glasses and bowls you use at home with a standard measuring cup and use the same amount each time you record your food intake. Be sure to have the person who does your cooking at home answer the questions in Appendix 2.4.

Summary of How to Record Portion Sizes

Record in Ounces (1 Cup = 8 ounces):
Beverages—all types (including alcoholic)

Record in Cups or Servings (Large Serving—Small Serving):
Potatoes, rice, etc.
Fruits, vegetables (cooked or canned)
Cereals
Soups
Casserole dishes

Record in Teaspoons or Tablespoons (3 Teaspoons = 1 Tablespoon):
Jelly, jam, sugar, syrup
Sauces, gravies
Salad dressing
Butter, margarine (or in pats)

Record by Number and Size:
Bread, rolls, crackers
Raw fruits and vegetables
Meat cuts, chicken, frankfurters, shellfish
Snack items—nuts, candy, etc.
Cookies

Record by Servings (Large Serving—Small Serving):
Pie
Cake, coffee cake
Pizza

Description of Mixed Dishes
For mixed dishes (such as stews, casseroles, etc.) record the total amount eaten, e.g.:

1 c. chicken stew
2 c. hamburger-macaroni casserole

For sandwiches, list ingredients separately, e.g., ham sandwich:

2 sl. whole wheat bread
2 oz. ham, trimmed
1 leaf lettuce
1 tsp. mayonnaise

APPENDIX 2.3: SAMPLE PAGE OF THREE-DAY FOOD RECORD

Day: Wednesday   Date: April 10, 1975

Time	What You Ate and How Much	Time	What You Ate and How Much
8 am	½ c. orange juice 1 c. oatmeal ½ c. whole milk 2 tsp. sugar 1 sl. white bread 1 tsp. butter 2 c. coffee, black	3 pm	1 c. coffee 1 tsp. sugar 5 pc. hard candy
10 am	2 fig bars 1 c. coffee 1 tsp. sugar	6 pm	1 can beer (12 ox.) 2 loin lamb chops, 2 oz. each ½ c. mashed potatoes with skim milk lettuce salad—1 c. 1 T. French dressing 1 pc. angel food cake
1 pm	2 sl. wheat bread 2 sl. salami 1 tsp. butter 1 leaf lettuce 1 med. apple 2 gingersnaps 1 c. whole milk	10 pm	10 pretzels 1 btl. ginger ale (6 oz.)

APPENDIX 2.4: FOOD PREPARATION NOTES

To be completed by the person preparing meals at home. Please answer all the following questions about the meals eaten at home during this three-day food record period.

1. Kinds of cooking fat used:

   Kind   Brand

2. Salad dressing used:

   Type   Brand

3. Was fat added to cooked vegetables? Yes____ No____ Kind: _____
4. Was spread used on bread, rolls, etc.? If yes, what kind?_____ Brand: ___
5. Type of fat used in baking:_____ Brand: _____
6. Was fat trimmed from meat before cooking? Yes____ No____ Partially____

APPENDIX 3: PHYSICAL ACTIVITY QUESTIONNAIRE*

This questionnaire is used by the Health Insurance Plan of New York to discriminate activity levels. The last off-job physical activity question was added; it is one used by Dr. Robert Bruce, of Seattle, and others to identify the active exerciser. A validated and more detailed and quantitative assessment of leisure time activity is available (76).

H.I.P. Job-Connected Physical Activity Questions
(Circle Assigned Score)

Question	Answer	
Time on job spent sitting	Practically all	0
	More than 50%	1
	About 50%	2
	Less than 50%	3
	Almost none	4
Time on job spent walking	Almost none	0
	Less than 50%	1
	About 50%	2
	More than 50%	3
	Practically all	4
Walking to and from job	None or less than 1 block	0
	1–2 blocks	1
	3–4 blocks	2
	5–9 blocks	3
	10–19 blocks	4
	20–39 blocks (1 mile, not 2)	5
	40+ blocks (2+ miles)	6
Transportation to and from job	None	0
	Car, bus, railroad, or ferry	1
	Subway	2
	Subway and one or more other modes of transportation	3
Lifting or carrying heavy things	Very infrequently or never	0
	Sometimes	3
	Frequently	6
Hours on job per week	Less than 25	1
	24–34	2
	35–40	3
	41–50	4
	51+	5

*From Shapiro S, Weinblatt E, Frank CW, et al: The H.I.P study incidence and prognosis of coronary heart disease. Preliminary findings on incidence of myocardial infarction and angina. *J Chronic Dis* 18:527, 1965.

H.I.P. Off-Job Physical Activity Questions
(Circle Assigned Score)

Item	Frequently	Sometimes	Very Infrequently or Never
Take walks in good weather	2	1	0
Work around house or apartment	2	1	0
Gardening in spring or summer	2	1	0
Take part in sports			
Active ballgame other than golf, bowling, pool, or billiards	4	3	0
Other	3	2	0

Dr. Bruce's question:
Do you engage in physical activity that causes you to sweat and become breathless at least once a week?

Yes 4   *No* 0

H.I.P. Classification of Physical Activity

The classifications of physical activity are limited to men. Both overall and job-connected physical activity classifications are applicable only to those men known to have been employed in the 5 years preceding the specified diagnosis (numerator) or the given mail survey (denominator).

Job-Connected Physical Activity (PAj). Four classes are defined in terms of the following ranges of accumulated scores for the six questionnaire items shown in the table.

PAj Class	Accumulated Score
1 Least active	1–10
2 First intermediate	11–14
3 Second intermediate	15–18
4 Most active	19–28

Off-Job Physical Activity (PAoj). Four classes are defined in terms of the following ranges of accumulated scores for the four questionnaire items shown in the table.

PAoj Class	Accumulated Score
1 Least active	0–1
2 First intermediate	2–3
3 Second intermediate	4–5
4 Most active	6–10

Overall Physical Activity (PAx). Three classes are defined in terms of the following specified combinations of job-connected and off-job physical activity classes:

PAx Class	PAj Class	PAoj Class
1 Least active	1	1 or 2
	2	1
2 Intermediate	1	3
	2	2 or 3
	3	1, 2, or 3
3 Most active	4	All classes
	Other	4

An alternative classification of overall physical activity (PAx') is defined as follows:

PAx' Class	PAj Class	PAoj Class
1 Least active	1 or 2	1 or 2
2 First intermediate	3 or 4	1 or 2
3 Second intermediate	1 or 2	3 or 4
4 Most active	3 or 4	3 or 4

APPENDIX 4: SMOKING QUESTIONNAIRE

1. (a) Do you smoke cigarettes now?

   Yes, regularly . . . . ☐

   No . . . . ☐
   <small>If No, go to question 2 (a)</small>

   Occasionally (usually less than one cigarette per day) . . . . ☐

   (b) Do you inhale?

   Yes . . . . ☐

   No . . . . ☐

   (c) What kind of cigarettes do you smoke?

   Manufactured, with filters . . . . ☐

   Manufactured, without filters . . . . ☐

   Hand-rolled . . . . ☐

(d) How many manufactured cigarettes do you usually smoke per day?

(e) About how many ounces (or grams) of tobacco do you use per week for rolling your own cigarettes?

(f) What is the maximum number of cigarettes that you have smoked per day for as long as a year?

   Record total number of manufactured and hand-rolled cigarettes, counting 1 oz of tobacco as 25 cigarettes and 1 g as 1 cigarette

(g) How many cigarettes did you smoke per day a year ago?

(h) How old were you when you began to smoke cigarettes?
   After answering this question, go to question 3 (a)

2. (a) Did you ever smoke cigarettes?

   Yes, regularly . . . .

   No, never . . . .
      If No, go to question 3 (a)

   Occasionally (usually less than one cigarette per day) . . . .

(b) What is the maximum number of cigarettes you ever smoked per day for as long as a year? . . . .
   Record total number of manufactured and hand-rolled cigarettes, counting 1 oz of tobacco as 25 cigarettes and 1 g as 1 cigarette

(c) Did you inhale?

   Yes . . . .

   No . . . .

(d) How old were you when you began to smoke cigarettes? . . . . . .

(e) When did you stop smoking cigarettes? . . . .
   Give year

(f) Why did you stop? _____

3. (a) Have you ever smoked cigars?

No .... ☐
If No, go to question 4 (a)

Used to, but not now .... ☐
If Not now, go to question 4 (a)

Now smoke occasionally (less than one per day) .... ☐

Now smoke regularly .... ☐

(b) About how many do you smoke per week? .... ☐

(c) Do you inhale?

Yes .... ☐

No .... ☐

4. (a) Have you ever smoked a pipe?

No .... ☐

Used to, but not now .... ☐

Now smoke a pipe occasionally (less than once a day) .... ☐

Now smoke one regularly .... ☐

(b) About how many ounces (or grams) of tobacco do you smoke per week? ☐

(c) Do you inhale?
Yes .... ☐

No .... ☐

6

Patient and Family Education

Nina T. Argondizzo, R.N.

In this era of enlightened consumerism in all areas of life, education plays a vital role. Health care personnel find this increasingly true as enrollments in prepaid health care plans increase and subscribers seek information about disease recognition and prevention. Current discussions involve the possibility of third-party payment for formally structured health education designed to improve adherence to therapeutic regimens; more familiar are patient and family teaching requirements during episodes of illness. The impact of coronary heart disease can create havoc in the lives of both patients and their families. Following an episode of myocardial infarction, the patient progresses through the stages of initial diagnosis, acute care in a coronary care unit, progressive care, convalescence at home, and return to work; at each stage the patient and family usually are exposed to some teaching-learning activities. Life as the family unit has known it is altered drastically. They need additional health education and information at various times in the health–illness continuum. Rehabilitation begins with diagnosis and continues until the patient has achieved optimal physical, psychosocial, and vocational potentials, and patient and family education becomes a key factor in facilitating movement toward this goal.

However, during the hospital phase of myocardial infarction many factors militate against learning and the retention of new knowledge, even during convalescence. It is difficult for the patient to anticipate the changes that will be faced on returning home. This is true also of the family; they do not know what to expect. On returning home, the patient depends on the physician for health care information. Patients who return for clinic appointments may have other health personnel to assist in transmitting information and answering questions. The in-hospital learning experience of the patient should serve as the basis for future teaching.

The physician must learn about the patient as a person. Of course, the physician is aware of the patient's disease, alterations in function, and perhaps emotional reactions to illness, but is the physician attuned to the important aspects of the patient's life and life-style from the patient's point of view? All the patient's activities are meaningful in the context of the care regimen. Relationships at home, at work, and in the community have specific bearing on whether or not patients perceive themselves as persons of worth as they attempt to integrate the experience of illness into their lives. Patients differ in their psychologic adaptations to illness, but generally they progress through several stages. Disbelief occurs initially, and denial may be prominent. During the stage of awareness, anger may be expressed openly as hostility or turned inward as depression. Acceptance and resumption of some control and finally resolution and adaptation follow as the patient begins to assimilate the experience, accept the loss, and reintegrate the personality. The manner in which a person reacts to the crisis of illness is determined by the coping mechanisms developed to resolve past crises. If the patient has a long-term illness, the process outlined here may be repeated over and over again. The myocardial infarction patient may experience fluctuations in these adaptive processes if complications develop or if myocardial infarction recurs. The stage of adaptation to illness may also affect the learning process.

Consideration should also be given to general components of the teaching–learning interaction. An old cliché states that if the learner hasn't learned, the teacher hasn't taught. More appropriately, if the learner hasn't learned, it is because the teacher has not assisted the learner to learn the things that are needed. No one really teaches someone else. The dynamic feature in the learning process is the experience of the learner, which is the interaction between individual learner and environment. The teacher is the facilitator who provides the environment from which the student gathers learning and who fosters the student's interaction to help maximize learning. More simply, the teacher helps the student utilize the available resources to meet goals and objectives. The main objective of education is to effect a change of behavior in the learner.

The educational objectives for learning behaviors may be divided into three domains: the cognitive, which is concerned with intellectual abilities; the affective, which concerns expressions of feelings as embodied in interests, attitudes, values, and appreciations; the psychomotor, which deals with motor skills. Within these domains there is a hierarchy of complexity of behaviors. Learning itself is complex, and much remains obscure about how people really learn. Nevertheless, the teaching–learning process should not be a haphazard venture for either teacher or learner. The behavioral objectives for the patient recovering from a myocardial infarction must indicate what the patient needs to know (cognitive), do (psychomotor), and value (affective) if rehabilitation is to be successful. Careful planning of educational content, creative and imaginative implementation of the plan, subsequent evaluation of results (i.e., change in behavior), and reorganization of the process when learning does not occur are the components of teaching–learning interaction.

To attain the desired effect, learning must be perceived by the patient to be personally meaningful. It must fill the gaps in information that prevent him from functioning as he desires. Theories of adult education state that the person will benefit most who is most involved in diagnosing personal learning needs, planning for meeting these needs, implementing the plan by participating in the learning experiences designed to meet the needs, and finally evaluating the success of the learning. Adult educators believe that the individual is the best evaluator of his or her own learning needs. Motivation and readiness to learn are ingredients necessary for behavioral change. When is the patient ready? In the hospital the patient's energies are concentrated on coping with the physical and emotional realities, the fright and anxiety attendant to life-threatening illness. Neither the patient nor the family are ready to learn intensively at that point. Nevertheless, simple and repeated presentation of information and preliminary planning for return home can help to allay anxiety and avert depression; patient and family are reassured by the concept of planning for the future. However, despite in-hospital teaching, many anxious and/or depressed patients will, when questioned about specific instructions given, respond, "I don't remember hearing that at all." For this reason the same information should be presented on several occasions.

However, many patients realize that once they are outside the hospital their need to know how to alter their lives and make the necessary changes will become more acute. The anxiety of not knowing how one will react when returning to home surroundings may be a spur to learning for patient and family, but either too much anxiety or too little can hinder the learning process.

Just what do patients and their families have to know? In consultation with the patient, plan what the patient needs to learn. In many instances, too much information is forced on the patient, or information is presented at an inappropriate stage of recovery. Much that is called teaching is merely telling or giving information or admonition; the latter can have negative effects if the patient gets more don'ts than dos. The emphasis in teaching should be prescription, not proscription. Instruction should be simple and understandable at the patient's level of education; it should be of short duration and should be repeated as necessary. Most important, conflicting information should not be given by the various health professionals caring for the patient. Remember that changes and adaptations occur over a period of time, and individual reorganization must repair the chaos caused when illness disrupts the usual patterns. The patient needs time to think about the changes deemed necessary and time to determine if and when they will be incorporated into a life-style the patient can tolerate.

The following topics should be included in the teaching plan: the patient's specific health problem, activity, nutrition, medications, smoking cessation, and community resources available for assistance during rehabilitation.

THE PATIENT'S HEALTH PROBLEM

The patient should be informed about the disease, the reasons for and the results of diagnostic tests, the clinical course, and the prognosis. Information about normal heart anatomy and function will be needed in order to understand the alterations that occur with atherosclerosis, as well as why there are symptoms, why myocardial infarction occurred, and how healing and recovery take place. Coronary risk factors must be discussed, with emphasis on the patient's alterable risk factors. If a pacemaker has been inserted, instruction must include measurement and recording of pulse rate, signs of battery failure, effects of electrical and other devices, the importance of carrying the pacemaker identification card at all times, etc. The significance of symptoms such as pain, dyspnea, fatigue, dizziness, and palpitations should be explained, with instructions for appropriate patient response to these problems. It should be made clear that depression is not uncommon when a patient returns home, nor is it uncommon for a patient to feel weak and tired; the patient should be reassured that these problems will lessen with time.

ACTIVITY

Specific activity instructions must be given; vague instructions to take it easy, rest, or relax promote anxiety. Activity instructions must cover several areas: rest, work, exercise, recreation, activities of daily living, sexual intercourse, and travel.

Rest

The amount and time of rest should be specified. The patient must be instructed to rest after activities that produce pain or other symptoms. The recommended hours of sleep should fit the patient's sleep pattern.

Work

How many hours of work each day should be permitted initially, and how should this be increased? Is work to be interspersed with rest? A detailed description of the patient's work pattern will be of assistance in tailoring the prescription for activity. If the job is sedentary, the patient may be instructed to move about periodically. If the job entails lifting, recommendations about limiting breath holding or the Valsalva maneuver may be appropriate. Work simplification methods may help the impaired homemaker continue in that role; having cooking utensils within easy reach can eliminate stretching and bending. What kind of work is permitted in the home? The amounts of cleaning, washing, ironing, lawn mowing, pruning, etc., should be indicated.

Activities of Daily Living

Personal hygiene requirements such as bathing, toileting, dressing, and shaving (including going up and down stairs for these activities) usually present no problem because these aspects of self-care have been practiced during hospitalization. Reasons for avoidance of extremes of temperatures should be explained. Patients should be told when they may go outdoors, ride in a car, and drive.

Exercise

Physical activity to increase physical capacity is widely used in rehabilitating patients after myocardial infarction and is discussed in Chapters 7, 8, and 9. The prescription must be precise. Commonly the first activity is walking on level ground; as the patient becomes stronger, the distance is increased and the time to accomplish the distance is decreased. Patients who must use cars to get to work may have limited opportunity to walk the prescribed amount. They can be instructed to park their cars in a distant area of a parking lot and use the walk back and forth to fulfill requirements. Another method is to get off the bus several blocks from the final destination and walk. Physical conditioning classes, which often are offered at community centers with medical supervision, can be used by patients who have progressed to increased activity.

Recreation and Leisure Activities

Patients usually have a variety of interests that can be enjoyed safely if they are not carried to the point of fatigue. Hobbies can help to occupy the early days at home until full activity is approached; e.g., art, handiwork, collections, and games such as cards, chess, backgammon, and Scrabble. Activities that are sedentary should be interspersed with activities requiring movement. Sports, when permitted, should not be highly competitive, nor should they be engaged in during extremes of temperature. Recreational activities of a social nature should be resumed slowly and spaced so that days do not become crowded with activity simulating the patient's preinfarction routine. The psychologic benefits of returning to a normal pattern are most salutory.

Sexual Intercourse

The usual advice given to the patient is to resume sexual activity with a familiar partner when the patient is able to perform the usual daily activities; the cardiac work of sexual activity is comparable to that of climbing several flights of stairs or walking several blocks briskly. Advice must be individualized and must be related to the level of sexual activity prior to infarction; the patient who has not been active sexually should not be pressed into taking up an activity long quiescent. The patient who experiences chest pain or discomfort can be instructed to take nitroglycerin prior to intercourse. Suggesting changes of position is inappropriate, as little difference in cardiac work has been documented. The patient's partner can be urged to be the more active participant initially. Counseling regarding resumption of sexual activity should be done with both partners present; they may understandably be fearful, but must be reassured that the incidence of coital deaths is minimal. Excesses of food and alcohol preceding sexual activity should be avoided.

Travel

Travel is a way of life for some people. Jetting across continents can present problems for the myocardial infarction patient: jet lag and fatigue, time changes affecting biologic rhythms, lifting suitcases, the bustling activity of an airport, long distances to walk in terminals, cabin pressurization, differences in altitudes, and the pressure of meeting tight schedules. The patient whose livelihood depends on travel requires special counseling about altering the pace of travel, resting at high altitudes, etc. The patient should know about the health care systems available at all destinations. Sufficient medication should be carried, as should a medical summary, a list of the patient's medications, and the physician's telephone number.

NUTRITION

Mealtimes are traditionally social times, and they should be as pleasant as possible. Instruction should be given in the general principles of adequate nutrition. For the patient with significant angina or congestive heart failure, it may be wise to alter eating habits and have the patient eat five or six small meals rather than the usual three. When special diets are ordered (e.g., low-calorie diet for weight reduction and maintenance of ideal weight), the rationale for their use and the specific preparation instructions are necessary. If salt-restricted or fat-restricted diets are indicated, the person who prepares the meals should be given instruction. Attention should be paid to alcohol intake in regard to caloric content and its potentially harmful effect on a damaged myocardium.

MEDICATIONS

Some patients may not have to take any prescribed medications, but many will, at least for a while. The points to be stressed are the reason for the medication, the dosage, the desired effects, and the importance of not altering the regimen prior to consulting the physician. Side effects to be reported and interactions with other medications and foods must also be discussed. The patient should be instructed to take medications in conjunction with some activity that always takes place at a standard time; it is better to order medication with breakfast, lunch, or dinner than at odd hours, particularly when the patient is trying to reorganize a life-style. Medications should be kept in an accessible, convenient place, not in a medicine chest two flights upstairs. Specific instruction is necessary for the patient taking digitalis (monitoring pulse), diuretics (fluid restriction, monitoring weight gain or loss), anticoagulant drugs (bleeding), antihypertensive agents (postural hypotension), etc. A review of nonprescription over-the-counter medications used by the patient is also important. Medication instruction will require the most repetition and support. "Taking pills" is a constant reminder to the patient of his vulnerability; consequently, when feeling good, the patient may "forget."

SMOKING

Despite receiving information via television, radio, newspapers, billboards, pamphlets, government warnings, etc., about the deleterious effects of smoking, many patients find it difficult to discontinue this habit. The physician should describe the risks of smoking and refer the patient to antismoking clinics, self-help guides, and other assistance programs for the inveterate smoker who would like to stop. The patient embarking on a campaign to stop smoking needs support from health care personnel. As with weight control, the nonsmoker role model is most effective in changing addictive behavior habits.

COMMUNITY AGENCIES THAT CAN ASSIST IN REHABILITATION

Some communities have work evaluation units, sheltered workshops, vocational rehabilitation counseling services, and supervised exercise programs. Individuals responsible for patient education should learn which services are available and how patients can gain access to them.

Educational Techniques, Programs, and Personnel

A busy physician cannot personally prepare and implement individual patient teaching plans. Valuable alternative strategies can provide for excellent patient and family education. The office nurse can readily take on the task. The nurse can function as a sounding board for patients and their families, eliciting their feelings about new or reinforced learning. Instead of asking "How is your diet?" and receiving an apathetic "Oh, all right, I guess," a better approach, but a more time-consuming one, is "Tell me about your diet." This encourages freer expression of feelings; clues are provided by what is said and how it is said, as well as by nonverbal cues from the patient. The educational algorithm used at Grady Memorial Hospital and the Emory University School of Medicine, Atlanta, Georgia, can be used to record what was taught and when and how, to determine the need for repetition, and to give some indication of patient adherence (see Appendix, p. 128). Although this algorithm was designed for use in a hospital setting, the portion devoted to posthospitalization care can be readily modified to fit the individual physician's specifications for keeping records.

To improve the patient's knowledge about medications, some hospitals have developed instruction cards for each medication the patient must take after discharge. These can also be used in office practice, tailored to the physician's specifications (see Appendix, p. 131).

To provide instruction about the patient's particular cardiac problem, pads of leaflets are available from the American Heart Association (Fig. 1) that show the relationships of the coronary arteries, cardiac chambers, and great vessels. Other materials available from the American Heart Association and other voluntary health agencies and local public health offices describe specific diets, coronary risk factors, rehabilitation following myocardial infarction, and many other aspects of cardiovascular problems. These materials are prepared for the public and are listed in catalogues available to interested health personnel for teaching purposes. Samples of general informational materials can be displayed in waiting rooms for interested patients, and specialized pamphlets can be given to specific patients. The value of learning from casual reading of health education material is yet to be determined. Audiovisual devices (videotapes and slide-cassette units) can be placed in offices for teaching or used by patients in waiting rooms. Research in audiovisual use reveals that 50% of what is seen and heard is remembered. These materials can be employed at the patient's individual rate of learning. However, a health professional must be available to discuss the material with the patient and answer questions. Before any educational material, written or otherwise, is given to the patient and family, it should be reviewed by the

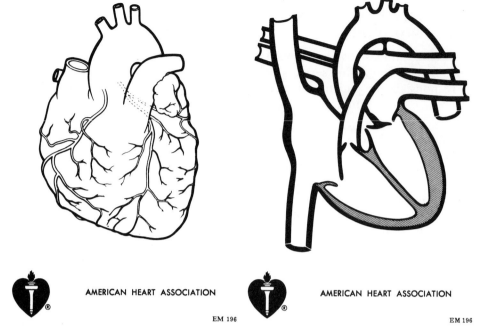

AMERICAN HEART ASSOCIATION

EM 196

AMERICAN HEART ASSOCIATION

EM 196

Figure 1. Pads of these leaflets may be obtained from the American Heart Association by local heart associations. The pads can then be stamped with the name of the local affiliate.

physician or his surrogate for accuracy, freedom from ambiguity, and pertinence for the patient.

The office nurse should be available to take telephone calls from patients who have concerns after returning home (e.g., the patient who didn't remember to ask or didn't remember being told about climbing stairs or some comparable problem). If need be, the hospital or office nurse could make a home visit to help plan for the patient's homecoming. A visit after the patient returns home permits observation to determine if learning has been effective in modifying behavior. Alternatively, community nurses (public health nurses or visiting nurse services) can fulfill this outreach service. The feedback in an office practice is limited, usually in response to questioning the patient and family about adherence to instructions; seeing the patient and family firsthand is preferable.

The physician without an office nurse might consider hiring, perhaps in conjunction with other physicians, a nurse educator on a part-time basis. Nurses who do not want full-time employment because of other responsibilities would welcome this type of position (they could teach patients with other problems as well). Professional health educators have also been used to teach in some group practice settings.

Maximal use of available personnel can be achieved by teaching patients in groups. The availability of patient and family education and discussion groups for those who have suffered myocardial infarction is increasing nationwide. The health personnel involved in initiating these groups usually have been nurses. However, collaboration among an interested group of physicians, nurses, social workers, and nutritionists would make for a better educational environment. The groups must be organized and must have educational goals; this differs from the situation in groups where people of like interests gather and socialize. The danger inherent in unsupervised groups (without a health professional as a resource person) is the sharing of myths, misinformation, and ignorance about health and health care. Although patients and families have common learning needs, the patient's position is unique. The patient may not progress at the same rate as the group, and peer pressure in such a group can be detrimental if the patient tries to conform. A trained leader can prevent competition and inappropriate group domination by a few individuals.

The organization and format of patient and family educational programs can vary, but often they are implemented in the following manner. The sponsoring group usually includes nurses, physicians, and other interested professionals such as nutritionists, social workers, and exercise physiologists. They meet as a faculty to formulate the curriculum and objectives and evaluate the program. There should be sufficient faculty to serve as group leaders of small group discussions, which can be most valuable in helping to change attitudes. Often a hospital will have a room available for use in the evenings, or schools or churches may have space available for classes.

The time schedule is typically 2 hr in the evening once a week for 6–8 weeks. The didactic part of the program is presented by one faculty member, e.g., the nutritionist when diet is discussed. Small groups are then formed for further discussion of the main topic or for discussion of other problems raised by group members. Exchange of information among group members about ways of handling problems is valuable and serves to bolster self-image. Refreshments may be provided; the atmosphere should be informal, open, and accepting in order to facilitate communication.

Topics for discussion include those previously mentioned: coronary risk factors, diet, medications, smoking, activity, early warnings of heart attack, how to enter the health care system, etc. One session should be saved for topics requested by the group. A topic included in many programs is emergency care, including cardiopulmonary resuscitation; most families learn this lifesaving technique with facility and are reassured by this knowledge.

A great advantage of group teaching is that increased learning takes place. If one person is shy and reticent about asking questions, answers may be provided if a less-inhibited person asks questions. A question asked by one person often triggers a question from another that might not have arisen in a one-to-one teaching interaction. Another advantage of a group of people meeting together after living through the same illness experience is the emotional support they afford one another. The "I was there, too" can never be matched by the physician or nurse saying "I know how you feel."

Community physicians should be informed when classes are being organized; most groups require that enrollees have the permission of their physicians to participate. Most classes are planned for patients who have had a myocardial infarction, but some physicians have asked that their high-coronary-risk patients be allowed to attend. Physicians report the patients and families who have participated in such programs adhere better to their prescribed regimens and accept changes in life-style.

The project described requires a cadre of knowledgeable, interested, competent persons. Nurses in various health care settings can participate in these educational endeavors. Faculty members in schools of nursing have an educational background and clinical expertise that can be valuable. Nurses in coronary care units often appreciate the opportunity to learn how their initial teaching serves as a basis for the continuing education of the patient and family. Observing comparatively successful results in the group motivates these nurses to improve their teaching as a vital component of care.

Local heart association nursing committees may assume leadership roles in such projects. Nurses in home health care agencies such as visiting nurse services and those employed in industry are experienced in counseling patients and families in the posthospital rehabilitative phase of long-term illnesses and are another competent resource.

Many school systems employ health educators and school nurse teachers who can be helpful in initiating patient education programs. Many colleges offer a variety of adult evening classes, and suggestions from the medical community to include health education in curriculum offerings are often well received.

Physicians who are members of community boards of education can suggest that information about health practices to prevent heart disease be included in the health education curriculum in elementary grades. The opportunity to alter life-style to promote health can and should begin early, and this health information eventually reaches parents as well.

Assessment and Advantages of Educational Programs

Does it make a difference? This basic question about health teaching is being answered favorably. Recent studies of the effects of counseling of poor adherers to medication have shown significant improvement. Similar favorable results in teaching segments of a population how to lower plasma cholesterol have been demonstrated by community diet education programs. The essential ingredients of these successful educational programs include demonstrations, specific instructions, guidance periodically repeated, self-monitoring by means of keeping records, and involvement of the participant. Organized education programs in inpatient and outpatient settings have produced significant changes in patients' knowledge of disease, medications, and diet, as well as better compliance with prescribed therapy. Studies have confirmed the validity of the activities of health care professionals who in the past taught patients because they believed that patients and families had the right to know about the health problems affecting their lives.

Concerned physicians attempt to use each interaction with patients as an opportunity to provide informal teaching and counseling, but brief encounters between anxious patients and busy physicians cannot result in intensive or sustained learning. Other options that focus on the educational needs of patients and families are available. By joining with colleagues in other health care disciplines the physician can fulfill the responsibility to teach patients with programs that reflect the high quality of care provided.

BIBLIOGRAPHY

Baden CA: Teaching the coronary patient and his family. *Nurs Clin North Am* 7:563, 1972

Braunwald E (ed): *The Myocardium: Failure and Infarction.* Hospital Practice Publishing, New York, 1974

Dunbar JM: Adherence to medication: An intervention study with poor adherers. *Circulation* 56:169, 1977

Haferkorn V: Assessing individual learning needs as a basis for patient teaching. *Nurs Clin North Am* 6:199, 1969

Hellerstein HK, Friedman EH: Sexual activity in the post-coronary patient. *Medical Aspects of Human Sexuality* 3:70, 1969

Knowles MS: *The Modern Practice of Adult Education.* Association Press, New York, 1970

Likoff W, Segal B, Galton L: *Your Heart.* JB Lippincott, Philadelphia, 1972

Linde BJ, Janz NM: The effectiveness of a comprehensive teaching program on the knowledge and compliance of cardiovascular patients. *Circulation* 56:146, 1977

Redman BK: *The Process of Patient Teaching in Nursing* (ed 3). CV Mosby, St Louis, 1977

Reeves RS, Foreyt JP, Scott LW, et al: Effectiveness of a low cholesterol eating plan for community groups. *Circulation* 56:114, 1977

Smyth K: Teaching patients. *Nurs Clin North Am* 6:571, 1971

Wenger NK, Mount F: An educational algorithm for myocardial infarction. *Cardiovascular Nursing* 10:3, 1974

Wenger NK: Coronary Care: Rehabilitation After Myocardial Infarction (Booklet EM-609). American Heart Association, Dallas, 1973

APPENDIX 1: PATIENT EDUCATION—CARDIAC REHABILITATION PROGRAM, GRADY MEMORIAL HOSPITAL

Problem: CASHD (Coronary Atherosclerotic Heart Disease)

	Content	Date & Teacher	Need for Further Teaching Yes No	Comments
ADJUSTMENT TO ICU	1. Purpose of CCU			
	2. Medications			
	3. I.V.			
	4. Monitor (sounds and leads)			
	5. Regulations of unit (visiting, smoking, flowers)			
	6. Activity (leg exercises)			
	7. Oxygen			
	8. X-ray			
	9. ECG			
	10. Blood tests			
	11. Diet (it changes)			
	12. Personal emergencies (ex.: bills, etc.)			
ADJUSTMENT TO TRANSFER FROM UNIT	1. Constant observation no longer necessary			
	2. Activity only with permission			
	3. Not to leave 6th floor without permission			

128

ADAPTATION TO DISEASE (AREA AND CLINIC)	1. Normal anatomy & physiology of heart
	
	2. Development of ASH⌐
	
	3. Heart Attack
	  A. Risk factors
	    1. General discussion
	    2. Those which apply to pt. (list below)
	      a.
	      b.
	      c.
	      d.
	  B. Warning signs
	
	  C. Healing stages—relation to activity
	
	4. Personal response to M.I.
	  A. Group discussion
	
	  B. Individual conference		

PLANS FOR POSTHOSPITALIZATION CARE	1. Diet
	  A. Group
	  B. Individual
	
	2. Medications (list)
	
	  A.
	  B.
	  C.
	  D.
	  E.
	  F.
	  G.
	  H. Medication card given
	3. Activity
	  A. General
	  B. Sexual
	  C. Work simplification
	
	4. Symptoms which should be reported
	
	5. Rehab. exercises
	
	6. Clinic appointments
	
	7. Community Resources		

OTHER AREAS OF TEACHING COVERED (LIST) (EX.: PACEMAKER, DIABETES, ETC.)				

List of Patient Education Materials

Place a X by those given to patient:

_____ Heart Attack (AHA EM 150)

_____ Heart Attack: How to Reduce Your Risk (AHA EM 517)

_____ After a Coronary (AHA EM 365)

_____ Why Risk Heart Attack? (AHA EM 414)

_____ About Your Heart and Your Blood Stream (AHA WM 286)

_____ Facts About Congestive Heart Failure (AHA EM 266A)

_____ If You Have Angina (AHA EM 448)

_____ Your Blood Pressure (AHA EM 33)

_____ Smoking and Heart Disease (AHA EM 343)

_____ How to Stop Smoking (AHA EM 487)

_____ Eat Well but Eat Wisely (AHA EM 478)

_____ Recipes for Fat-Controlled, Low Cholesterol Meals (AHA EM 455A)

_____ Be Good to Your Heart (Ga. Dept. of Public Health)

_____ Cut Down on Your Salt

_____ Foods (booklet developed by Cardiac Clinic dietician)

_____ High Blood Pressure (developed by Cardiac Clinic nurse)

_____ Now That Your Heart Is Healing (developed by Cardiac Clinic nurse)

_____ Your Pacemaker (developed by Cardiac Clinic nurse)

Please list any other patient education material given to the patient.

130

APPENDIX 2: THE NEW YORK HOSPITAL
PATIENT MEDICATION INSTRUCTION CARD*

Dear Patient:

Your physician has prescribed warfarin sodium (Coumadin). The purpose of this medication is to thin your blood and inhibit the formation of harmful blood clots in your blood vessels. The dosage schedule that your physician has prescribed should be followed very closely. To insure successful management of your condition it is essential to follow these instructions:

1. Avoid situations that may result in injury to yourself; for example: cuts, bruises, or contact sports.
2. Never increase, decrease, or change your dose without specific instructions from your physician.
3. Inform any physician that you visit that you are on warfarin sodium.
4. Avoid the use of aspirin or aspirin containing products (Anacin, Excedrin, Bufferin, Alka Seltzer or Empirin Compound). Use Tylenol, Nebs, or Valadol.
5. Avoid the use of harsh laxatives such as Dulcolax, citrate of magnesia, cascara sagrada, or Exlax. Use mild laxatives if needed, such as milk of magnesia, Colace, or mineral oil.
6. If you are in need of a cold, cough, laxative, headache, or pain remedy, seek the advice of your physician or inform your community pharmacist that you are on warfarin sodium and ask him to suggest a remedy.
7. Purchase a medic-alert bracelet that states you are taking warfarin sodium or an anticoagulant.
8. Keep your clinic appointments. Report these signs to your physician if they occur:
    1. Excessive bruising, black and blue marks or tiny red spots on your skin.
    2. Pinkish or reddish colored urine.
    3. Black, red or tar colored stools.
    4. Excessive nose bleeds.
    5. Red colored sputum or vomit.
    6. Bleeding gums.
    7. Excessive menstrual bleeding.
    8. Unusual dizziness, episodes of fainting or weakness.

Dr. ——————————————————————— at The New York Hospital,

phone ————————————————————————————————

*Permission for use was given by the Patient Care Committee, The New York Hospital, 525 East 68th Street, New York, N.Y. 10021.

7

Clinical Exercise Physiology

C. Gunnar Blomqvist, M.D., Ph.D.

PHYSICAL PERFORMANCE CAPACITY

Physical performance capacity is a complex entity that has three major components:

· capacity for energy output: aerobic and anaerobic mechanisms
· neuromuscular function: strength, technique, coordination
· psychologic factors: motivation, tactics

This framework is equally applicable to analysis of individual capacity and analysis of the highly variable demands imposed by different forms of physical activity. Studies of running have demonstrated that successful long-distance running is primarily a matter of high aerobic capacity. Football players usually rely on anaerobic mechanisms for energy output; for them, superior neuromuscular function and psychologic factors are much more important than high aerobic capacity.

Exercise physiology deals with all components of human physical performance capacity. Mechanisms relating to energy output, particularly oxygen demand and oxygen supply during exercise, are of primary interest to the physician dealing with cardiovascular disease. This chapter will focus on oxygen transport and cardiovascular function, but it will also consider oxygen demand and skeletal muscle physiology.

Skeletal muscle has a greater metabolic range than any other organ. Its metabolic rate may increase 50-fold during transition from rest to maximal exercise. The peak rate of oxygen delivery, i.e., the capacity of the lungs and the cardiovascular system to transfer oxygen from ambient air to working muscle, is usually regarded as the principal factor limiting physical activity that involves large muscle groups and that lasts for more than a few minutes. Work of shorter duration is supported by anaerobic mechanisms, and oxygen transport during that work is not as critical.

Aerobic capacity or *maximal oxygen uptake* is defined as the level of oxygen uptake at which, in a given individual, an increase in work load no longer produces an increase in oxygen uptake. The classic concept of oxygen transport and utilization regards *cardiac output* as the main determinant of maximal oxygen uptake. *Ventilatory capacity* and *diffusing capacity* of the lung, unless significant lung disease is present, are not limiting factors except at high altitudes. This view has recently been challenged by physiologists who consider the *oxidative capacity* of skeletal muscle (the ability to utilize oxygen) the primary determinant, at least in the absence of significant cardiovascular or pulmonary disease. This controversy has not yet been completely resolved. Peripheral mechanisms are clearly much more important than was recognized only a few years ago. On the other hand, there are powerful arguments in favor of oxygen transport capacity rather than skeletal muscle metabolism being the limiting factor. Increased oxygen content of inspired air is associated with an increase in maximal oxygen uptake. Quantitative studies of enzyme activity in skeletal muscle have suggested that the oxygen utilization capacity of skeletal muscle exceeds the delivery capacity of the cardiovascular system.

SKELETAL MUSCLE PHYSIOLOGY

Skeletal muscle physiology has been a particularly fruitful area of investigation during the past few years. New techniques, including biopsy methods for human studies and various chemical and histochemical methods, have provided new insights into the acute response to exercise and the effects of physical training.

The functional unit within a skeletal muscle is the *motor unit,* groups of muscle fibers innervated by a single motor nerve fiber. The individual skeletal *muscle cell or muscle fiber* usually extends from tendon to tendon. Each fiber contains a number of parallel *myofibrils* running longitudinally and consisting of a series of *sarcomeres.* The sarcomere, the basic contractile unit, is demarcated by narrow membranes or Z lines transecting the myofibrils. Thin rods of *actin* extend in both directions from the Z lines and are in the central part of the sarcomere paralleled by thicker rods of *myosin.* Muscle contraction is caused by a sliding movement of the peripheral actin filaments into the central array of myosin rods, with the formation of cross-bridges. Energy is supplied by transfer of energy-rich phosphate bonds from adenosine triphosphate (ATP), transforming ATP to adenosine diphosphate (ADP) in the presence of calcium and magnesium ions. ATP is the universal intracellular carrier of chemical energy. The ATP-ADP system is driven by the enzyme ATPase. ATPase actually consists of myosin, with magnesium serving as an activator.

The amount of ATP stored in muscle and available as an energy source can support activity for a few seconds at most. Muscle stores of creatine phosphate (CP) provide an immediately available reserve of high-energy phosphates, but the total amount of CP is also small. The combined stores of ATP and CP are depleted during a 100-yard dash. Continued muscular activity requires replenishment of ATP via *oxidative* (aerobic) or *glycolytic* (anaerobic) metabolic pathways. The principal energy exchange processes are outlined in Table 1.

Table 1. Energy Exchange Processes in Skeletal Muscle: Principal Pathways

Anaerobic
1. $ATP \rightleftharpoons ADP + P +$ free energy
2. *creatine phosphate* $+ ADP \rightleftharpoons$ *creatine* $+ ATP$
3. *glycogen or glucose* $+ P + ADP \rightarrow$ lactate $+ ATP$

Aerobic
4. *glycogen or glucose* $+ P + ADP + O_2 \rightarrow CO_2 + H_2O + ATP$
5. *free fatty acids* $+ P + ADP + O_2 \rightarrow CO_2 + H_2O + ATP$

Glycogen, glucose, and free fatty acids are the major fuels. Proteins have generally been regarded as unimportant contributors to skeletal muscle metabolism, but recent studies have suggested that amino acids may to some extent be used as fuel and may also have a regulatory function. Glucose and glycogen may be metabolized either aerobically or anaerobically. Complete aerobic oxidation to water and carbon dioxide yields more than 10 times as much ATP and energy as the anaerobic or fermentation pathway, which produces pyruvate and lactate.

The duration and intensity of exercise determine which pathways and fuels will be utilized. Equal amounts of energy are derived aerobically from fats and carbohydrates at rest. Free fatty acids remain important during low-level steady-state exercise, but the proportion of energy derived from carbohydrates increases steeply at an effort level of 65–75% of maximal capacity. Only carbohydrates are burned during maximal work. These changes are reflected in the respiratory quotient (R.Q.), i.e., the CO_2/O_2 concentration ratio of expired air (Fig. 1). R.Q. is approximately 0.8 at rest and 1.0 during maximal work. The selective utilization of fuel is linked to *relative work load*, or actual oxygen uptake

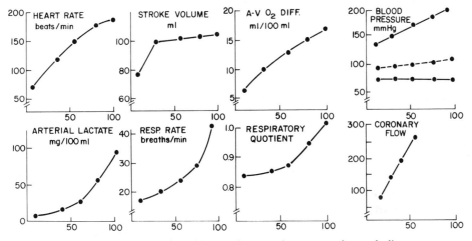

Figure 1. Principal features of cardiovascular, respiratory, and metabolic responses to exercise. Data points represent sitting rest, three levels of submaximal exercise, and maximal exercise. Values are plotted against relative load, i.e., actual oxygen uptake as percentage of maximal oxygen uptake. Blood pressure data represent systolic, mean, and diastolic brachial artery pressures. Coronary flow measurements are given as milliliters per minute per 100 g cardiac muscle. [Based on data of Saltin et al. (4), Nelson et al. (7), and Holmberg et al. (8).]

Table 2. Relative Contributions of Anaerobic and Aerobic Processes to Total Energy Output During Maximal Exercise[a]

Work Time	Total Energy Output (kcal)	Relative Contribution (%)	
		Anaerobic Processes	Aerobic Processes
10 sec	24	83	17
1 min	50	60	40
2 min	75	40	60
5 min	150	20	80
10 min	270	9	91
30 min	695	3	97
60 min	1215	1	99

[a]From Gollnick (2), with permission.

measured as percentage of the individual's maximal oxygen uptake, rather than to absolute levels. This means that the well-trained subject at any given submaximal level of exercise will utilize more fat and less carbohydrate than the untrained person. The physiologic advantage of using fat as fuel is obvious in view of the relative sizes of the energy stores of the body (Table 2).

The glycogen content of skeletal muscle is a limiting factor during continuous work at high submaximal intensities, e.g., 70–80% of maximal capacity. Maximal work time is closely related to glycogen content of muscle at onset of exercise, and glycogen concentration approaches zero at the point of exhaustion. Drastic changes in carbohydrate content of the diet may cause up to a 50% change in normal resting glycogen content of about 1.5 g/100 g muscle, with corresponding changes in endurance time. Extremely high glycogen levels, above 4 g/100 g muscle, can be produced by a sequence of glycogen depletion by exercise to exhaustion followed by a diet rich in carbohydrates.

Anaerobic metabolism of glucose and glycogen is the main source of energy early during exercise when the ATP and CP stores have been depleted but muscle blood flow has not reached the level necessary to sustain aerobic metabolism, i.e., during the initial 1–2 min of exercise. Anaerobic metabolism also helps support exercise at supramaximal levels and bridges the gap between the energy demand and the energy actually available from maximal utilization of aerobic processes. Recent studies have demonstrated that, contrary to previous belief, anaerobic metabolism also normally occurs during exercise at high work-load levels in the absence of muscle hypoxia. Arterial lactate levels (Fig. 1) usually remain only slightly above resting levels during exercise intensities up to 60–75% of maximal capacity, but they show a steep rise at higher work-load levels.

Anaerobic metabolism can be utilized only to a limited extent. The maximal total anaerobic energy output is about 30 kcal. Relative contributions of anaerobic and aerobic processes to the total energy output during maximal exercise of increasing duration are listed in Table 3. The exact mechanisms limiting anaerobic metabolism are still poorly defined. Lactate does not appear to

Table 3. Energy Stores Available for
Muscular Work[a]

Source	Energy (kcal)[b]
ATP	1.2
Creatine phosphate	3.6
Glycogen	1,200
Fat	50,000

[a]From Åstrand (1), with permission.
[b]Total kilocalories; body weight 75 kg (165 lb);
muscle weight 20 kg (44 lb).

have intrinsic toxicity, but there is a strong correlation between lactate accumulation and acidosis. Typical arterial pH and lactate values in a sedentary individual after maximal exercise are pH 7.30 and lactate 100 mg/dl. The intracellular pH in muscle is lower and is at a level that may temporarily inhibit glycolysis and contractility. The term anaerobic metabolism has often carried the connotation of dangerous overload. It is true that the contribution from anaerobic mechanisms increases at high work-load levels, but anaerobic metabolism is clearly part of the physiologic response to exercise. It is impossible to define a specific level of effort below which exercise is aerobic and above which it is anaerobic. Athletes may reach arterial lactate concentrations well above 200 mg/dl and pH levels below 7.0 without adverse effects.

Human skeletal muscle contains two distinct fiber types that differ with respect to metabolism and contractility. Red fibers are rich in myoglobin and mitochondria and have high oxidative capacity. Their contractile response is slow, and they have low myofibrillar myosin ATPase activity. White fibers have a low myoglobin content and fewer mitochondria. Their oxidative capacity is low, but their glycolytic capacity is high. Their contractile response is fast, and they have high myosin ATPase activity. The two fiber types are distributed in a mosaic pattern. Most animal muscle contains a third fiber type, a fast-twitch red fiber, and there are muscles or portions of muscles that contain only one fiber type.

The ratio of red fibers to white fibers in humans varies greatly from individual to individual. As would be expected because of the basic fiber characteristics, the best athletes in endurance sports have a very high proportion of red fibers, whereas athletes successful in sports requiring great speed and high-intensity work of short duration have mainly white fibers. To what extent this distribution is genetically determined has not been settled. The oxidative capacity of both red and white fibers can be greatly increased by physical training, but glycolytic capacity and contractile properties are not modified.

There are also important differences between red and white fibers with respect to innervation. The two fiber types are recruited selectively during exercise. Red fibers are supplied by small neurons with a low threshold of activation and are used preferentially during exercise of low intensity. White fibers are innervated by larger neurons with a high threshold, and they resist activation until exercise reaches high intensities. Both fiber types are active during very high intensities of exercise.

MAXIMAL OXYGEN UPTAKE

Maximal oxygen uptake is an important point of reference in exercise physiology. It is a stable and highly reproducible characteristic of the individual that serves as a measure of the functional capacity of the cardiovascular system.

Physiologic Variations

Differences in body size, age, sex, and habitual level of physical activity or physical conditioning account for much of the physiologic variation in maximal oxygen uptake. Measurements of maximal oxygen uptake may be given either in absolute terms such as liters per minute or as milliliters per kilogram of body weight per minute to facilitate comparison of persons of various body sizes. Maximal oxygen uptake expressed as liters per minute measures the maximal amount of external physical work that a subject can perform over a given period, provided the work involves large muscle groups and lasts for more than 2 min. Maximal oxygen uptake expressed as milliliters per kilogram of body weight per minute defines with similar qualifications the capacity for locomotion, and it is the accepted unit of measurement when used as an index of cardiovascular function. The absolute magnitude of maximal oxygen uptake (liters per minute) in normal subjects is strongly correlated with body weight. An even higher correlation is found with lean body mass. An abnormally low maximal oxygen uptake (in terms of milliliters per kilogram of body weight per minute) in an overweight subject may thus reflect obesity rather than a functional limitation due to heart disease. On the other hand, the value normalized with respect to total body mass rather than lean body mass accurately reflects one's ability to transport one's own body.

The effect of age on maximal oxygen uptake is highly significant (Fig. 2). There is a peak between 15 and 20 years of age and a gradual decline with advancing age. The average maximal oxygen uptake of a 60-year-old man is about two-thirds the mean value at age 20 years. This age trend seems to be universal and has been demonstrated in a variety of populations. Endurance

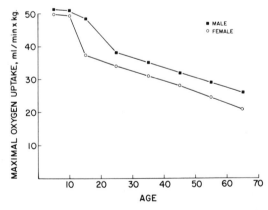

Figure 2. Maximal oxygen uptake by age and sex. The 95% confidence limits are closely approximated by the mean ± 25%. [Based on data of Åstrand and Rodahl (1) and AHA Committee on Exercise (9) and including several series.]

athletes (e.g., long-distance runners and cross-country skiers) who continue training and competition through their forties and fifties do not escape the decrease, but their values tend to remain well above the mean for less active populations.

There is little difference in maximal oxygen uptake with respect to sex in children 6–12 years old. Mean values for adolescent girls show a precipitous fall at 12–14 years of age, declining to about two-thirds to three-fourths of the values for boys of the same age, possibly because of changes in habitual levels of physical activity at the time of puberty. Further changes in women with increasing age parallel those seen among men. The lower average values for adult women are partially explained by the fact that muscle mass tends to be a smaller fraction of total body weight in women. Hemoglobin values are also lower in women, and this results in decreased oxygen-carrying capacity of arterial blood.

Ample evidence exists that the habitual level of physical activity is an important factor in determining maximal oxygen uptake. A decrease in activity causes a prompt fall in maximal oxygen uptake. A 20–25% drop below control value may occur after 3 weeks of bed rest in young normal subjects. Any increase in habitual physical activity that includes at least moderately heavy work involving large muscle groups will produce some increase in maximal oxygen uptake. The magnitude of the increase is determined by several factors, among which are the intensity, frequency, and duration of exercise and the initial level of maximal oxygen uptake. Age has some effect on the response; changes tend to be smaller in older age groups, but significant effects of physical training have been observed in men over 60 years of age. Long periods of hard physical training before full growth has been attained appear to be more effective than similar programs after 18–20 years of age, perhaps by means of increasing the dimensions of the circulatory system. Most short-term training experiments have produced increases in maximal oxygen uptake of about 20%.

Mean maximal oxygen uptake in populations of moderately active, healthy 20-year-old men is about 45 ml/kg/min, with a standard deviation of 10–15% of the mean. Strenuous physical training may produce at most a 35% increase in maximal oxygen uptake. Virtually all Olympic champions in endurance events have a maximal oxygen uptake between 75 and 80 ml/kg/min. Values above 55 ml/kg/min are rarely recorded among subjects who do not train regularly. These data suggest that it takes an exceptional genetic background combined with hard physical training to produce a gold-medal-winner in an Olympic endurance event.

Maximal Oxygen Uptake in Patients With Cardiovascular Disease

Maximal *systemic cardiac output* is the determinant of maximal oxygen uptake in most patients with cardiovascular disease. In others (e.g., patients with angina pectoris or claudication) failure of *regional blood flow* to meet increased demands during exercise will cause the patient to discontinue work before he has reached his potential maximal cardiac output. Occasionally an inefficient *distribution of blood flow* results in a low maximal oxygen uptake despite maximal normal cardiac output. Some patients with hyperkinetic hemodynamic syndrome (neurocirculatory or vasoregulatory asthenia, DaCosta's syndrome) fall into this category. A more common cause of disparity between maximal cardiac output and oxygen uptake is *low oxygen-carrying capacity* of the blood, as in anemia.

The level of oxygen uptake associated with angina and/or ischemic ST-segment depression, ventricular dysrhythmias, or signs of cerebral ischemia, i.e., symptoms and signs of inadequate regional perfusion, is the functional equivalent of the level producing a true maximal oxygen uptake in a normal subject, but it is appropriate to indicate the difference by using the term *peak oxygen uptake* rather than maximal oxygen uptake. Peak or maximal oxygen uptake is also referred to in the clinical literature as *physical work capacity*.

Comparisons between measured and expected maximal or peak levels of oxygen uptake may be used to quantitate the functional impact of cardiovascular disease, taking into account known sources of variation among normal subjects. The use of oxygen uptake as an index of performance capacity rather than work load has important practical advantages. Oxygen uptake serves as a common denominator for results obtained by different exercise test methods, e.g., treadmill and bicycle exercise. The energy demands of various forms of occupational and recreational physical activities can also be expressed in terms of oxygen uptake.

Measurement of maximal oxygen uptake is a poor test for diagnosing the presence or absence of heart disease. The level of maximal oxygen uptake in a given patient is likely to reflect the interactions among the premorbid functional capacity, the severity of the disease, and the effects of various compensatory mechanisms. In other words, the relationship between measured and expected maximal or peak oxygen uptake quantitates the *functional impact* rather than the anatomic extent or severity of the disease process. Groups of patients with various forms of acquired and congenital heart disease generally have subnormal mean maximal oxygen uptake, but the proportion of individuals with frankly abnormal values is variable. Most patients with angina pectoris become symptomatic at a level corresponding to 50–60% of expected maximal oxygen uptake for age and sex. Patients with healed myocardial infarctions without angina usually have higher work capacity and average about 75% of normal values. Less than 20% of patients with patent ductus, but virtually 100% of patients with tetralogy of Fallot, have abnormally low work capacity. Patients with rheumatic heart disease have an average oxygen uptake about two-thirds of normal.

There is only a tenuous correlation between the extent of arterial disease, as revealed by coronary angiography, and peak oxygen uptake (Figs. 2–4). Average work capacity declines progressively with the number of major vessels involved, but the degree of physical impairment cannot, in the individual patient, be used to predict the degree of anatomic involvement. The same is true for a variety of estimates of the severity of lesions in other forms of heart disease, e.g., pressure gradients, valve areas, and magnitudes of shunts.

This relative lack of correlation between anatomy and performance, or hemodynamic measurements at rest and physical work capacity, is surprising only if the pathophysiologic aspects are ignored. A severe stenosis of a single coronary artery may cause angina pectoris at very low work-load levels, whereas an occasional patient with triple-vessel disease but adequate collateral vessels may have nearly normal work capacity. A high left ventricular end-diastolic pressure at rest may reflect increased stiffness of the ventricular wall rather than failure, and the patient may show little impairment. Similarly, a patient with normal left ventricular function at rest (as judged from left ventricular end-diastolic pressure and ejection fraction) may be severely limited because of angina and may have a much lower work capacity than a patient with severe left ventricular dysfunction.

NORMAL AND ABNORMAL CARDIOVASCULAR RESPONSES TO EXERCISE

Systemic Circulation

Transition from rest to maximal exercise in the average young healthy man causes a 10-fold increase in metabolic rate. Oxygen uptake increases from about 0.3 to 3.0 liters/min during maximal treadmill or bicycle exercise. The increased peripheral oxygen demand during exercise is met by *increased transport* and *increased extraction* of oxygen from arterial blood.

Oxygen transport and utilization may be described in terms of a rearranged Fick equation: oxygen uptake = cardiac output × total arteriovenous oxygen (A-V O$_2$) difference, where cardiac output = heart rate × stroke volume. Typical values at sitting rest and during maximal exercise in a normal young sedentary subject are illustrated in Table 4.

Cardiac output increases almost by a factor of four, from about 5.2 to 19 l/min, primarily by a threefold increase in *heart rate*. The magnitude of the increase in *stroke volume* is a function of which body position is selected as representative of the resting control state. Stroke volumes at rest supine and during mild upright exercise are similar and are within 20% of maximal stroke volume. The stroke volume at standing rest in normal subjects averages less than 65% of the maximum. The value for stroke volume at sitting rest falls between the values for the supine and standing positions.

The relationship between oxygen uptake (or work load) and *heart rate* during exercise at submaximal levels is approximately linear in normal subjects (Figs. 1 and 3). The maximal heart rate is a function of age. Average maximal heart rate is 190 beats/min in normal 25-year-old subjects. There is a linear decrease with increasing age to an average of 160 beats/min at age 65 years, i.e., a decline of about 0.75 beat/min per year after the age of 25 years.

Table 4. Circulatory Data at Rest and During Maximal Exercise in a Normal Sedentary Young Man

	Oxygen Uptake (ml/min) =	Heart Rate (beats/min) ×	Stroke Volume (ml) ×	A-V O$_2$ Difference (ml/dl blood)
Sitting rest	300	75	75	5.2
Maximal exercise, upright	3000	190	100	15.8

Extraction of oxygen is about three times as effective during maximal exercise as at rest. The increasing A-V O_2 difference (the difference in oxygen content between arterial and mixed venous or pulmonary artery blood) with increasing load reflects a redistribution of blood flow. Blood is shunted away from the nonworking muscles, the skin, and the splanchnic area and delivered to exercising muscles. There is a progressive decrease in hepatic and renal blood flow with increasing work loads.

Total *systemic peripheral resistance*, or the ratio between mean arterial pressure and cardiac output, decreases progressively with increasing levels of exercise. Measurement of systemic blood pressure, as in peripheral arteries, shows a progressive increase in systolic pressure during exercise, with a much smaller increase in mean pressure (Fig. 1). Diastolic pressure usually falls, but it may show a small increase. Peripheral systolic pressures exceeding 200 mm Hg are frequently seen in normal young subjects during maximal work. The pulse pressure is exaggerated in the periphery, i.e., systolic pressure is higher and diastolic pressure is lower in the brachial artery than in the proximal aorta. The increase in *mean arterial blood pressure* from sitting rest to maximal exercise is usually less than 20 mm Hg and is of the same magnitude in the aorta and in the periphery.

Cardiovascular control during exercise involves the central nervous system as well as local mechanisms. The onset of exercise (and in many cases the anticipation of effort) causes inhibition of parasympathetic activity or vagal withdrawal, and increased sympathetic drive. These changes in autonomic balance result in an increased heart rate and an increased inotropic state, with increased force and velocity of myocardial fiber shortening. The details of the neural pathways involved in the rapid adaptation to exercise are still controversial. Two mechanisms probably are involved: a central mechanism with direct action of the motor cortex on the cardiovascular center, *cortical radiation; and reflex mechanisms* involving receptors in the exercising muscles. It is likely that the muscle receptors (which do not include the muscle spindles) are activated by local metabolites, perhaps the increased potassium concentration caused by muscle activity. A combination of vasoconstrictor and vasodilator stimuli causes redistribution of blood flow from inactive to active tissues. Sympathetic vasoconstrictor fibers act on the vessels of the splanchnic organs and the skin. There is also general venoconstriction. There probably are no specific vasodilator fibers in skeletal muscle. Rather, reflex sympathetic vasoconstriction is rapidly overcome by local autoregulatory vasodilation, probably mediated by the decreased oxygen tension and increased potassium concentration associated with muscle activity. Circulating catecholamines contribute to some extent to the adaptation to exercise. Patients with transplanted hearts are able to respond to exercise, but both the heart rate increase at onset and the return to resting level post exercise are delayed.

Typical maximal data for a normal young sedentary subject, a champion long-distance runner, and a patient with moderately severe left ventricular dysfunction following myocardial infarction (limited by cardiac output and not by angina pectoris) are shown in Table 5. Differences with respect to maximal heart rate and A-V O_2 differences are small. *Stroke volume* is the main determinant of maximal cardiac output and maximal oxygen uptake. Heart rates and A-V O_2 differences tend to be similar also at submaximal levels if the load is

Table 5. Typical Maximal Data in a Patient With Moderately Severe Coronary Heart Disease (Left Ventricular Dysfunction but No Angina Pectoris), a Normal Sedentary Subject, and a Long-Distance Runner

	Oxygen Uptake (liters/min)	Heart Rate (beats/min)	Stroke Volume (ml)	Cardiac Output (liters/min)	Total A-V O_2 Difference (ml/dl)
Patient	1.5	175	50	8.8	17.0
Sedentary normal man	3.0	190	100	19.0	15.8
Runner	5.6	180	180	32.5	17.0

measured as relative load, i.e., when the actual oxygen uptake is expressed as percentage of maximal oxygen uptake rather than as absolute units. The basic similarity in the approach to maximal levels in normal subjects and patients with heart disease (excluding limitations due to regional circulation, e.g., angina) has been well documented. The respiratory and metabolic responses to exercise, except for moderate hyperventilation at low work loads in cardiac patients, are also similar when related to relative levels rather than absolute levels. The principal features of the response to progressive levels of exercise as they appear in a normal young subject are shown in Fig. 1.

Patients with myocardial or valvular disease have, as a group, low cardiac output at rest and subnormal increases in output for any given increase in oxygen uptake. The degree of abnormality correlates with the clinical severity of the disease, but individual patients frequently show values within the normal range both at rest and during mild exercise. Maximal or near-maximal exercise often uncovers cardiac output restrictions that are not apparent at rest or at low work-load levels.

The stroke volume response to exercise is often inappropriate in patients with heart disease. The increase in stroke volume on transition from sitting rest to upright exercise may be smaller than normal. The stroke volume often decreases rather than increases when the patient progresses from light to heavy exercise.

There is a highly efficient distribution of blood flow in patients with restricted cardiac output. The total A-V O_2 difference and total systemic resistance tend to be high, indicating tight control of the peripheral circulation. Nevertheless, patients with inability to maintain stroke volume during exercise, particularly patients with severe mitral stenosis or markedly impaired myocardial function, frequently develop exertional hypotension. Hypotension is unusual in patients with valvular regurgitation unless associated with myocardial dysfunction. Exertional hypotension in aortic stenosis may be related to activation of left ventricular baroreceptors and inhibition or reversal of the usual vasoconstrictor responses in inactive tissue.

Heart rate and A-V O_2 difference at any given submaximal oxygen uptake vary inversely with maximal oxygen uptake. During a bicycle ride or treadmill walk requiring an oxygen uptake of 1.0 liter/min, the athlete (Fig. 3) is likely to have a heart rate of 70 beats/min and an A-V O_2 difference of 7 ml/dl blood.

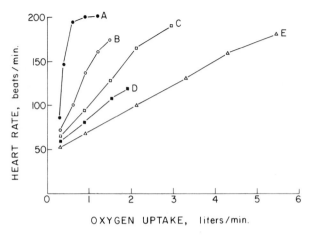

Figure 3. Heart rates at rest and during submaximal and maximal exercise. A: Patient with severe mitral stenosis and atrial fibrillation. B: Patient with a healed myocardial infarction, moderately severe left ventricular dysfunction. C: Normal sedentary subject. D: Patient with cardiomegaly and severe left ventricular dysfunction. E: Champion long-distance runner.

Corresponding figures for the normal sedentary subject are 110 beats/min and 12 ml/dl blood. Figure 3 also illustrates typical heart rates during exercise at several submaximal work loads and maximal work load in a patient with severe mitral stenosis and atrial fibrillation, a patient with sinus rhythm and a healed myocardial infarction, and a patient with severe left ventricular dysfunction. Maximal oxygen uptakes varied from 1.2 to 5.5 liters/min, and heart rates during exercise at a work load requiring an oxygen uptake of 1 liter/min ranged from 70 to 195 beats/min.

The heart rate/work load relationship approaches linearity in normal subjects. Maximal oxygen uptake can be predicted with fair accuracy from a single paired observation of heart rate and oxygen uptake at a submaximal load. The slope of the heart rate/oxygen uptake regression is highly correlated to the heart rate at the test load. The oxygen uptake intercept at the appropriate average normal age-specific maximum heart rate is taken as an estimate of maximal oxygen uptake. It follows that in normal subjects the heart rate during exercise provides an index of relative load, i.e., the heart rate may be used to estimate work load as a fraction or percentage of individual maximal load. A work load of 25% of the subject's maximal capacity usually produces a heart rate equal to 50% of maximal, i.e., 90 beats/min if the maximal heart rate is 180 beats/min. Corresponding heart rates for work loads of 50% and 75% are about 65% and 85% of maximal heart rate, or 120 and 155 beats/min.

Patients with heart disease have a less predictable relationship between work load or oxygen uptake and heart rate. Atrial fibrillation is particularly likely to cause a nonlinear heart rate/work load relationship and a high maximal heart rate, sometimes well above 200 beats/min. A disproportionately large increase in heart rate at submaximal loads and an ability to tolerate increasing work loads after a maximal heart rate has been reached often are seen in patients with atrial fibrillation who are taking little or no digitalis, but occasionally this is also observed in patients who otherwise appear to be adequately digitalized. Conversion to sinus rhythm results in increased stroke volume and cardiac output, lower heart rate, and increased physical work capacity. For reasons not yet understood, sinus rhythm in patients with severe myocardial dysfunction and cardiomegaly is often associated with an attenuated heart rate response to exercise and a markedly reduced maximal heart rate.

Angina pectoris presents a special case. The heart rate response to work-load levels below the threshold of myocardial ischemia is usually normal and linear, but it is impossible to predict the heart rate/work level at which angina and ischemic electrocardiographic abnormalities will appear. The range of variation with respect to the heart rate increase that is required to precipitate angina is extremely wide. Some patients who are asymptomatic at rest may regularly get angina at a heart rate of 85–90 beats/min, and others may not experience angina until a heart rate of 170 beats/min is reached.

Coronary Circulation

The principal determinants of myocardial oxygen demand are *ventricular wall tension, heart rate,* and *contractility.* The product of wall tension and heart rate is often referred to as *internal work.* Wall tension is proportional to the product of ventricular pressure and volume. *External work,* the product of load and fiber shortening, is measured clinically as stroke work or the product of stroke volume and mean aortic or left ventricular systolic pressure. Changes in stroke volume have little effect on myocardial oxygen demand. Mean systolic pressure is closely related to wall tension. This means that the external work of the left ventricle can largely be disregarded as a determinant of myocardial oxygen demand when internal work is taken into account.

Contractile state or the velocity of fiber shortening is an important factor, but its contribution is difficult to evaluate in the intact subject. An increase in contractility is often associated with a decrease in ventricular volume that minimizes the expected increase in myocardial oxygen demand.

Exercise markedly affects all major determinants of myocardial oxygen demand. The relationships between exercise and heart rate and exercise and blood pressure have been discussed in detail. Changes in left ventricular volume do occur during exercise in normal subjects, but they probably are of relatively small magnitude. End-systolic volume tends to decrease during exercise, reflecting an increase in contractile state. End-diastolic volume is usually smaller during mild upright exercise than at rest in the supine position, but it increases above resting control levels during maximal exercise. More significant volume changes may well occur during exercise in patients with heart disease, but there is little solid information on human left ventricular volumes during upright exercise.

The increased *peripheral oxygen demand* during exercise is met by increased skeletal muscle blood flow and increased extraction of oxygen. The myocardium extracts a much larger fraction of the available oxygen at rest, i.e., about two-thirds, as compared to one-fourth in the systemic circulation. This means that an increased *myocardial oxygen demand* mainly has to be met by an increase in coronary blood flow. In the normal heart, coronary blood flow closely parallels the in-

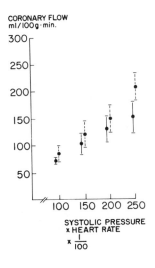

CORONARY FLOW
ml/l00g·min.

Figure 4. Relationship between coronary flow and the product of systolic pressure and heart rate. Mean values and standard deviations for control subjects (dotted bars) and patients with coronary disease (solid bars). [Data from Holmberg et al. (8).]

creased myocardial oxygen demand during exercise. Coronary vascular resistance, which in the normal heart is mainly at the arteriolar level, decreases markedly. Flow rates at rest are about 60 ml/100 g of left ventricular myocardium per minute. Values exceeding 300 ml/100 g/min have been reported in normal young subjects during heavy upright exercise. Coronary artery disease is associated with significant vascular resistance to flow, at the arterial level as well as at the arteriolar level. Flow rates at rest usually are not affected by large-vessel disease until the obstruction approaches 50% of the vessel diameter (corresponding to a 75% reduction of cross-sectional area), i.e., the conventional arteriographic limit for significant obstruction. However, the increased flow rates and decreased arteriolar resistance during exercise are likely to unmask significant obstruction to flow in less severe coronary arterial disease.

Coronary blood flows at different levels of exercise in a normal subject are shown in Figure 1. Figure 4 compares the relationships between myocardial oxygen demand and coronary blood flow in normal subjects and in patients with significant coronary disease. Total coronary blood flow is usually normal in patients at rest even if regional underperfusion is present. Exercise clearly demonstrates a restricted coronary blood flow. Myocardial oxygen uptake in the normal heart (which is an excellent estimate of myocardial oxygen demand, since the myocardium is virtually unable to utilize anaerobic metabolic pathways) and coronary blood flow are closely correlated to the product of heart rate and systolic blood pressure. The *rate-pressure product* provides a measure of internal myocardial work but ignores the effects of changes in contractile state and ventricular volume. Nevertheless, the validity of the rate-pressure product has been well established by direct measurements of coronary blood flow and myocardial oxygen uptake in normal subjects under a variety of experimental conditions, and also by empirical studies in patients with angina pectoris. Patients with typical effort angina have a well-defined threshold of myocardial ischemia, as measured by the rate-pressure product. Only interventions with marked effects on contractility and ventricular volume, e.g., treatment with β-adrenergic blocking agents, invalidate the rate-pressure product. Work capacity is increased, but the apparent threshold of ischemia (i.e., the rate-pressure product at the onset of ST abnormalities and angina) is lowered, by propranolol. This is most likely due to unaccounted-for increases in left ventricular volume and wall tension at any given systolic blood pressure.

The rate-pressure product is easily measured, and with the limitations noted, it provides an excellent index of myocardial oxygen demand.

RELATIONSHIP BETWEEN STANDARDIZED AND NONSTANDARDIZED EXERCISE

Most of our current concepts of cardiovascular function during exercise are based on laboratory studies performed during treadmill or bicycle exercise of relatively short duration. Several factors, including *prolonged duration of work, environmental temperature,* and *emotional factors,* modify the basic relationship between oxygen uptake and circulatory response that is evident during standardized exercise. Submaximal heart rates are often higher during nonstandardized work than during standardized work for identical levels of oxygen uptake, particularly during work involving small muscle groups. Blood pressure tends to vary inversely with environmental temperature.

Dynamic work (walking, running) causes only a moderate increase in arterial pressure, but the blood pressure in a normotensive subject may increase markedly during heavy *isometric exercise.* A sustained handgrip contraction at half-maximal strength, which is the equivalent of an adult man carrying a 40–50-lb load, often produces an increase from 120/75 to 220/130 mm Hg. *Arm work* frequently represents a mixture of dynamic and isometric effort, and systolic and diastolic blood pressures are significantly higher during arm work than during leg work at any given level of oxygen uptake. Heavy isometric exercise is more likely to precipitate ventricular dysrhythmias than is heavy dynamic exercise.

Occupational work tends to be intermittent in nature. Periods of strenuous activity, if present, tend to be of short duration. Cardiac output and oxygen uptake do not reach a steady state until about 2 min after the beginning of work at a submaximal rate, and the blood pressure response is also gradual. Myocardial work is lower than during a steady-state effort. Therefore persons with low physical work capacity and low maximal oxygen uptake can often tolerate surprisingly high work loads provided that the peaks are of short duration and adequate rest periods are interspersed. Untrained persons can ordinarily sustain continuous work at levels corresponding to 50% of capacity for no longer than 1 hr. Studies were made of workers in occupations demanding heavy labor who were motivated by a piecework pay system but who were free to regulate their pace within reasonable limits. They tended to select an average work intensity during actual working hours corresponding to 40% of maximal capacity. For a full 8-hr period, including customary rest periods, an average level of 30% of capacity is considered a reasonable upper limit for safe employment.

Frequently, peak loads of short duration that contribute little to the average level of energy expenditure will rule out a given job for patients with angina pectoris or exercise-induced arrhythmias who would have no difficulties at a work-load level equal to the 8-hr average for the job. Thus, both peak loads and average loads must be taken into consideration when evaluating a patient's capacity to meet job requirements.

REFERENCES

General Exercise Physiology

1. Åstrand PO, Rodahl K: *Textbook of Work Physiology.* McGraw-Hill, New York, 1977

Skeletal Muscle Physiology

2. Gollnick PD, Hermansen L: Biochemical adaptations to exercise: Anaerobic metabolism. In Wilmore JH (ed): *Exercise and Sport Sciences Reviews, Vol. 1.* Academic Press, New York, 1973, p. 1
3. Holloszy JO: Biochemical adaptations to exercise: Aerobic metabolism. In Wilmore JH (ed): *Exercise and Sport Sciences Reviews, Vol 1.* Academic Press, New York, 1973, p 45

Maximal Oxygen Uptake and Circulatory Response to Exercise

4. Saltin B, Blomqvist G, Mitchell JH, et al: Response to exercise after bed rest and training. *Circulation* 37–38 (Suppl 7):1, 1968
5. Mitchell JH, Blomqvist G: Maximal oxygen uptake. *N Engl J Med* 284:1018, 1971
6. Rowell LB: Human cardiovascular adjustments to exercise and thermal stress. *Physiol Rev* 54:75, 1974

Myocardial Oxygen Demand and Coronary Blood Flow

7. Nelson RR, Gobel FL, Jorgensen CR, et al: Hemodynamic predictors of myocardial oxygen consumption during static and dynamic exercise. *Circulation* 50:1179, 1974
8. Holmberg S, Serzysko W, Varnauskas E: Coronary circulation during heavy exercise in control subjects and patients with coronary heart disease. *Acta Med Scand* 190:465, 1971

Test Procedures

9. AHA Committee on Exercise (Chairman AA Kattus): Exercise Testing and Training of Apparently Healthy Individuals. American Heart Association, New York, 1972, p 1

8
Exercise Testing and Prescription

Herman K. Hellerstein, M.D.

Barry A. Franklin, Ph.D.

Physical fitness tests are useful in many areas of medical practice and research. They extend the clinical significance of information obtained from other sources (detailed history, thorough physical examination, resting electrocardiogram, chest x-ray, and other basic laboratory analyses). They are commonly used to diagnose relative myocardial ischemia and ischemic heart disease and to investigate physiologic mechanisms of cardiac symptoms.

Our studies of a large number of subjects in a variety of occupations have indicated that cardiovascular responses to the stresses of exercise in the controlled environment of a testing laboratory differ from those in the world of work (1,2). These marked differences challenge the usefulness of exercise tests in formulating work prescriptions, unless certain modifications are introduced. The physical stresses of occupational energy expenditure usually are low, involving submaximal muscular effort of brief duration, rarely sustained at high levels for more than 2–3 min, i.e., intermittent and not continuous. In addition, there are rest periods for 30–45% or more of the total working shift (1,2). Persons at work perform muscular effort while fully clad, often after ingestion of meals, coffee, tobacco, and prescribed medications. Major muscle groups in the upper extremities, rather than in the lower extremities, are called on extensively. The physical and emotional environments are rarely as well controlled as in the exercise laboratory. Factors other than aerobic expenditure (e.g., extremes of temperature; noises; dusts; mental, intellectual, emotional, and cognitive demands; interpersonal relationships; deadlines; supervision; monetary and other societal pressures) constitute the major occupational stresses in most societies. Contemporary exercise tests rarely simulate real life situations. The aerobic

Supported in part by grants from the U.S. Department of Health, Education, and Welfare, Office of Human Development Services, Rehabilitation Services Administration, grant 13-P 55917, and grants from Mr. Leo Demsey, Mr. and Mrs. Francis M. Fine, Mr. and Mrs. Marvin Itts, Mr. and Mrs. William Lipman, Mr. and Mrs. Harry Mann, and Mr. Maurice Saltzman.

stresses of exercise tests exceed those of most occupations and fail to account for most of the important determinants of successful performance of work. However, standard test conditions (adequate sleep, fasting, privacy, controlled temperature, graded submaximal or maximal effort of the lower extremities in the presence of considerate and trained supervising personnel and nearby safety provisions) have many advantages, especially in regard to reproducibility and quantitative assessment of cardiovascular function.

The objective of exercise tests is to evaluate quantitatively and accurately the following functions:

- chronotropic capacity
- aerobic capacity of the body ($\dot{V}O_2$), i.e., oxygen uptake and central and peripheral utilization
- myocardial aerobic capacity ($M\dot{V}O_2$)
- associated changes in electrical functions of the heart

The last includes impulse initiation, ectopic activity, atrioventricular and intraventricular conduction, and ventricular repolarization (ST-T changes). Responses to exercise tests are useful in the evaluation of various types of therapy. From the viewpoint of a W.H.O. Expert Committee on Rehabilitation, "the primary purpose of an exercise test is to determine the responses of the individual to efforts at given levels and from this information to estimate probable performance in specific life and occupational situations"(3). Exercise tests, although not predictive of circulatory responses in the world of work at equal energy levels, provide reasonable information about $M\dot{V}O_2$ and tolerance to increases in heart rate and blood pressure at work. However, some work situations may impose demands greater than those produced by peak effort in exercise laboratories.

In the following discussion we shall review several types of tests, their utilization, and also provide suggestions for their modification in order to enhance their value in the counseling of normal and cardiac subjects in regard to vocational, recreational, and physical training activities.

The approach to exercise testing should be integrative of the many mechanisms that come into play during exercise. The ability to exercise at high levels of effort efficiently depends not only on the integrity of these mechanisms but also on their integration (4). As was discussed in Chapter 7, the determinants of performance include the following: aerobic capacity, i.e., oxygen intake (ventilation, diffusion); transport by adequate cardiac output; oxygen utilization by peripheral skeletal musculature and organs; central nervous system function; hemoglobin (mass and type); and electrical function of the heart. Indeed, exercise tolerance may be limited by malfunction of one mechanism, thus precluding the attainment of peak or maximal performance even though the other mechanisms are functioning well. Increasing the intensity of effort may stress the adaptation of the various mechanisms to the limit; for example, serious multiform ventricular arrhythmias may preclude the attainment of a true peak or maximal aerobic performance. For this reason, as many as possible of these mechanisms should be evaluated at each of several loads of increasing intensity (4).

TEST PROCEDURES

Indications and Contraindications to Performance of Exercise Tests (Table 1)

The evaluation of function is a continuing process throughout all stages of an illness, from the acute stages to return to normal living. Traditionally this has been accomplished by questioning the individual regarding tolerance to specific activities in the hospital and later at home and work. More objective information has become available from direct electrocardiographic monitoring in intensive care facilities and later indirectly from portable electromagnetic recorders. Supervised exercise testing has been demonstrated to be safe within the first several weeks of acute myocardial infarction (5).

Supervised exercise testing is indicated in the absence of contraindications whenever it is clinically important to obtain quantitation of cardiovascular func-

Table 1. Indications and Contraindications for Exercise Testing and Participation in Programs Planned to Enhance Physical Fitness

Indications	Contraindications	
	Cardiovascular	Others
Normal subjects, especially highly coronary prone, general deconditioning, neurocirculatory asthenia, before and after surgery*	Severe (80–90%) stenosis of three major coronary arteries	Acute illness
	Rapidly progressing angina	Uncontrolled diabetes mellitus, thyrotoxicosis, other metabolic instability
	Impending infarction	
Arteriosclerotic heart disease*	Recent infarction within first week or two	Severe electrolyte imbalance
Intermittent claudication*	Massive ventricular aneurysm	Morbid obesity
Pulmonary disease*		Deforming arthritis*
	Congestive failure, uncontrolled, manifest	Disabling skeletal muscle disorders
	Arrhythmias: uncontrolled ventricular tachycardia, second- or third-degree A-V block, fixed ventricular rate pacemaker, untreated atrial fibrillation, ventricular premature beats at rest that increase with exercise	Psychosis
Caution: drugs: reserpine, propranolol, guanethidine, ganglionic blockers, procaine amide, quinidine, digitalis		Recent pulmonary embolism
		Severe pulmonary hypertension
		Severe varicose veins with thrombophlebitis, phlebothrombosis
		Severe anemia
	Valvular disease: uncompensated moderate to severe aortic valvular or subvalvular outflow obstruction	Central nervous system disease,* recent transient cerebral ischemia
		Acute infectious diseases
	Uncontrolled hypertension	Dissecting aortic aneurysm
	Acute myocarditis	Acute febrile illness

*Selected cases.

tions, from the earliest stages of illness (after the first or second week of acute myocardial infarction) to later in convalescence and recovery.

Indications for Halting an Exercise Test in Progress

Commonly used criteria for discontinuing an exercise test consist of attaining a predetermined end point of submaximal performance or evidence of peak or maximal performance or emergence of evidence of a disease process or potential hazard.

Arbitrary End Points

Submaximal end points include attainment of arbitrarily designated values: 85% of age-predicted maximal heart rate, external work load that raises heart rate to 150–170 beats/min, respiratory exchange ratio (R.Q.) above unity, blood pressure above 220–240 mm Hg, etc.

Clinical Signs

Clinical signs include marked dyspnea, pallor, cold sweat, central nervous system dysfunction, ataxia, staggering, confusion in responding to questions, head-nodding. *Physical signs* include failure of blood pressure to rise with increasing work loads, hypotension, excessive increase of systolic blood pressure, and electrocardiographic signs: ventricular arrhythmias, frequent multiform ventricular premature beats, recurring couplets, salvos or paroxysms or sustained supraventricular or ventricular tachycardias, bundle branch block, second- or third-degree atrioventricular (A-V) block, ST-T displacement of more than 3–4 mm (0.3–0.4 mV).

Symptoms

Symptoms include increasing chest or leg pain or other pain or discomfort (with or without electrocardiographic changes), lightheadedness, dizziness, or indications that the subject can continue no longer.

Peak performances in such tests are improperly classified as maximal. A physiologic maximal test is defined as a test in which the subject is unable to increase oxygen intake with further effort. These tests are more appropriately designated *symptom-limited tests* (by chest or leg pain, excessive dyspnea, intolerable fatigue) or *"signomatic" tests* (multiform ventricular ectopic rhythms, impairment of intraventricular conduction, hemiblock, complete bundle branch block, marked ST-T displacement, syncope, staggering, incoordination). The external work that produces such responses is more properly designated peak performance or peak work load.

CLASSIFICATION OF EXERCISE TESTS

Exercise tests may be classified in regard to the equipment used, magnitude (maximal or submaximal), duration, number of stages, end points, muscle

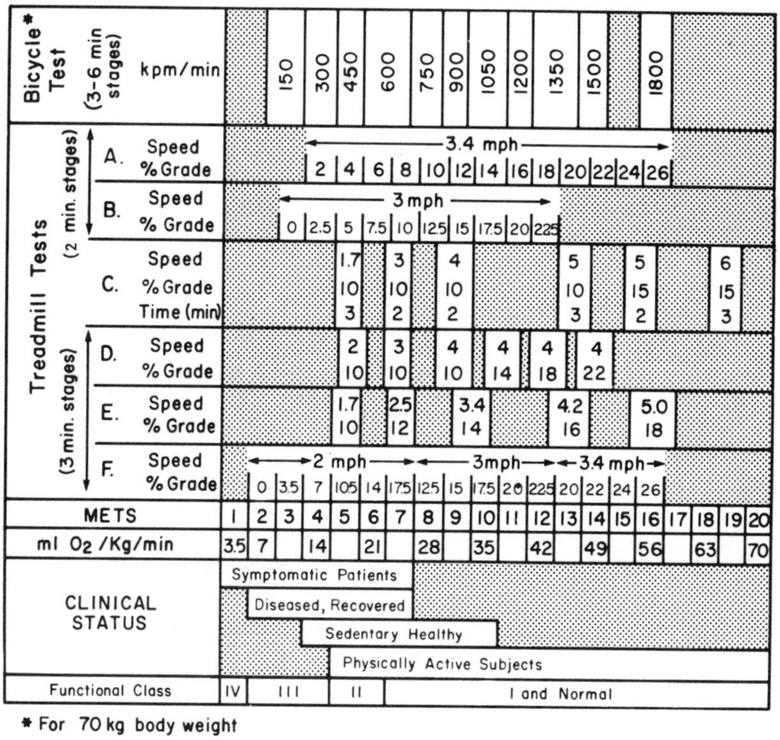

Bicycle* Test (3–6 min stages) kpm/min	150	300	450	600	750	900	1050	1200	1350	1500	1800

Treadmill Tests (2 min stages)

A. Speed 3.4 mph; % Grade: 2 4 6 8 10 12 14 16 18 20 22 24 26

B. Speed 3 mph; % Grade: 0 2.5 5 7.5 10 12.5 15 17.5 20 22.5

C. Speed / % Grade / Time (min):
- 1.7 / 10 / 3
- 3 / 10 / 2
- 4 / 10 / 2
- 5 / 10 / 3
- 5 / 15 / 2
- 6 / 15 / 3

Treadmill Tests (3 min stages)

D. Speed / % Grade: 2 / 10, 3 / 10, 4 / 10, 4 / 14, 4 / 18, 4 / 22

E. Speed / % Grade: 1.7 / 10, 2.5 / 12, 3.4 / 14, 4.2 / 16, 5.0 / 18

F. Speed / % Grade: ←2 mph→ ←3 mph→ ←3.4 mph→ 0 3.5 7 10.5 14 17.5 12.5 15 17.5 20 22.5 20 22 24 26

METS	1	2	3	4	5	6	7	8	9	10	11	12	13	14	15	16	17	18	19	20
ml O_2/Kg/min	3.5	7		14		21		28		35		42		49		56		63		70

CLINICAL STATUS:
- Symptomatic Patients
- Diseased, Recovered
- Sedentary Healthy
- Physically Active Subjects

Functional Class	IV	III	II	I and Normal

* For 70 kg body weight

Figure 1. Estimated oxygen and met requirements of commonly used treadmill and bicycle ergometer exercise protocols. Methods: A & B, Balke (6); C, Ellestad (7); D, Kattus (6); E, Bruce (9); F, National Exercise and Heart Disease Project (70).

groups involved, position of the body, and types of effort (dynamic, static, isotonic, or isometric).

Standardized exercise tests have the advantages of reproducibility and quantitation of physiologic responses to external work loads of accurately known demands or power. Detailed descriptions of currently popular tests that employ steps, treadmill, or bicycle ergometer are readily available (6–9) and therefore will not be described in detail here. Figure 1 shows several commonly used exercise protocols.

Realistic Performance Tests of Cardiovascular Function

Our on-the-job studies have revealed shortcomings in the design and application of the results of standardized exercise tests originally intended for diagnosis of myocardial ischemia. Exercise tests should be realistic. The objective of the test and the type of subjects being evaluated should determine its design. The exercise mode should be chosen to evaluate the performances of muscle groups and skills used in past, current, or projected activities. Tables 2A and 2B summarize the equipment and purposes of various types of tests. Such a listing constitutes a virtual pharmacopoeia of exercise tests. Realistic performance tests should also take into consideration the type and duration of skeletal muscle

Table 2A. Indications for Various Types of Exercise Tests

Type of Test	Equipment	Objectives, Evaluations, and Applications
Rhythmic, isotonic Lower extremities	Bicycle, steps, treadmill	To determine submaximal, maximal, peak aerobic capacity, max $\dot{V}O_2$ legs Occupations: mail carrier, police officer, supervisors, field workers Recreation and training: walking, jogging, running, climbing, soccer, golf
Upper extremities	Arm cycle ergometer, wall pulley, wheel arm crank	To determine submaximal, maximal, peak aerobic capacity, max $\dot{V}O_2$ of upper extremities Occupations: sawing, manufacture, machine operation, typing, pianist, dentist, surgeon, music conductor Recreation and training: swimming, canoeing, games, volleyball, pool, billiards
Upper and lower extremities	See above	Performance of activities involving entire body Occupations: manual labor, ditch digging, shovelling, gardening, ladder climbing Recreation and training: basketball, handball, mountain climbing, cross-country skiing, tennis, football, fencing, squash, paddleball, horseback riding, dancing
Isometric Hand grip	Hand dynamometer, sphygmomanometer, weights, handbag filled with weights	Cardiovascular responses to isometric activities (heart rate, blood pressure, electrocardiogram) Occupations: hand and arm effort: saws, levers, portage, jackhammer operator; controls operator in steel mill or factory, firefighter, control of fire hose Recreation and training: weight lifting, water skiing
Orthostatic Postural	Changes from supine and upright postures	Change in heart rate, blood pressure, and electrocardiogram with postural changes Occupations: mechanics, plumbers Training: floor exercises
Hyperventilation	Sphygmomanometer, electrocardiograph	To distinguish effects of increased minute ventilation due to muscular effort, respiratory effort per se, or hypocapnia

154

Table 2A. (Continued)

Type of Test	Equipment	Objectives, Evaluations, and Applications
Valsalva maneuver (Flack test)	Mouthpiece attached to sphygmomanometer	Cardiovascular responses to increased intrathoracic pressure may reveal syncope in patients with chronic lung disease, or in cardiac patients with hypersensitive carotid sinus reflex Closed-glottis activities: in occupations requiring sustained or near-isometric activity: use of wrenches, levers, wind instruments Recreation and training: push-ups, leg raising, body-contact sports: wrestling, football

Table 2B. Modes of Testing

Continuous	Maximum or peak testing of physically active normal young subjects and a few older subjects, especially in epidemiology surveys Rarely simulates on-the-job performance
Intermittent	Testing of physically inactive younger and older normal subjects, known cardiac patients Similar pattern of effort occurs during work
Medications	To compare performances with and without medication, as in prescribing recreational or training target levels, and where it is inadvisable to discontinue or interrupt therapy
Clothing (worn in occupation or recreation)	To study effects of apparel and impairment of heat exchange Occupation: firefighter, steel mill work Recreation: underwater diving, surfing, etc.

contraction used to stress the cardiovascular system and its applicability to the anticipated vocational, recreational, or training activities of the individual. In addition to the standardized isotonic, so-called steady-state, exercise of the lower extremities, non-steady-state exercise, isometric exercise, hyperventilation, Valsalva maneuver (Flack test), and carotid sinus reflex evaluation are frequently indicated. For example, a subject with a hypersensitive carotid sinus reflex may be able to perform dynamic isotonic exercises such as walking, jogging, or using an arm cycle ergometer, but the subject would be more appropriately evaluated by static isometric contractions, as in handgrip, weight lifting, or carrying, either alone or in combination with isotonic effort.

Regardless of the instrumentation and protocols used, certain principles have been developed that merit wide acceptance and repetition. A good clinical test of function should be safe and simple, should require no special training or undue motivation, and should have realistic energy requirements comparable to those of contemplated activities. An exercise tolerance test should not be performed sooner than 2 hr after a light meal, unless the additive effects of food are being evaluated. The same proscription applies to alcohol, tea, coffee, cola drinks, etc.

The minimal parameters that should be monitored include blood pressure (cuff method), heart rate, and multiple-lead electrocardiograms at rest; these should be monitored during each work load and during recovery. Other valuable parameters that are not yet widely available include ventricular systolic intervals (heart sounds, carotid pulse, and electrocardiogram) to estimate ejection fraction; cardiac output (CO_2 rebreathing, nitrous oxide, or impedance method); and myocardial contractility (echocardiogram, isotopes, etc.).

Informed consent should be obtained prior to the test. Safety precautions, trained personnel, and emergency equipment should be in the immediate vicinity (see Chapter 9). Following performance of the test, the subject should not leave the premises until heart rate, blood pressure, and electrocardiographic parameters have returned to a range based on pretest levels.

RHYTHMIC ISOTONIC EXERCISE TESTS

Intensity and Duration of Tests

If the purpose of a test is to determine the maximal power output ($\dot{V}O_2$ max of arms or legs), it will be necessary for the power output to be constant long enough for most of the variables to reach a relatively constant or steady-state value. In general, this occurs within the first 3–4 min after an increase in external work load. However, a longer period (5–6 min) of exercise at a constant work rate is required in order to maintain a steady state long enough for more elaborate measurements (e.g., cardiac output and gaseous changes) to be valid (4). From the clinical standpoint, a 3-min stage at each work level usually is adequate, except for individuals whose occupations require longer periods of sustained effort.

Non-Steady-State Tests

If the purpose of a test is to determine the response of the individual to *non-steady-state exercise* (Fig. 1, A–C), the design should be different. The duration of the test effort should be short, perhaps 30–60 sec, and the intensity should be considerably greater than in steady-state protocols for individuals who work in sudden spurts of energy and are required to respond at high submaximal or maximal intensity. Non-steady-state exercise tests are useful in evaluating sprint runners and persons whose occupations require a similar but less intense effort, as in the case of a police officer in pursuit of a lawbreaker, or a rescue-squad worker ascending several flights of stairs in a burning building. The energy sources for sustained effort are released mainly through oxidative mechanisms; thus they differ from those for brief high-intensity activities, which act mainly through glycolytic mechanisms (10). The circulatory responses of the same individual to high levels of energy expenditure with and without preceding warm-up will vary considerably. For example, normal subjects exercising maximally for 30 sec without warm-up developed electrocardiographic signs of ventricular ischemia, but they did not do so when exercise was preceded by 2 min of jogging-in-place warm-up. This implies that different adaptive mechanisms were called on (11).

Multistage Steady-State Exercise Test Protocols

In multistage steady-state tests each stage lasts approximately 3–6 min, and the stages are progressively increased in intensity (Fig. 1, D–F, bicycle). Measuring energy expenditures of tests makes it possible to compare populations evaluated by various tests. The major differences among protocols involve the magnitudes of the increments in energy requirements for each stage and the methods by which they are produced. The latter include change in speed or grade or both in treadmill testing and change of external load with constant pedaling speed or constant load with change of pedaling speed or both in mechanical-resistance bicycle ergometer testing.

Comparable values of $\dot{V}O_2$ max can be obtained by several protocols (12), e.g., several stages with a few large increments of brief duration or many smaller increments of longer duration. Some protocols are unacceptable to many subjects (with the exception of athletes) because they are unaccustomed to the large increments of sustained effort required at each stage, as well as lactic acidosis, muscle cramps, etc. Obviously, acceptance by patients should influence the choice of protocol. In addition, the test protocol should be related to the requirements of the activities under consideration, as was mentioned earlier. Few occupations and training techniques require sudden large increments of effort. Another disadvantage of protocols with large increments is the difficulty of obtaining high-quality electrocardiographic tracings and blood pressure measurements during effort. The obvious disadvantage of smaller increments is the greater time required to reach an end point.

The type of equipment used in multistage steady-state exercise of the *lower extremities* is not critical, particularly in evaluation of middle-aged subjects and those with heart disease. In both groups of subjects the hemodynamic stress of bicycle exercise at any given submaximal oxygen uptake is greater than that of treadmill exercise; although cardiac output is the same, heart rate is approximately 6–10 beats faster, implying a lower stroke volume during bicycle exercise. Although $\dot{V}O_2$ max is approximately 250 ml/min higher with treadmill exercise than with bicycle ergometer exercise, this difference is not significant clinically. If provisions are taken to avoid isometric hand grip on the handlebars during measurement of blood pressure, erroneously high systolic blood pressure readings will be avoided. The peak systolic blood pressure responses of subjects on bicycle ergometer exercise testing and on treadmill exercise testing are comparable, generally reaching 196–200 mm Hg regardless of the method of testing (13).

ARM ERGOMETER EXERCISE

Exercise testing and training of both upper and lower extremities is a concept that merits considerably more attention in cardiac rehabilitation and in clinical evaluation of myocardial ischemia. Many patients with angina pectoris experience chest pain at relatively low work loads during upper-extremity activities but are asymptomatic during leg exercise. This disparity is particularly important for subjects who rely mainly on their upper extremities occupationally, as in machine operation and control in industry. Since cardiac rehabilitation is concerned with the total individual, and since training is muscle-specific, exercise that involves upper and lower extremities is indicated for both testing and training. If the patient is to be prepared for greater leisure activity and for greater occupational physical performance, all muscle groups should be stressed. In our studies of occupations we found that the upper extremities usually are involved to a greater extent than the lower extremities (1,2).

Method of Arm Ergometer Exercise Test. The following protocol has been used in our laboratory for the past 4 years. The same safety precautions and measurements are employed as in leg testing. We use a mechanical bicycle ergometer (EX 1 Schwinn Ergometer Bicycle for Legs) that is slightly modified for the use of arms (14). Other investigators have found that the Monark bicycle ergometer works just as well. The arm ergometer is mounted on a table at a height of 68–70 cm. Arm extension is standardized by seating the subject and adjusting a specially constructed breastplate support so that the forearms are fully extended at right angles to the body at maximal reach. Full extension of the forearms is analogous to adjustment of a bicycle seat so that when bicycling is done in an upright position the leg is fully extended when the pedal is down. For the arm ergometer, a constant speed of 60 rpm is maintained throughout the test. Although, unlike the Monark ergometer, the Schwinn ergometer is designed to be rate-independent, the heart rate can fluctuate considerably according to pedal revolution speed, even though physical work and $\dot{V}O_2$ remain constant. This may be attributed to increased proprioceptor stimuli with increased joint motion. The patient is seated in such a manner that the midpoint of the sprocket is shoulder-high for each individual. The testing protocol consists of intermittent progressive multistage exercise. Each exercise stage is 4 min long, with 2 min of rest in between. Tests are performed in an air-conditioned laboratory at least 2 hr after a light meal. Subjects are instructed to minimize their activity prior to testing. An initial test is recommended as a pretrial for the purposes of test familiarization and reducing anxiety on subsequent visits. Warmup consists of 3 min of arm pedaling at zero work load. The work load is then increased by 150 kpm/min at each level until 1200 kpm/min is attained. (Kpm = kilopond-meter, the work done when a mass of one kilogram is lifted one meter against the force of gravity.) For the rare subject who reaches this level, the work load is thereafter increased by 300 kpm/min at each stage.

Maximal or peak effort is defined as that level at which the subject is no longer able to maintain the correct pedal speed, notwithstanding encouragement. The electrocardiogram is monitored continuously, and six precordial V leads and AVF, or scalar X, Y, and Z leads, are recorded at 1-min intervals. Arm blood pressure (cuff method) is measured immediately following the last minute of exercise at each work load and also in the second minute of the rest period between work loads.

Observations. Studies comparing circulatory and metabolic responses to peak efforts of the upper extremities and the lower extremities showed that $\dot{V}O_2$, minute ventilation, heart rate, systolic blood pressure, heart rate $\times$ systolic blood pressure product, lactate production, and respiratory exchange ratio were significantly greater and that the anaerobic threshold expressed as percentage $\dot{V}O_2$ max was lower during arm exercise at the same work load, as well as when compared to the level of maximal arm exercise (14–17). However, regression equations between percentage maximal heart rate and percentage $\dot{V}O_2$ max revealed no differences between arm exercise and leg exercise for the same relative work load. We previously reported almost identical equations for normal persons, cardiac patients, and athletes performing treadmill or leg bicycle ergometer exercise (14):

· percentage $\dot{V}O_2$ max (arms) = 1.2 (% maximal heart rate) $- 29.3$
· percentage $\dot{V}O_2$ max (legs) = 1.3 (% maximal heart rate) $- 36.3$

$\dot{V}O_2$ max with leg exercise was 45–50% higher than that with arm exercise. This indicates that measurement of physical work capacity, as defined by maximal body aerobic capacity, cannot be based on arm work alone. However, considering that the measured volume of the upper extremity is only 30% of that of the lower extremity, it appears that $\dot{V}O_2$ max per volume for arm exercise is twice that of the legs. The significantly greater $\dot{V}O_2$ max with the legs may be attributed to their greater muscle mass, or perhaps leg musculature contains more high-oxygen-extraction tissue than does arm musculature. When considered per milliliter of segment volume of the extremity, $\dot{V}O_2$ is greater in the arms. Explanations of this finding are still speculative. Perhaps more high-oxygen-extraction fibers are present in the arm muscles. The question whether the percentages of fiber types in an individual can vary in different limbs has not been settled. Another possible explanation is that arm ergometer exercise recruits muscle groups of the back, shoulder, and chest that when added to arm musculature greatly increase the muscle mass being used.

Clinical Significance. The results of arm exercise tests have important implications for diagnosis and prescription of therapeutic training. Mechanical efficiency, defined as the ratio between output of external work and caloric expenditure, is lower during arm work, since oxygen uptake at a given external work load is significantly greater for arm work than for leg work. Myocardial efficiency likewise is lower during arm work; viz., the peak arm effort, or heart rate times systolic blood pressure (HR $\times$ SBP product), a measure of $M\dot{V}O_2$, is disproportionately higher than that for leg work at the same effort. The calculated $M\dot{V}O_2/\dot{V}O_2$ ratio for peak leg work is significantly lower than that for peak arm work. Thus myocardial efficiency during arm work is lower than during leg work, not only at submaximal arm work but also at peak arm work, which is submaximal in relation to the legs. Patients with coronary disease are able to perform considerably less external work (35% decrease) before experiencing angina when the exercise is performed with the arms rather than the legs.

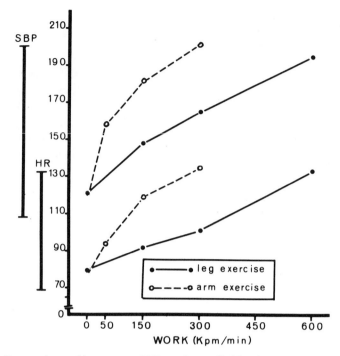

Figure 2. Comparison of heart rate (HR) and systolic blood pressure (SBP) responses at rest and during submaximal arm and leg bicycle ergometer exercise in patients with ischemic heart disease. At each work level the HR and SBP responses were greater during arm exercise. [Adapted from Schwade et al. (18).]

The relatively greater myocardial stress and lower efficiency during arm work may account for the high prevalence of induced ischemic changes in patients with coronary disease. In a recent article Blomqvist and associates (18) reported that 26 of 33 patients showed identical end points for arm and leg exercise tests (Fig. 2). These end points were manifested in fatigue, shortness of breath, chest pain, abnormal electrocardiograms, and insignificant differences in HR × SBP products. They concluded that arm ergometer exercise is a satisfactory alternative diagnostic test with respect to eliciting myocardial ischemia.

The finding that the physiologic cost for a given amount of external work is not necessarily constant is important in prescribing exercise. An exercise prescription based on the bicycle ergometer cannot be assumed to be appropriate when the individual is performing the same amount of work with the arms. An individual who relies principally on arm musculature in daily activity needs to be concerned primarily with training these muscle groups. In such subjects, because of the lack of crossover effects from training the legs, the upper extremities should also be trained. The finding of similar regression equations for arm and leg exercise, in terms of percentage maximal heart rate and percentage $\dot{V}O_2$ max indicates that in regard to maximum rate the exercise prescription can be based on a single regression equation regardless of the muscle groups involved and the condition of the subject.

ISOMETRIC EXERCISE TESTS

An isometric exercise is defined as muscle contraction without major shortening of the muscle fibers during the peak of contraction. The myocardial demands imposed by isometric effort or high-resistance effort may exceed those for low-resistance, isotonic, dynamic exercise. The magnitude of the cardiovascular response to isometric exercise is proportional to the percentage of maximal strength rather than absolute strength of the contracting muscle. In contrast, cardiovascular response to dynamic isotonic exercise is linearly related to the work performed.

Maximal Voluntary Handgrip Contraction

Handgrip exercise can be performed by squeezing the inflated cuff of a sphygmomanometer and sustaining the pressure at some percentage of maximal voluntary hand contraction (e.g., 50%) or by using a handgrip dynamometer. Significant increases in heart rate and systolic and diastolic pressures occur during sustained isometric exercise. Static exercise performed to the limit of fatigue produces a pressure load on the left ventricle, as is reflected by a high HR × SBP product, that is disporportionate to the oxygen uptake of the body during the effort. As was mentioned in Chapter 7, the energy requirements are met by glycolytic mechanisms rather than by oxidative mechanisms. At the same time, the electrocardiogram can show changes in rhythm and ST-T changes that reflect increased myocardial oxygen demand. Subjects who perform isometric exercise in the course of their occupations every day may develop significant ST-T displacement and ventricular arrhythmias, and in cardiac patients with hypersensitive carotid sinus reflexes, marked sinus bradycardia or even standstill may occur. When isometric exercise is combined with dynamic exercise, the effects are additive (19).

Clinical Significance. Realistic testing should include an evaluation of the effects of isometric exercise when appropriate. This applies to individuals involved in occupations with isometric requirements (carrying luggage or other weights, operating a jackhammer, carpentering, etc.) as well as to those involved in physical training and recreational activities (push-ups, weight lifting, downhill skiing, water skiing, etc.). Rather than arbitrarily proscribing such activities, the physician should test the individual's responses to such predominantly isometric activities and give advice about how to minimize adverse responses; for example, a yoke or shoulder strap for carrying weights can be used to avoid the Valsalva maneuver.

Valsalva Maneuver

The Valsalva maneuver is another type of static exercise to measure cardiovascular function. It can elicit marked changes in heart rate and blood pressure and electrocardiographic changes (20,21). Cardiovascular responses to increased intrathoracic pressure and straining with a closed glottis are important in recreation and in occupations requiring sustained or near-isometric activity. This includes the use of wrenches and levers, playing wind instruments, participating in body-contact sports, etc.

Equipment and Method. The equipment required for measurement of the Valsalva maneuver consists of a standard aneroid or mercury manometer attached to a mouthpiece by connecting tubing. A needle placed in the tubing provides a small leak during the expiratory strain, which maintains the glottis open and thereby prevents subjects from maintaining the pressure with either cheek muscles or the tip of the tongue.

Subjects are studied in the semirecumbent or sitting position. They should be instructed in how to maintain an expiratory pressure of 40 mm Hg for 10–15 sec. The pressure should rise sharply at the onset and fall abruptly at the termination of the strain period. Following a training period, each subject should perform two Valsalva maneuvers separated by a rest period of at least 1 min. Before and during each maneuver the heart rate should be recorded continuously by means of an electrocardiograph throughout the strain period and for 15 sec following release of the strain.

Interpretation. In normal subjects the blood pressure rises and the heart rate slows reflexly with the onset of straining (phase 1); the blood pressure falls and the heart rate sympathetically rises during the period of sustained straining (phase 2); with sudden release of straining (phase 3) the blood pressure drops and the heart rate increases; in phase 4 there is an overshoot of blood pressure that induces a marked reflex bradycardia, usually within 5–9 beats. In the presence of advanced heart disease, reduced myocardial reserve, or significant valvular obstruction there is no increase in blood pressure and hence no bradycardia in phase 4. The heart rate changes induced by the Valsalva maneuver can be quantitative and expressed as the Valsalva ratio (the ratio of maximal tachycardia to maximal bradycardia). The Valsalva ratio is calculated as the ratio of maximal R-R interval to minimal R-R interval; intervals associated with premature beats should be excluded. A Valsalva ratio of 1.50 has been suggested as a lower limit of normal. In one study 96% of 200 normal subjects had ratios of 1.50 or higher (21). The ratio is inversely related to left ventricular diastolic-pressure and mean pulmonary wedge pressure (21). The Valsalva ratio is significantly reduced in the presence of pulmonary congestion, obstructive mitral and aortic valvular disease, ischemic heart disease, and cardiomyopathy. The Valsalva maneuver may elicit complex arrhythmias, reflex cardiac standstill, or syncope in patients with a hypersensitive carotid sinus reflex or chronic obstructive lung disease.

Summary. Measurement of the changes in heart rate induced by the Valsalva maneuver provides a rapid, safe, and inexpensive method of evaluating cardiac function and permits the prediction of certain hemodynamic variables (20,21).

HYPERVENTILATION TEST

The subject usually performs the hyperventilation test before undergoing an exercise test. While in the same position in which the multistage exercise test will be performed, the study subject is instructed to breathe rapidly and deeply for 30 sec, but not as vigorously as in a maximal breathing test. Prior to, during, and for 30 sec after the hyperventilation a continuous recording is made of the electrocardiographic leads that will be used in the exercise test.

Interpretation. Normal responses consist of a feeling of lightheadedness, slight hypotension, tachycardia, peaking of the P waves, prolongation of electrical systole, and a lowering of the amplitude of the T waves. Abnormal responses include tightness in the chest, confusion, persistence of the previously cited symptoms and signs for more than 5–10 min, arrhythmias, ST-T displacement, bundle branch block, or variable degrees of A-V block. The electrocardiographic changes produced by hyperventilation are probably due to changes in acid-base balance, hypocapnia, and associated intracellular shifts of potassium rather than to the oxygen cost of the effort of hyperventilation per se. Recent studies of the cost of ventilation have suggested that no more than 250–350 ml of oxygen are expended during 30 sec of hyperventilation (22). This is less than the oxygen demand of the first stage of practically all exercise testing protocols. The electro-cardiographic changes of hyperventilation are taken into consideration in evaluating electrocardiographic responses during peak or maximal effort.

EXERCISE TESTING OF PATIENTS WITH ACUTE MYOCARDIAL INFARCTION DURING HOSPITALIZATION

In the past decade the period of bed rest after acute myocardial infarction has been shortened, ambulation has been instituted earlier, and hospitalization has been reduced from 6 weeks to 3 weeks or less (5,23,24). The pace of resumption of physical activity in the intensive care unit and later in the hospital room can be based on clinical observations of the patient's tolerance to low levels of activities such as dangling the legs, self-care, and ambulation. The guidelines include symptoms (weakness, chest pain, dizziness, diaphoresis), circulatory signs (new murmurs, gallops, dyspnea, hypotension, excessive tachycardia for the low levels of efforts, i.e., above 115–120 beats/min, and dysrhythmias in the form of multiform ventricular premature beats, salvos, tachycardia, or marked ST-T displacement) (25).

   Low-level ergometric testing of the convalescing ambulatory uncomplicated infarction patient prior to hospital discharge provides objective quantitative information on functional status and degree of recovery that can be used to formulate guidelines for clinical management later at home (5). Generally these patients will have advanced beyond self-care, and the detrimental effects of bed rest will be minimal. They should be ambulatory within the hospital room before being eligible for discharge from the hospital 10–14 days after acute infarction.

Methods. Although the intensity of the test should be considerably lower than the first several stages of conventional exercise tests, the same recording methods, supervision procedures, and safety precautions are indicated. The equipment includes sphygmomanometer, electrocardiograph, and treadmill or bicycle er-gometer (5). Before, during, and after the test the patient's signs, symptoms,

Table 3. Guidelines for Stopping Low-Level Exercise Tests of Acute Myocardial Infarction Patients

---

Signs and symptoms
    Chest pain, discomfort
    Severe dyspnea, extreme fatigue
    Dizziness, faintness, lightheadedness
    Apprehension, cyanosis, confusion
    Incoordination, ataxia
    Heart rate above 115 beats/min
    Decrease or failure to increase heart rate and systolic blood pressure
    New murmurs or gallops

Electrocardiographic signs
    Frequent ventricular ectopic beats, salvos, bigeminy, multiform or R on T phenomena, tachycardia
    Paroxysmal atrial or supraventricular tachycardia or fibrillation
    Second- or third-degree A-V block
    ST-T displacement more than 2 mm from preexercise level

---

heart rate, and blood pressure are recorded, and continuous electrocardiographic monitoring is carried out. The purpose of the low levels for hospital exercise tests is to determine the tolerance of the patient to activities comparable to those that will be performed at home during convalescence, generally less than 3–4 mets; thus the low-level exercise tests have been designed to impose comparable work loads of less than 3–3.5 mets, equal to 10–13 ml of oxygen per kilogram per minute. In the absence of the signs and symptoms listed in Table 3, a patient occasionally can be tested to higher levels (4–5 mets). Figure 3 presents several exercise protocols for low-level testing.

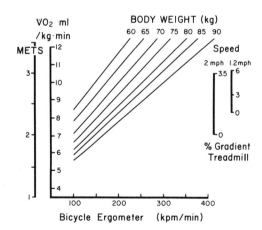

Figure 3. Estimated oxygen and met requirements of three low-level exercise protocols suitable for testing patients with acute myocardial infarction prior to discharge from the hospital. Comparable work loads can be obtained from stages 2 and 3 of the NEHDP (70), from Sivarajan et al. (5), and from bicycle ergometer load corrected for body weight.

The treadmill test consists of walking continuously on a treadmill at a speed of 1.2 mph (1.9 km/hr) for 3 min each at zero, 3%, and 6% gradients (5). The bicycle ergometer test consists of pedaling 60 rpm for 4 min at each of two work levels adjusted for body weight to impose a peak load of 3 mets. There is a 2-min rest period between work loads.

Guidelines for Stopping the Exercise Test. The criteria for stopping these tests are more rigorous than those for stopping peak or maximal performance tests (Table 3).

Interpretation of Results. The responses to low-level testing prior to discharge provide objective information about the functional capacity and the therapeutic needs of the individual patient. Delaying discharge from the hospital or retesting after administration of antiarrhythmic drugs or nitrites may be indicated for patients who show significant arrhythmias or ST-T displacement during low-level testing.

Early activation and supervised ambulation reduce the deconditioning effects of bed rest and account in part for the lower occurrence of subjective complaints of weakness, depression, anxiety, and low self-esteem. The finding that within 2–3 weeks after myocardial infarction most subjects with uncomplicated infarctions can increase their HR × SBP products shows that they can increase myocardial oxygen uptake to meet the metabolic demands imposed by the exercise test (5). The results of the exercise test, coupled with information about the individual's activities of daily living at home, facilitate individualized prescriptions for medications and physical activities and lead to better control of the pace of convalescence prior to return to work.

EVALUATION OF TEST RESPONSES

Responses to exercise tests can be expressed in terms quantitating chronotropic, aerobic, and myocardial aerobic capacities and changes in electrical function. They are useful in evaluating various types of interventions and therapy.

Chronotropic Reserve and Impairment

One of the major adaptive mechanisms of the heart is to increase the heart rate in order to increase cardiac output to meet the increasing demands of the body during exercise. Measurement of peak or maximal effort may be used to assess the age-related reduction in chronotropic capacity, the threshold at which dysrhythmias occur, and information about myocardial oxygen capacity. Since myocardial oxygen uptake has been found to be related to the HR × SBP product, the response of an individual to physical or occupational stress can easily be expressed in terms of heart rate, HR × SBP product, or estimated myocardial oxygen uptake (MVO_2). The age-predicted maximal heart rate can be estimated in one of two ways: 220 − age in years; 215 − (0.66 × age in years) (6,7,9). Maximal heart rate decreases with age, but it decreases even more with heart disease. Impairment of chronotropic capacity due to heart disease can be calculated by the following formula:

$$\text{percentage chronotropic impairment} = \frac{a - b}{a} \times 100$$

where a is age-predicted maximal heart rate and b is heart rate attained at peak or maximal effort.

Aerobic Capacity ($\dot{V}O_2$) and Impairment

The oxygen cost of peak or maximal effort is a measure of functional aerobic capacity. To determine the degree of functional aerobic impairment it is necessary to relate the individual subject's performance to values for healthy individuals of the same age, sex, and habitual physical-activity status. Subjects can be classified as sedentary if they do not exert themselves sufficiently to develop sweating at least once a week. Table 4 presents $\dot{V}O_2$ max values for sedentary and active males and females of various ages (26).

Table 4. $\dot{V}O_2$ max of Healthy Active and Sedentary Men and Women[a]

| Age (years) | Men | | Women | |
	Active 69.7–0.612 years	Sedentary 57.8–0.445 years	Active 42.9–0.312 years	Sedentary 42.3–0.356 years
20	57.5	48.9	36.7	35.2
22	56.2	48.0	36.0	34.5
24	55.0	47.1	35.4	33.8
26	53.8	46.2	34.8	33.0
28	52.6	45.3	34.2	32.3
30	51.3	44.5	33.5	31.6
32	50.1	43.6	32.9	30.9
34	48.9	42.7	32.3	30.2
36	47.7	41.8	31.7	29.5
38	46.4	40.9	31.0	28.8
40	45.2	40.0	30.4	28.1
42	44.0	39.1	29.8	27.3
44	42.8	38.2	29.2	26.6
46	41.5	37.3	28.5	25.9
48	40.3	36.4	27.9	25.2
50	39.1	35.6	27.3	24.5
52	37.9	34.7	26.7	23.8
54	36.7	33.8	26.1	23.1
56	35.4	32.9	25.4	22.4
58	34.2	32.0	24.8	21.7
60	33.0	31.1	24.2	20.9
62	31.8	30.2	23.6	20.2
64	30.5	29.3	22.9	19.5
66	29.3	28.4	22.3	18.8
68	28.1	27.5	21.7	18.1
70	26.9	26.7	21.1	17.4

[a]From Bruce (26), with permission.

Functional aerobic impairment (FAI) can be calculated from the following formula:

$$\text{percentage FAI} = \frac{\text{age-, sex-predicted } \dot{V}O_2 - \text{attained } \dot{V}O_2}{\text{age-, sex-predicted } \dot{V}O_2} \times 100$$

The degree of FAI can be categorized as mild, moderate, or marked, which in our experience equals approximately 15–25%, 26–40%, and 41–51% FAI, respectively.

The concept of FAI is particularly useful in making serial evaluations of individuals as well as comparisons with peers (26). For example, a 50-year-old sedentary man with a peak $\dot{V}O_2$ of 28.0 ml/kg/min had an FAI of 21.3%: [(35.6 − 28.0)/35.6] × 100 = 21.3%. Seven years later his peak $\dot{V}O_2$ increased to 30 ml/kg/min as a result of participating in a supervised exercise program. Although the change was only 2.0 ml/kg/min, i.e., 7.1%, the age-corrected FAI had decreased from 21.3% to 7.6%. In other words, his functional aerobic capacity had increased from 78.7% at age 50 years to 92.4% at age 57 years!

Myocardial Aerobic Capacity (M$\dot{V}O_2$)

Several investigators (27,28) have shown excellent correlations between measured myocardial oxygen consumption [milliliters of oxygen per 100 g of left ventricle (LV) per minute] and two of its major determinants: heart rate alone, $M\dot{V}O_2 = 0.28 \text{ HR} - 14$ ($r = 0.88$); HR × SBP product, $M\dot{V}O_2 = [(0.14 \times \text{HR} \times \text{SBP})/100] - 6.3$ ($r = 0.92$) (Fig. 4). Heart rate per se has limitations for use in assessing $M\dot{V}O_2$, especially when blood pressure is disproportionately elevated; this may occur during upper-extremity effort, in conjunction with emotions, etc. Our studies both on the job and in the laboratory (1,2,14) have demonstrated that upper-extremity effort elicits greater responses than lower-extremity effort of equal magnitude in terms of heart rate, blood pressure, minute ventilation, oxygen uptake, respiratory exchange ratio, and ST-T changes. For example, a 72-kg man develops a heart rate of 130 beats/min and a blood pressure of 170/90

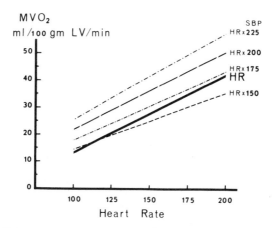

Figure 4. Myocardial oxygen consumption, M$\dot{V}O_2$, estimated from heart rate and from HR × SBP product.

mm Hg while consuming oxygen at 900 ml/min during upper-extremity work (12.5 ml/kg/min); he has a heart rate of 130 beats/min and blood pressure of 130/80 mm Hg while consuming oxygen at 1.5 liters/min during leg effort (20.8 ml/kg/min). The $M\dot{V}O_2$ estimated from heart rate alone will be 22 ml/100 g LV/min with an $M\dot{V}O_2/\dot{V}O_2$ ratio of 17.6:1 for arm work and 10.6:1 for leg work. A better estimation of true $M\dot{V}O_2$ load can be obtained by incorporating the effects of systolic blood pressure responses and heart rate and then relating that to total body oxygen consumption (28). The $M\dot{V}O_2$ calculated from HR × SBP products will be 24.6 and 17.4 ml/100 g LV/min for arm exercise and leg exercise, respectively, and the $M\dot{V}O_2/\dot{V}O_2$ values will be 19.7 and 8.4, respectively.

An increase in HR × SBP product indicates that the subject is able to increase myocardial oxygen consumption to meet the metabolic demands imposed by a given level of activity. The maximal HR × SBP product can be considered to be a measure of cardiovascular adequacy, namely, myocardial aerobic capacity. The maximal HR × SBP product or calculated $M\dot{V}O_2$ decreases with age, mainly because of the decrease in heart rate, and it decreases even more with the advent of heart disease (9). In the latter, symptoms or electrocardiographic changes during exercise tests may preclude attainment of a maximal HR × SBP product.

The relative changes in oxygen consumption of the heart and of the body at rest and at peak effort can be expressed in various ways: the ratio of calculated $M\dot{V}O_2$ to estimated oxygen uptake of the body ($M\dot{V}O_2/\dot{V}O_2$); the ratio of HR × SBP product to estimated oxygen uptake of the body. The $M\dot{V}O_2/\dot{V}O_2$ ratio provides insight into relative cardiac efficiency: the higher the ratio, the greater the energy input:output ratio or cost:benefit ratio and the lower the efficiency. For example, if a subject develops a heart rate of 175 beats/min and a systolic blood pressure of 200 mm Hg at 3 mph and 22.5% gradient, the $M\dot{V}O_2$ will be 42.7 ml/100 g LV/min (Fig. 4), and the $\dot{V}O_2$ will be 42.0 ml/kg body weight (bw)/min, or 4.2 ml/100 g bw/min. The ratio of $M\dot{V}O_2/\dot{V}O_2$ will be 42.7:4.2 = 10.2. However, if the same subject were less fit and developed the same heart rate and blood pressure at 2 mph and 17.5% gradient, $\dot{V}O_2$ would be 24.5 ml/kg bw/min or 2.45 ml/100 g bw/min, and $M\dot{V}O_2/\dot{V}O_2$ would be 17.4 (Fig. 5). The latter ratio

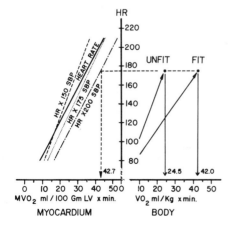

Figure 5. Changes in the ratio of myocardial oxygen consumption to body oxygen consumption ($M\dot{V}O_2/\dot{V}O_2$) of subject with identical HR × SBP response (heart rate 175 beats/min, systolic blood pressure 200 mm Hg) whose peak performance decreased from 42.0 ml/kg bw/min (fit) to 24.5 ml/kg bw/min (unfit). The $M\dot{V}O_2/\dot{V}O_2$ ration increased from 10.2 to 17.4.

indicates an excessive metabolic expenditure of the myocardium for the external work performed by the body of the unfit subject.

The ratio $M\dot{V}O_2/\dot{V}O_2$ at peak effort, in our experience, as well as that calculated from published data (28), ranges between 7 and 10.5 for healthy young and middle-aged adults with less than 9% FAI. Higher values from 11 to 25 have been found in subjects with significant degrees of FAI, viz., 25% in unfit normal and cardiac subjects. These findings are to be expected, since heart rate and blood pressure are higher in such subjects at lower levels of effort.

The peak ratio $(HR \times SBP \times 10^{-2})/\dot{V}O_2$ shows changes similar to those of $M\dot{V}O_2/\dot{V}O_2$ in fit and unfit subjects. For example, the ratio $(HR \times SBP \times 10^{-2})/\dot{V}O_2$ for a 40-year-old man with no FAI is 9.3; with 25% FAI the ratio is 12.4, and with 35% FAI the ratio is 14.2, as calculated from the data of Bruce et al., (29).

Myocardial Aerobic Impairment

The percentage of myocardial aerobic impairment (MAI) can be calculated by relating the individual's $HR \times SBP$ product at peak effort to values for healthy individuals of the same age and sex (9).

Bruce's experience (29) was that age-predicted maximal $[(HR \times SBP)/100](Y)$ can be calculated from the formula $Y = 364 - (0.58 \times \text{age in years})$.

percentage MAI =

$$\frac{\text{age-predicted max } (HR \times SBP) - \text{attained max } (HR \times SBP)}{\text{age-predicted max } (HR \times SBP)} \times 100$$

For example, if a 50-year-old man develops a peak heart rate of 145 beats/min and a systolic blood pressure of 180 mm Hg in symptom-limited peak performance of $\dot{V}O_2$ 24.5 ml/kg bw/min, his FAI will be 31.2%: $[(35.6 - 24.5)/35.6] \times 100$. His percentage MAI will be 22.1%: $[(335 - 261)/335] \times 100 = 22.1\%$. This degree of MAI becomes more meaningful when his maximal $(HR \times SBP)/100$ product or calculated $M\dot{V}O_2$ is related to his body's $\dot{V}O_2$ and to that of a healthy man his age, i.e., $\dot{V}O_2$ max of 35.6 ml/kg bw/min. The ratio of the maximal $(HR \times SBP)/100$ product to $\dot{V}O_2$ of the patient is $261/24.5 = 10.7$, and that of a healthy man his age is $335/35.6 = 9.4$. The ratios of calculated $M\dot{V}O_2/\dot{V}O_2$ will be $30.24/2.45 = 12.3$ and $40.6/3.56 = 11.4$, respectively.

EXERCISE-PRODUCED CHANGES IN ELECTRICAL FUNCTIONS OF THE HEART: IMPULSE INITIATION, ATRIOVENTRICULAR AND INTRAVENTRICULAR CONDUCTION, ECTOPIC ACTIVITY, AND VENTRICULAR REPOLARIZATION (ST-T COMPLEXES)

Since the primary objective of exercise tests is to evaluate cardiovascular function quantitatively, the changes in chronotropic, aerobic, myocardial aerobic, and electrical parameters are valuable in assessing the responses to various types of therapy. With the advent of quantitative exercise electrocardiography (30–35), a new dimension, time, has been added to the testing of cardiac function. "Previously, follow-up studies of presumed normal or abnormal populations were dependent on either incidence rates of new coronary events or mortality data. Both types of evaluation require relatively long time intervals to obtain significant numbers. In addition presumed normal populations contain many subjects with sub-clinical heart disease which can only be uncovered by exercise testing or coronary arteriography" (33). Traditionally the electrical changes (especially ST-T depression either horizontal or downsloping) have been considered to be diagnostic of coronary heart disease (37) and quantitatively prognostic of morbidity and mortality (38).

The etiologic nonspecificity of exercise-induced ST-T depression (and ventricular arrhythmias) has been demonstrated by the occurrence of similar changes in patients with a variety of diseases but with normal coronary arteries: anemia, hyperthyroidism, vasoregulatory disorders, myocarditis, asymmetrical septal hypertrophy, valvular disease, cardiomyopathy, prolapse of the mitral valve, hypertension, drug therapy, etc. (39). The ST-T depression in such conditions can be considered to be electrophysiologically specific, representing an imbalance between myocardial oxygen supply and demand elicited by exercise.

The predictive value of exercise depends on the degree of ST-T displacement (depression, elevation) and the pretest risk of coronary artery disease (40). The latter per se is an important determinant of the predictive value of any exercise test result in the individual patient. The greater the pretest risk of coronary disease (number and types of coronary risk factors), the more likely that exercise ST-T displacement will be greater, and the better the correlation with severity of coronary atherosclerosis. Rifkin and Hood (40) urged that the concept of positive and negative responses to exercise be abandoned altogether and that individual tests be interpreted in terms of a continuum of risk based on the extent of ST-T depression. Thus the risk of coronary disease associated with a given level of ST-T depression must be interpreted according to the level of pretest risk of coronary disease.

In this context, quantitation of repolarization changes can be used to evaluate the adequacy of relative myocardial oxygen supply at various levels of effort and in serial tests, regardless of the etiology of the heart disease.

Methods of Assessing ST-T Displacement

ST-T displacement can be quantitated manually or more precisely with the aid of a computer.

ST-Junction and ST-Segment Method

In an ST-junction (STJ) and ST-slope plot (31,33) the STJ displacement is measured in millimeters from the reference level of the ends of the P-R segments of two consecutive beats. The slope of the first 80 msec of the ST segment is expressed in millivolts per second. Lester et al. (31) plotted the slope and STJ displacement and classified the zones of normal, borderline and abnormal responses (Fig. 6). Normal responses show a marked increase in ST slope that exceeds the STJ with increasing levels of effort. In the abnormal category, the STJ displacement is 0.1 mV or more with a zero or negative slope. The responses during multistage tests can be plotted and the levels noted at which borderline or

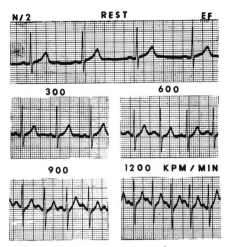

Figure 6A. Exercise electrocardiogram of a 45-year-old man with no history of heart disease who runs an average of 6 miles each week.

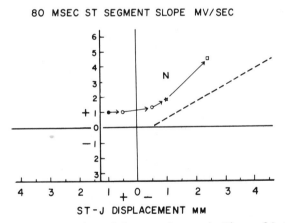

Figure 6B. Graphic representation of the exercise test in Figure 6A. Note that at progressive work levels both the STJ displacement and the slope of the ST segment increase. The test remains normal even at near-maximum performance. N, B, and A represent zones of normal, borderline, and abnormal responses, respectively.

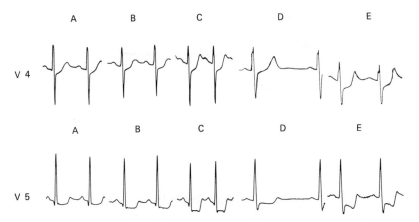

Figure 6C. Exercise electrocardiograms (V4 and V5, sections A, B, and C) of a 52-year-old man with significant stenosis of three coronary arteries and progressive displacement of the ST junction and the ST segment. Note that the ST segment is negative in V5 but positive in simultaneously recorded lead V4. Similar findings are shown in sections D and E in the exercise electrocardiograms of another subject with coronary artery disease and angina pectoris.

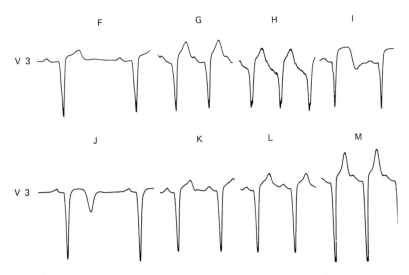

Figure 6D. Exercise electrocardiogram (V3) of two middle-aged men with large anteroseptal myocardial infarctions, excellent aerobic capacities, and minimal symptoms even at high levels of effort. Note the increase of positive STJ displacement with progressive levels of effort. Neither subject has a ventricular aneurysm.

172

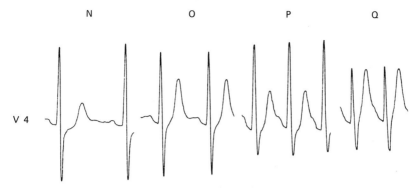

Figure 6E. Exercise electrocardiogram of a 56-year-old man with recent walk-through angina pectoris. Note that the STJ displacement subsides and the slope of the ST segment increases with progressive levels of effort.

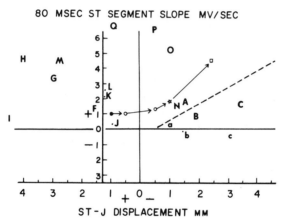

Figure 6F. Graphic representation of the exercise tests of subjects whose electrocardiograms are shown in Figures 6A through E. The response of the subject in Figure 6A remains in the N (normal) zone; that of the subject in Figure 6C shows that V4 starts in the normal zone and moves progressively to the so-called borderline zone, while simultaneously recorded V5 moves from the borderline to the abnormal zone. Subjects in 6D show progressive STJ elevation and increase of the slope of the ST segment with movement into the left upper section of the graph. This occurs in subjects with areas of myocardial dyskinesis or akinesis (discussed in text).

abnormal responses occur. The electrocardiograms of follow-up tests can be evaluated in the same manner and comparison made for the same leads at identical work loads. Deterioration of exercise electrocardiograms can be judged by a change in category.

ST Index

McHenry and Fisch obviated the need to plot the STJ and ST slope by expressing their relationship in the form of an ST index, which is the algebraic sum of the STJ depression in millimeters and the ST slope in millivolts per second (37). A negative index is considered as being abnormal, assuming that the magnitude of the ST depression is at least 1.0 mm. Slow-upslope criteria are reliable only during exercise or in the immediate recovery period (37).

ST Depression 80 msec After STJ

In the presence of technical problems in obtaining noise-free recordings, quantitative measurements of the ST slope may be difficult. An alternative method that attains greater accuracy is to measure the magnitude of ST depression at 0.08 sec after the J junction. Degrees of ST-segment depression can conveniently be classified as 0.5 mm, ≥ 0.5 mm, ≥ 1.0 mm, ≥ 1.5 mm, ≥ 2.0 mm, etc. (9,37).

ST-T Area Displacement Method

The area below reference level can be measured precisely by computer; it can be measured less precisely, but still adequately, by estimating the number of millimeter squares in the area below the reference level (Fig. 7). Each millimeter square equals 4 μV-sec. An ST-T area of approximately 8 μV-sec or more has been shown to be abnormal (32).

Positive ST-T displacement (elevation) is more common in transmural anterior myocardial infarctions than in inferior or posterior myocardial infarctions. Such ST-T elevation occurs in areas of myocardial dyskinesis or akinesis (37). On the other hand, ST-T elevation in the absence of a previous transmural myocardial infarction suggests critical stenosis of one or more major coronary arteries.

Interpretation

The exercise ST-T response has greater value when quantitated and related to the development of chest discomfort or pain, the level of effort at which it occurs, and the duration of its persistence after completion of the exercise test. For comparisons after therapeutic interventions, the time, heart rate, blood pressure at onset of ST displacement, with or without angina, and other important parameters such as complex arrhythmias, bundle branch block, new murmurs, or S_3 or S_4 gallops should be recorded. "The development of standard methods of multi-level exercise tests of physical fitness and standardized methods of recording and quantitative analysis of the exercise ECG has made it possible to compare an individual with himself over a time interval. This is now feasible not only in regard to the ECG and to the heart rate response traditionally used by effort physiologists as a measure of aerobic capacity, but also in regard to exercise blood pressure whose product with heart rate is an indirect measure of myocardial oxygen consumption" (33).

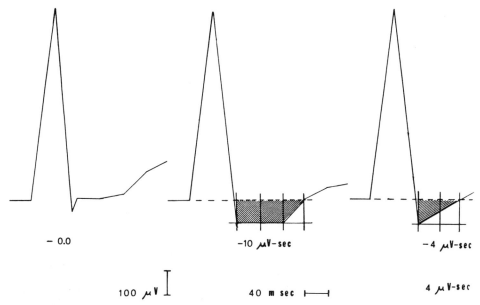

Figure 7. ST-T area displacement method of Sheffield et al (32). On the left there is no depressed ST interval. In the center there is a depressed ST area of exactly 2.5 squares, corresponding to 2.5 units on standard chart paper. At 4 μV-sec per square unit, this equals -10 μV-sec. On the right there is a depressed ST area equal to exactly half of 2 square units (equal to -4 μV-sec). [Reproduced by permission from Sheffield et al. (32).]

It seems reasonable to assume that improvement in the exercise electrocardiogram is related to enhancement of physiologic function. Since inadequacy of oxygen supply to the myocardium produces displacement of the ST segment and changes its slope, improvement in the exercise electrocardiogram of the conditioned subject suggests that the myocardial oxygen needs have been satisfied. This may occur either by augmentation of oxygen supply or by reduction of need. Reduction of myocardial oxygen need for the same work load is suggested by the reductions in exercise heart rate and blood pressure after exercise training. An increase in ST-T displacement at lower work loads, heart rate, systolic blood pressure, or HR × SBP product is consistent with deterioration of cardiovascular function. Such patients with significant impairment of aerobic capacity and marked ST-T displacement with or without angina pectoris are not likely to benefit from maximal medical therapy (37); they should be considered as candidates for cardiac catheterization, coronary angiograms, and possibly coronary bypass or other surgery. Eligible for similar management are atherosclerotic heart disease (ASHD) subjects who have combinations of three nonelectrocardiographic parameters that have more ominous prognostic significance than ST-T depression (29). The triad of cardiomegaly, failure to raise systolic blood pressure above 130 mm Hg, and peak exercise response below 3 mets probably occurs in fewer than 5% of ASHD subjects.

In our experience, changes in exercise electrocardiograms were related to changes in physical fitness, especially in ASHD subjects with initial borderline or abnormal exercise electrocardiograms. Improvement in exercise electrocardiograms occurred in 79% of ASHD subjects with initial borderline or abnormal exercise electrocardiograms whose physical fitness improved; improvement was characterized by a decrease in STJ displacement and an increase in the slope of the 0.08-sec ST segment. The opposite changes in STJ displacement and ST-segment slope occurred in subjects who showed deterioration in exercise electrocardiograms and physical fitness (33).

Electrocardiographic Lead Systems

The heart is a three-dimensional anatomic structure whose electrical functions are likewise three-dimensional. For this reason it is important to use leads that reflect not only the X but also the Y and Z components. The addition of precordial leads, especially V-1 to V-3 and V-4, or Z scalar lead, provides invaluable information in the diagnosis of infarction with predominant Z components, i.e., anteroseptal, anterior, and true posterior myocardial infarctions. The use of a single unipolar or bipolar V-5 lead is associated with a large number (approximately 11%) of false negative responses, i.e., subjects who show abnormal responses when monitored with multiple leads. Since the V-5 or C-5 lead reflects 'predominantly an X component of the heart's electrical activity, it is advisable to enhance sensitivity with additional leads that also reflect changes in the Y and Z axes, i.e., AVF, II, III, scalar Y leads, and V-1, V-2, V-3, or scalar Z leads. A single bipolar lead like CM5 or CB5 may be sufficient for detection of myocardial "ischemia during exercise in patients with a *normal* ECG at rest. However, in patients with abnormal ECGs at rest, multiple leads remain necessary since the ST changes during exercise in these patients occur in all directions, and may therefore be missed by a single lead" (35).

Exercise Arrhythmias

Arrhythmias that appear during exercise tests must be considered as potentially dangerous and may merit test termination, unless they subside as the test proceeds. Ventricular ectopic rhythms during exercise tests are more common than supraventricular beats, and they increase significantly with age (from 15–35% of men below 35 years of age to 50–60% of men between 45 and 55 years of age) (41). Paired or multiform ventricular premature beats, salvos, or couplets, or ventricular tachycardia, occur more commonly in cardiac patients and at significantly lower heart rates than in normals (9). Since these ventricular arrhythmias may be harbingers of ventricular fibrillation, exercise should be terminated. Subjects without heart disease rarely develop ventricular premature beats below 70% of age-predicted maximal heart rate (9,37). The concurrence of chest pain and complex ventricular arrhythmias, even in the absence of ST-T displacement, likewise is an indication to halt the exercise test.

Complete bundle branch block may occur during an exercise test and may be related to a specific heart rate, disappearing predictably when the rate decreases. The degree of preexercise A-V block may increase or decrease with exercise. Subjects with complete A-V block and narrow QRS complexes generally are able to attain a higher heart rate than subjects with broad QRS complexes.

Since most of the potentially hazardous arrhythmias cited are not accompanied by symptoms and may not occur regularly at a specific heart rate, antiarrhythmic medications and exercise training should be prescribed at an intensity below the arrhythmia threshold.

EXERCISE PRESCRIPTION

The exercise recommendation should be treated with the same seriousness and caution employed in prescribing a pharmacologic agent. Consideration must be given to numerous factors, including the patient's age, sex, health status, current medications, orthopedic and musculoskeletal integrity, degree of motivation, individual recreational preferences, and, most important, diagnostic and functional evaluation (results of the exercise tolerance test). The following information derived from the multistage exercise test is vital to the exercise prescription: estimated or measured peak oxygen uptake; peak attained heart rate; limiting symptoms and their physiologic accompaniments; occurrences of symptomatic or asymptomatic ischemic electrocardiographic changes, dysrhythmias, or excessive blood pressure responses. The prescribed exercise intensity should be above the threshold level needed to demonstrate a conditioning response, yet below the level that evokes significant clinical symptoms or significant electrocardiographic abnormalities.

The format for the physical conditioning session should include a warm-up period (10 min), an endurance phase (15–30 min), and a cool-down period (5–8 min), with an optional recreational game (10–15 min) (42). The endurance phase should be prescribed in specific terms of intensity, duration, frequency, and type of activity.

Warm-up Period

The warm-up period permits adaptation to the transition from rest to exercise. Physiologically it facilitates gradual circulatory adjustment and minimizes oxygen deficit and the formation of lactic acid; it increases muscle and core temperature, which enhances muscular efficiency and oxygen dissociation (43); it decreases total pulmonary vascular resistance and increases pulmonary circulation; it increases the rate of nerve conduction and decreases muscle viscosity; it decreases susceptibility to injury; it decreases the occurrence of ischemic electrocardiographic changes and arrhythmias following sudden exertion (11). Thus the warm-up period has preventive value and enhances performance.

Warm-up exercises should include both musculoskeletal (i.e., static stretching, flexibility, muscle-strengthening exercises) and cardiopulmonary activity. Exercises may be modified to incorporate tossing a ball or other movement skills for greater variety. The cardiopulmonary warm-up should involve total body movement to include a level of activity (i.e., alternate walking-jogging, swimming-recovering, moderate cycling) slightly below (i.e., within 20 beats/min) that employed during the endurance phase. The cardiopulmonary warm-up permits gradual elevation of the heart rate to the appropriate training level.

Endurance Phase

The endurance phase serves to stimulate the oxygen transport system directly. Some of the dynamic activities that improve endurance include walking, jogging (in place or moving), running, cycling, skiing (downhill or cross-country), swimming, skipping rope, ice skating, rowing, climbing stairs, and stepping onto a bench.

The three critical elements of the endurance phase (intensity, duration, and frequency) have now been quantified (44). The interrelationships among these factors permit an inadequacy in one to be partially or totally compensated for by appropriate changes in one or both of the other factors. Proper adjustment of these factors plays a major role in achieving an effective but safe exercise dosage. Improvement generally shows a positive correlation with conditioning frequency, intensity, and duration and a negative correlation with the subject's age, initial fitness, and habitual level of activity.

Intensity

The intensity of effort relative to the subject's initial aerobic power is perhaps the most important factor influencing the response to a training regimen (45). Despite some recent studies favoring control of the total amount of exercise stress (i.e., a predetermined number of heartbeats above resting level), conditioning of relatively high intensity, even when performed for a shorter period of time, appears to elicit greater improvement than prolonged moderate-intensity training. The threshold intensity of training that is sufficient to produce a measurable beneficial training effect probably lies between 25% and 50% of $\dot{V}O_2$ max. For younger men a threshold intensity of more than 50% $\dot{V}O_2$ max has been recommended (46,47). However, the training stimulus threshold (intensity) appears to have a wide variance, with some evidence suggesting that it increases in direct proportion to the initial level of fitness. Thus the higher the initial level of fitness ($\dot{V}O_2$ max) the higher the threshold and thus the intensity necessary to elicit a significant response (44).

The optimal intensity of exercise (which is usually related to the speed of walking, jogging, bicycling, or swimming) should be in the range of 57–78% $\dot{V}O_2$ max (Fig. 8). In this relative range several key physiologic and biochemical changes occur, indicating that the aerobic metabolism is being stressed: the respiratory exchange ratio approaches unity (Fig. 9), and there are increases in blood lactate, fibrinolytic activity, urinary catecholamine excretion, capacity to oxidize fatty acids, release of fatty acids from adipose tissue, capacity to regenerate ATP by oxidative phosphorylation, protein content of the mitochondrial fraction of skeletal muscle, etc., desirable changes that are associated with favorable adaptation and improvement (13).

A key point is that exercise intensity does not have to be exhaustive to accomplish a substantial training response. Improvement in $\dot{V}O_2$ max increases curvilinearly with increasing intensity of exercise to a peak of approximately 78% $\dot{V}O_2$ max, with little additional increase thereafter (Fig. 10). Cardiovascular function in middle-aged men showed no greater improvement at a training intensity of 94% $\dot{V}O_2$ max than at 83% $\dot{V}O_2$ max (48).

High-intensity conditioning (95–100% $\dot{V}O_2$ max) is not desirable for most

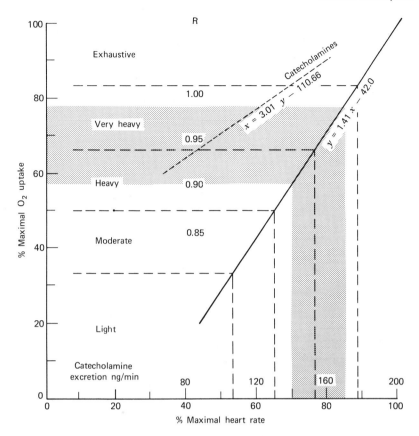

Figure 8. Relationship between percentage maximal oxygen intake and percentage maximal heart rate for normal and cardiac subjects. Y = 1.41 × −42.0. Shaded area represents 70% to 85% of maximal heart rate, equal to 57% and 78% of maximal oxygen intake, respectively.

subjects, not only because it cannot be sustained long enough to develop endurance but more important because it increases the risk of cardiovascular complications (i.e., arrhythmia, ischemic manifestations, myocardial infarction, and cardiac arrest). A recent review of 15 cases of cardiac arrest occurring during supervised exercise revealed that 12 men had been training in excess of 80% of maximal heart rate and 9 men had been exceeding 85% in earlier training sessions (49). Manifestations of excessive effort during or following exercise training are listed in Table 2 of Chapter 9.

Target Heart Rate Concept

Advantages and Limitations. Although the same exercise frequency and duration may be prescribed for most participants, the exercise intensity must be *individually* prescribed to equate relative cardiovascular stresses among individuals. Because of the linear relationship between heart rate and oxygen intake during dynamic exercise tests involving large muscle groups, the heart

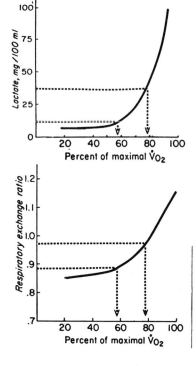

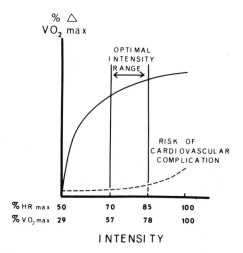

Figure 9. Relationship between intensity of exercise expressed as percentage of maximal oxygen intake and changes in respiratory exchange ratio (R) and serum lactate. Between the range 57% and 78% maximal oxygen intake (which corresponds to 70% and 85% of maximal heart rate), a significant increase occurs in lactate, and R approaches unity.

Figure 10. Relationship between gain in aerobic capacity (expressed as $\dot{V}O_2$ max, %Δ) and intensity of exercise (expressed as %HR max or %$\dot{V}O_2$ max). As the intensity of exercise exceeds 85% maximal heart rate, the relative risks of arrhythmias, angina pectoris, and other ischemic manifestations increase abruptly, whereas the improvement in aerobic capacity levels off. [Adapted from Dehn and Mullins (53).]

rate can be used to estimate oxygen intake during other efforts involving the same muscles. The target training zone of 57–78% maximal aerobic power corresponds to approximately 70–85% maximal (symptom-limited) heart rate (Fig. 8). For example, an individual whose exercise test shows a maximal (symptom-limited) heart rate of 182 beats/min will have a training heart rate range of 127–155 beats/min. The training heart rate selected within this range is often referred to as the target heart rate (THR). Figure 1 in Chapter 9 shows a convenient means of calculating THR.

The THR concept has several important advantages for controlling exercise intensity. For example, a THR (e.g., 140 beats/min) that is established during physical conditioning can be applied outside the gymnasium to new and different activities. The THR has a built-in regulator for changes in fitness, thus enabling the individual to maintain the same relative intensity throughout an exercise program. As the patient becomes better conditioned, the speed of jogging or swimming or cycling must be slowly increased to compensate for the decrease in heart rate produced by conditioning; the THR initially achieved by a given level of effort can later be reached only by greater exertion. THR also provides for extremes in environmental conditions. For example, in hot or humid weather less work will be required to achieve a specific THR, even though the work of the heart (myocardial oxygen uptake) remains unchanged. The subject who is trained to monitor THR will also be able to detect arrhythmias (ventricular premature beats) and will have been advised to slow down the training pace and/or seek medical advice.

However, use of THR alone as an inflexible measure of intensity, particularly in patients with coronary heart disease, is both naive and unwarranted. The fallacy in using only the heart rate as a guide is the implication that there are no other conditions that may restrict a person's performance. Recent changes in clinical status and/or physical appearance are reasons to reduce exercise intensity, irrespective of THR. Specific examples include intercurrent illness, orthopedic injury, anemia, cerebral dysfunction (i.e., dizziness), pallor or cyanosis, medication changes, and surgery. In addition to monitoring heart rate, measuring blood pressure may be particularly important in known hypertensive patients and in those persons who show disproportionately high blood pressure responses to multilevel steady-state exercise. Blood pressure and heart rate should be monitored during training as well as in exercise testing, since both are important determinants of myocardial oxygen consumption. Finally, a primary limiting factor may be the occurrence of arrhythmias before and during exercise. In our experience we have found individuals who had this limitation. One patient who was able to attain a heart rate of 150 beats/min had repeated episodes of several seconds of asymptomatic ventricular flutter. As we train and follow an increasing number of cardiac patients, we find that complex arrhythmias are potentially prognostic of sudden death, usually occurring at rest.

Attainment of THR. The success of exercise training depends in large part on regulating the intensity of effort to attain the prescribed THR. Two weeks of unannounced spot checks of the training heart rates of our coronary patients (National Exercise and Heart Disease Project) demonstrated that the average deviation from THR was 4.9 beats/min (SE ± 0.6). Heart rates were monitored "instantaneously" using Physio-Control Lifepak-4 defibrillator paddles that provided recordings of heart rates and electrocardiogram waveforms. Patients were not told when monitoring electrocardiogram strips would be recorded; they were instructed to proceed at the usual walking or jogging speed designed to achieve the THR. Our experience indicates that the intensity of training can be regulated in supervised nontelemetered gymnasium reconditioning programs.

Obtaining the Pulse. Physicians have traditionally measured heart rate by timing the pulse of the radial artery at the wrist. Although the carotid pulse may be easier to obtain, patients should be instructed not to press too hard with the palpating fingers, as this may produce marked bradycardia or even asystole in the presence of a hypersensitive carotid sinus reflex.

The question is frequently asked: "How long should the pulse be counted to obtain the heart rate during exercise?" As soon as an individual starts to exercise, the heart rate accelerates; within 3–4 min it reaches a fairly steady plateau that varies with subsequent adjustment in pace. It is this steady level of heart rate during exercise that should be measured. Since it is difficult to count the heart rate during vigorous activity, the heart rate taken within 10 sec of cessation of exercise can be used as a valid measure of the heart rate during activity. In our experience, the heart rate decreases by 7–9 beats/min within 10 sec after cessation of exercise. For this reason, if the heart rate taken within 10 sec of exercise proves to be the THR (e.g., 150 beats/min), the actual working rate most likely will be in excess of the THR by 7–9 beats/min (i.e., 157–159 beats/min)! The THR should be adjusted downward slightly when the 10-sec recovery pulse is employed.

Limitations of Age-predicted Maximal Heart Rate and Absolute Heart Rate as Indices of Maximal Oxygen Intake and Training Intensity. When the maximal heart rate is not determined for the individual subject, the intensity prescription is often based on a percentage of the age-predicted maximal heart rate. The disadvantage of this approach lies in the variation of the age-predicted maximal heart rate, usually a standard deviation of about 10 beats/min. Consequently a training heart rate range of 40 beats/min is necessary to include 95% of the population. One could therefore easily overestimate or underestimate the optimal training level and reduce the safety and/or the possibility of achieving positive training effects.

When the highest tolerated work load is significantly reduced, a degree of uncertainty may be expected in the use of age-predicted maximal heart rate as an index of oxygen intake and as a guide for training intensity. In a large number of ASHD subjects the limiting factor may be the highest attained heart rate, which is often significantly reduced even in the absence of ischemic ST-T changes and will vitiate estimation of $\dot{V}O_2$ max. Thus in middle-aged normal persons the average predicted maximal heart rate is 165–170 beats/min, and in ASHD subjects of similar age it may be 140 beats/min or less. Even though "strain" does not appear, the reduced ceiling on the heart rate may determine the level of training. An extreme example is the ASHD subject who has marked sinus bradycardia at rest (36 beats/min) and at tolerated work level attains a maximal heart rate of 96–100 beats/min.

The restriction in the rise of the heart rate may be due to intrinsic disease of the sinoatrial or A-V nodes, or it may be due to the appearance of signs and symptoms that preclude exercising at a higher work level, e.g., exertional hypertension, hypotension, ventricular ectopic activity in salvos or paroxysms, sinoatrial block or high degrees of A-V block, 3–4 mm of ST-T displacement, severe angina pectoris, or other severe symptoms. In these cases the age-predicted maximal heart rate should be considered unrealistically high; extrapolation from low values is unwarranted, and heart rate cannot be considered as a measure of $\dot{V}O_2$ max. Instead, the heart rate at which any of the above signs or symptoms cause termination of the test can be designated the maximal safe heart rate, and an average of 70% with peaks to 85% of this value can be used as guidelines in training prescription (13).

Although the intensity of training would appear to be too modest, significant improvement has been obtained in such subjects. This method is realistic and probably is safer than the method of Karvonen, in which the intensity of training is based on a percentage of estimated chronotropic reserve.

Karvonen's Method. The training heart rate equals the difference between maximal age-adjusted heart rate (max AAHR) and resting heart rate (RHR), multiplied by 60–70%, plus RHR (46): training heart rate = (max AAHR − RHR) (60–70%) + RHR. For example, if a 45-year-old man with max AAHR of 175 beats/min and RHR of 62 beats/min attained a peak heart rate of 120 beats/min, at which time he developed 4 mm of ST-T displacement and severe chest pain and the test was terminated, the theoretical available maximal heart rate (heart rate reserve) would be 113 (175 − 62). The training heart rate according to Karvonen's formula would be (175 − 62) (60%) + 62 = 130. The training heart rate of 130 beats/min exceeds the attained peak heart rate and would indicate an unrealistic and potentially dangerous work load. *At no time should the training intensity and heart rate exceed those of the exercise test.* Our recommendation for this subject would be an average training heart rate of 84 beats/min (70% of 120) and a peak heart rate of 102 beats/min (85% of 120) (see Table 3 in Chapter 9). These values would correspond to 38% and 69%, respectively, of his actual heart rate reserve plus his resting heart rate; i.e., 84 = (120 − 62) (X) + 62 and 102 = (120 − 62) (X) + 62, where X is percentage available heart rate reserve. Furthermore, the training heart rate range of 84–102 beats/min represents 19.4–35.4% of the *theoretical* maximal heart rate, viz.:

$$84 = \frac{(175 - 62)(X) + 62}{100} \qquad X = \frac{84 - 62}{113} \times 100$$

$$X = 19.4\% \text{ theoretical maximal heart rate reserve}$$

$$102 = \frac{(175 - 62)(X) + 62}{100} \qquad X = \frac{102 - 62}{113} \times 100$$

$$X = 35.4\% \text{ theoretical maximal heart rate reserve}$$

Gualtiere and associates confirmed that ASHD subjects with restricted maximal heart rates and work capacity show significant improvement when trained at 16–43% of theoretical maximal available heart rate (50).

In our opinion, the Karvonen formula has only limited application in normal individuals and especially in cardiac patients unless reliable values of resting heart rate and the individual's peak heart rate are obtained.

Arbitrary Training Heart Rates. Establishing an intensity prescription on the basis of absolute heart rates, e.g., 120 or 150 beats/min, ignores the fact that maximal heart decreases, so that *a particular heart rate represents different percentages of maximal heart rate and maximal oxygen intake for subjects of different ages. Thus a heart rate of 150 beats/min represents 77%, 81%, 86%, and 91% of age-predicted maximal heart rate for men 24, 35, 45, and 55 years of age, respectively.*

Duration

In order to achieve the desired cardiovascular effects, the subject should perform dynamic exercise for a period long enough to stimulate energy production predominantly through the aerobic, as opposed to the anaerobic, energy pathways. Although the requirements of the first few minutes are met primarily from anaerobic energy sources, the anaerobic component rapidly becomes less important with increasing duration of exercise. Prolonged or sustained exercise is required to activate and condition the aerobic energy pathway that supplies energy for most daily activities.

Although the minimal duration for effective conditioning has not been established, it seems likely that more than 2 min of exercise are necessary to stress the aerobic energy pathways and elicit aerobic adaptation. Significant improvement occurred in blind subjects trained with four periods of bicycle ergometer exercise each lasting 3 min and followed by 3-min rest periods (51). Thus the effectiveness of short work periods depends on an interval approach. By alternating periods of work and rest, a substantial total work load can be achieved (44). However, several investigators have reported significant improvement in subjects trained for continuous periods as brief as 10–12 min each day (52).

The duration of exercise necessary to produce a significant conditioning response varies inversely with intensity: the lower the intensity of exercise the longer the duration necessary. Conversely, the greater the intensity (up to about 80% $\dot{V}O_2$ max) the shorter the duration necessary to achieve the same benefits. At a given intensity (i.e., 75% $\dot{V}O_2$ max), improvement increases as the duration of the session is prolonged to 30 min (Fig. 11), but there is little additional benefit thereafter (53). Thus exercise training for 10–15 min improves $\dot{V}O_2$ max, but 30-min sessions are even more effective (54). Moreover, 45-min sessions do not produce a greater increase in $\dot{V}O_2$ max (48), but they do increase the risk of orthopedic complications (Fig. 11) (55).

Continuous Versus Intermittent Exercise. There is considerable controversy whether exercise training should be continuous or intermittent (interval). Each approach has certain advantages. The former enhances endurance; the latter, with its work–rest pauses, increases strength. In the conditioning of cardiac patients, interval training has several important advantages:

· The patient can achieve a larger total work load per session with less fatigue. The recovery periods with interval work minimize the lactate accumulation associated with continuous work. For a given submaximal work load, oxygen pulse is higher and respiratory exchange ratio, minute ventilation, and heart rate are lower with intermittent exercise.

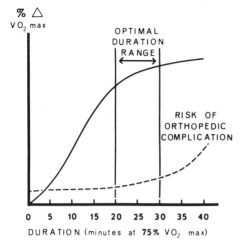

% △
VO₂ max

OPTIMAL
DURATION
RANGE

RISK OF
ORTHOPEDIC
COMPLICATION

0   5   10   15   20   25   30   35   40
DURATION (minutes at 75% VO₂ max)

Figure 11. Relationship between exercise duration (minutes at 75% $\dot{V}O_2$ max) and increase in aerobic capacity ($\dot{V}O_2$ max, %Δ). Prolonged workouts beyond 30 min increase the risk of orthopedic complications, with slight additional improvement in aerobic capacity. [Adapted from Dehn and Mullins (53).]

· The severely limited patient with angina can accomplish a larger total work load prior to increasing symptoms.

· Larger numbers of training stimuli are presented to the heart during each session because of the repeated increases in stroke volume, venous return, and intracardiac pressures. The suggestion has been made (56) that the maximal stroke volumes needed to evoke a training effect are developed only in the recovery intervals. The increase in oxygen pulse noted during exercise recovery (13), implying an increase in stroke volume and/or peripheral A-V oxygen extraction, may substantiate this belief.

· Intermittent exercise, incorporating a variety of upper- and lower-extremity exercise devices, is better suited to enhancement of the total fitness necessary for a return to occupational and leisure-time activities.

Frequency

Figure 12 shows the relationship between exercise frequency (sessions/week) and increase in aerobic capacity ($\dot{V}O_2$ max). Once-a-week conditioning is not enough to elicit an increase in $\dot{V}O_2$ max in young men. However, older men or cardiac patients, having lower initial $\dot{V}O_2$ max, may respond to slightly less than twice-a-week exercise. A twofold increase in $\dot{V}O_2$ max occurs when the exercise frequency increases from two times per week to four times per week. Additional benefits of more frequent training (5 sessions/week or more) appear to be minimal, whereas the incidence of orthopedic injury increases markedly (55). Thus three or four evenly spaced workouts per week appear to represent the most cost-effective training frequency in normal individuals.

Our experience with 254 ASHD subjects participating in three 1-hr training sessions per week revealed that subjects who trained an average of 2.2 to 3 sessions/week or more showed significantly greater improvement in aerobic capacity and electrocardiographic response to exercise than their counterparts who averaged 1.0 to 2.0 sessions/week (57). Surprisingly, subjects who attended 3.5 to 5.0 sessions/week showed no greater improvement than those who attended 2.2 to 3.0 sessions/week. Nevertheless, normal subjects have been shown

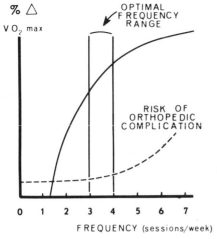

Figure 12. Relationship between exercise frequency (sessions/week) and improvement in aerobic capacity (VO_2 max, %Δ). The risk of orthopedic injury increases markedly for high-frequency training (≥ 5 sessions/week), with slight additional improvement in aerobic capacity. [Adapted from Dehn and Mullins (53).]

to have increased aerobic capacity after training twice a week at higher intensities than cardiac subjects (80% and 92% of maximal heart rate) (48).

Types of Training Activities

Cardiovascular function and physical work capacity are best enhanced through dynamic aerobic activities involving sustained movement of large muscle groups of the upper extremities and torso as well as those of the lower extremities. Walking, jogging, swimming, bicycling (mobile or stationary), rowing, cross-country skiing, and running games (tennis, handball, squash, basketball) are included in this category. Because of the relative consistency of energy expenditure in persons participating in walking, jogging, and cycling, these activities lend themselves particularly well to exercise prescription. Furthermore, recent work (58) has shown them to be equally efficient modes of training. The relative merits and limitations of several commonly employed training modes will be discussed in the following sections.

Walking and Jogging. Walking and jogging are the most accessible and most easily regulated exercises that are effective in developing cardiorespiratory endurance. The inherent neuromuscular limitations on the speed of walking (and therefore the rate of energy expenditure) establish it as the most appropriate form of activity for the early stages of an unsupervised conditioning program. The advantages of a walking program include a low dropout rate, an easily tolerable working intensity, and few orthopedic problems of the legs and knees. In contrast, jogging (particularly at high intensity) is associated with increased orthopedic and musculoskeletal problems. Adequate warm-up, a schedule of moderate intensity (60–80% VO_2 max), proper footwear, and avoidance of hard and uneven surfaces should eliminate most such problems. Investment in a pair of shoes designed for running (with thick sole, well-supported arch, and elevated heel) is probably the single most important consideration.

Swimming and Aquatic Exercise. Swimming is also an excellent aerobic exercise, particularly for the upper extremities. It has the advantage of enhancing venous return because of body position and hydrostatic pressure, and it also reduces concern for thermal regulation because of the water's cooling effect (59). However, swimming activity may be difficult to prescribe because energy expenditure is highly dependent on skill. An inexperienced swimmer will expend more energy thrashing across the pool than his skilled counterpart. Despite this, swimming has been used during the initial phase of cardiac reconditioning. The inaccessibility of swimming pools and the lack of swimming skill among older generations are the major disadvantages of swimming as a training activity.

Aquatic exercise has the advantage that it is particularly useful as an activity for patients with neurologic and musculoskeletal disorders. Special aquatic exercises may include torso and extremity movements in shallow water, thus taking advantage of the buoyancy of the water to minimize orthopedic trauma and the resistance of the water to augment the work load. Training of specific muscles of the upper body can be achieved by various arm strokes.

Bicycling. Bicycling programs are versatile because they offer the flexibility of outdoor (mobile bicycle) or indoor (stationary bicycle) training. An additional advantage is that the stationary bicycle can be modified for arm cranking. However, certain precautions are necessary to ensure safety and effectiveness. Care should be taken to ensure proper adjustment of seat height and handgrips. There should be a slight bend in the knee when the pedal is in the down position. Improper seat height will result in decreased efficiency during pedaling. Handlebars should be positioned so that the body is relaxed and is leaning slightly forward. Sustained tight gripping of the handlebars should be avoided so that isometric contraction will not be superimposed on dynamic exercise. The intensity of effort can be controlled by speed, grade, or resistance adjustments.

Skipping Rope. Skipping rope is a practical and enjoyable means of cardiovascular conditioning. A jump rope is inexpensive; it can be taken on trips and can be used indoors or outdoors; it offers many variations in technique and provides exercise for both arms and legs. Ten minutes of vigorous rope skipping yield cardiovascular improvement similar to that achieved with 30 min of jogging (60). However, skipping rope does require coordination; if it is done inefficiently (due to improper technique or incorrect rope length) it may cause the heart rate to exceed the target training level. Cardiac patients who use rope skipping as a fitness activity are advised to step over the rope one foot at a time, as opposed to jumping with the feet together. This technique should minimize orthopedic problems while preventing increases in heart rate above the recommended training level. The step-over method is similar to the foot motion used in jogging.

Calisthenics. Recent fitness publications have denigrated the value of calisthenic exercise as a cardiovascular conditioner. Consequently, calisthenic exercise has been eliminated in many adult fitness programs in all but the initial warm-up phases. Two criticisms are frequently cited: calisthenics are ineffective in raising the heart rate and total body oxygen demands to those threshold (intensity) levels needed to elicit a training effect; calisthenics cannot be maintained long enough (duration) to reach the steady state required to produce a training effect.

Although certain calisthenic exercises fit this description (i.e., toe touching), many others can be used effectively to develop cardiorespiratory endurance (57).

Graded rhythmic calisthenics involving continuous movement of the large muscle groups, preferably the antigravity muscles, can result in a significant training effect if performed for an adequate period of time. The key lies in alternating rapidly from exercising one group of muscles to exercising another so as to maintain the heart rate at or near the target training level. Furthermore, calisthenics involving total body movement (e.g., straddle hops or jumping jacks, hops, sailor's hornpipe) will most effectively serve this purpose.

Our experience in the training of 254 convalescent and postconvalescent ASHD subjects demonstrated that calisthenic exercise can be of sufficient intensity and duration to elicit a training effect (57). Monitored heart rates during early training demonstrated that an average heart rate of 120 beats/min was attained during 30 min of calisthenics; this is 73% of predicted maximal heart rate for men 50 years old, which is equivalent to 60% of maximal oxygen intake. The peak heart rate of 140 beats/min during running sequences corresponded to approximately 80% of maximal heart rate and 70% of maximal oxygen intake (Fig. 13).

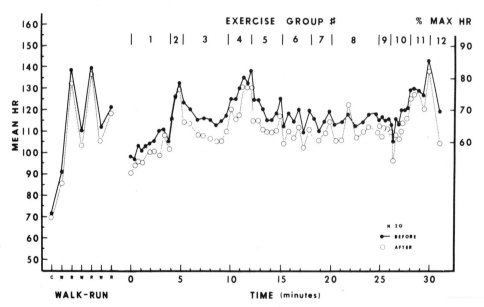

Figure 13. Average heart rates of walk-run sequences (W = walk, R = run, C = control) and consecutively performed calisthenics done routinely in the CWRU-CJCC study. The electrocardiograms of 20 subjects (average age 48) were telemetered before (solid lines) and several months after (dotted lines) participation in the training program. Note that the average heart rate was about 120 beats/min, representing 70% of their highest exercise test heart rate. Exercise numbers: (1) shoulder exercises, standing, warm-up; (2) hops, walk steps; (3) arm sweeps, standing; (4) hops, sailor's hornpipe; (5) body bends; (6) leg exercises, supine; (7) leg-arm-hip exercise, sitting on floor; (8) leg exercises, lying on side; (9) leg exercises, bicycle movements, supine; (10) sit-ups; (11) push-ups, not performed by all subjects; and (12) shoulder exercises, standing, cool-off. [Reproduced by permission from Hellerstein (57).]

Weight Training. Cardiac patients who need to develop strength for orthopedic reasons may use a low-resistance, high-repetition weight training program. However, patients should be cautioned to breathe properly, exhaling with each contraction, so as to avoid performing a Valsalva maneuver. Strength and muscular endurance training with light weights and high repetitions has some merit in cardiac patients who desire to return to occupations requiring moderate manual labor or frequent lifting. Since the magnitude of the pressor response to isometric work is directly related to the percentage of maximal voluntary contraction (MVC) (19), any increase in strength (MVC) should result in a lower blood pressure response to any given submaximal isometric load, since it represents a lower percentage of MVC.

Marathon Running. Reports documenting the unusually large coronary arteries (61) and superb cardiac performance (62) of marathon runners have led to speculation (63) that marathon running may promote "immunity to coronary heart disease." Marathon running has partaken of a cardiovascular mystique perpetuated by the familiar quotation that "no active marathoner has ever died of myocardial infarction" (63). The most recent extension of this belief has been advocacy of marathon running for cardiac rehabilitation patients.

Marathon running has many limitations that preclude its general use for cardiac rehabilitation (64):

· Marathon running offers little crossover of training benefit to the upper extremities (see the subsequent section on training specificity).
· Marathon running has limited application to the general ASHD population; fewer than 7 of 1000 patients who survive myocardial infarction can achieve by training the aerobic capacity ($\dot{V}O_2$ max) necessary to complete a marathon in 5 hr or less.
· Marathon running poses the risk of activity-induced cardiac arrest in a setting where cardiopulmonary resuscitation personnel and emergency equipment may be unavailable. Recent reports have documented fatal myocardial infarction in conjunction with marathon running (65) and training (66).
· The frequency, intensity, and duration of training required for marathon running far exceed the threshold necessary for development of an optimal training effect (44).

Other Daily Activities. In addition to a specific conditioning program, patients should be encouraged to perform greater activity in everyday living. Modification of previously sedentary habits through appropriate changes in attitude and behavior is important. Specific suggestions include avoiding elevators, walking instead of riding a vehicle, and parking farther away from stores when shopping. The merit of staircases as sources of exercise also deserves emphasis, since they are immediately available to every apartment dweller and office worker. A study of an at-work stair-climbing program in healthy men showed that a work load of 5500 kgm/day (approximately 25 flights for a 70-kg man) resulted in a significant increase in aerobic capacity (67). Similar or greater improvements may occur at reduced total work in cardiac patients with low baseline fitness levels.

Training Specificity

Training-induced lowering of heart rate and blood pressure response to arm exercise would appear to be desirable from a clinical standpoint. However, the effects of training on physiologic responses to arm exercise remain unclear. Few training studies have been conducted to date (68,69). Leg and arm training have been shown to have little (69) or no (68) transfer effect on arm and leg working capacity, respectively (Fig. 14); thus in subjects training by means of lower-extremity exercise, arm performance did not improve, and vice versa. The

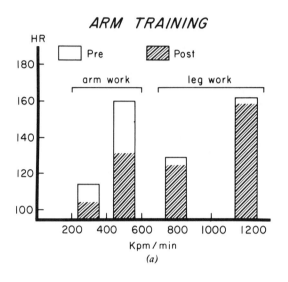

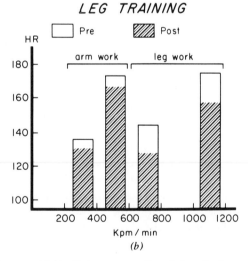

Figure 14. Training specificity. Importance of peripheral adaptation to training of arms (*a*) and legs (*b*). Arm training on the bicycle ergometer reduced heart rate during arm work but not during leg work. Similarly, leg training was associated with lower heart rate responses during leg exercise but not during arm exercise. [Adapted from Clausen et al. (68).]

implication is that a substantial portion of the conditioning response derives from peripheral adaptations (increased A-V oxygen extraction by exercising muscle) as well as cardiac adaptations.

The absence of cardiovascular crossover benefits of training between the upper extremities and the lower extremities has significant implications for the design of cardiac exercise training programs. Since few recreational and occupational activities require sustained lower-extremity activity (1,2), the rationale of restricting exercise to the lower extremities (e.g., walking-jogging format) appears questionable (64).

The principle of specificity of training has largely been ignored in the planning of most adult fitness and cardiac exercise training programs. Many cardiac reconditioning programs, with the exception of the ongoing National Exercise and Heart Disease Project (70), are based solely on leg training (i.e., walking, jogging, or stationary cycling). Such programs are limited in scope; they ignore the small group (approximately 8%) of patients who have significant limitations (orthopedic problems, arthritis, peripheral vascular disease) to performance of lower-extremity activity (64), and they fail to consider that daily living activities employ all major muscle groups (total fitness concept). An individual whose occupation requires mostly arm work needs to be concerned with training these muscle groups, with the expectation that the heart rate and blood pressure response will decrease with training. Since one of the primary objectives of cardiac rehabilitation is to prepare the individual for a return to an occupation and leisure-time physical activity, a physical conditioning program should include exercise for the arms and torso as well as the legs.

Specific recommendations include various trunk and upper-extremity exercises to supplement the chosen dynamic exercise mode. Examples of upper-body programs to be used in conjunction with jogging, walking, or cycling are sports such as volleyball, paddleball, or basketball or specific calisthenic exercises aimed at arm, shoulder, and trunk movement. Additional recommended exercises include rowing, arm ergometry, wall pulleys, shoulder wheels, gardening, raking, and sawing wood.

Cool-down Period

Disregard of the need for a cool-down period may be the most common cause of cardiovascular complications after exercise (49,53). During exercise, normal vasoconstriction yields to vasodilation in the active muscles to accommodate the increased volume of blood necessary to satisfy metabolic demands. The potential for accumulation of blood is nicely balanced by a milking action of the muscle on the veins that augments venous return and stroke volume. When exercise is suddenly stopped, the free flow into the limbs continues despite inactivation of the skeletal muscle pump. Compensatory adjustments in peripheral resistance secondary to the rapid fall in cardiac output may not occur instantaneously. Consequently, blood may accumulate or pool in the lower extremities until normal vasoconstriction is reestablished. The subsequent decrease in venous return may induce fainting or arrhythmias because of inadequate blood flow (and oxygen) to the brain and heart.

The best way to prevent pooling of blood in the limbs is to maintain the massaging action of the muscles through continued movement. A cool-down period (5–10 min) involving walking or low-intensity exercise usually permits appropriate circulatory readjustment and return of heart rate and blood pressure to near preexercise values, allows dissipation of heat load, and promotes more rapid removal of lactic acid than does stationary recovery (71).

Recreational Games

The inclusion of various enjoyable recreational activities in the conditioning format usually enhances program adherence. In cardiac reconditioning programs the games portion has a single objective—fun. Participation should be predicated on enjoyment of the game for its own sake (72); winning or losing should be secondary to play (42). However, care should be taken to ensure that games are modified to decrease the energy cost and heart rate response. Modifications should minimize skill requirements and competition and maximize the feeling of successful participation. To this end, the imaginative exercise leader may suggest a smaller court size, frequent player rotation, intermittent play, minor rules changes, and adjusted scoring rules (72). For example, volleyball played allowing one bounce of the ball per side facilitates longer rallies, provides additional fun, and minimizes the skill required to play the game. Many other team games and individual sports can be modified in similar fashion.

ADHERENCE

Since adherence to the training program plays an important role in determining the magnitude of the conditioning response, the factors that affect adherence

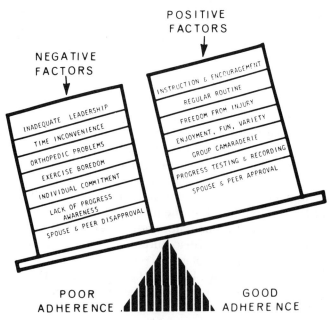

Figure 15. Factors affecting adherence to a physical conditioning program. Negative factors often outweigh positive factors, resulting in poor adherence.

must be considered in any prescription. Exercise testing and training are often overemphasized at the expense of the counseling, leadership, education, and motivation phases of the program. As a result, negative factors often outweigh the positive factors contributing to sustained participant interest (Fig. 15); adherence declines, and the effectiveness of the program diminishes.

Adherence to long-term exercise programs can have a wide range, from poor to excellent (57,73). Designers of the more successful programs have recognized and made provision for the following important factors: comprehensive program design; preliminary and follow-up evaluations (retesting), with feedback of results; exclusion of subjects with specific contraindications; supervision; recreational aspects and camaraderie stimuli; regularity of sessions; positive attitudes of spouses toward the program (74); freedom from injury (55); reward system, with recognition and symbols of participation.

ENVIRONMENTAL FACTORS

Dynamic exercise in cold weather is relatively safe if proper clothing is worn to avoid exposure of the lower neck and chest to abnormally high rates of cooling. Excessive cooling may trigger reflexes that can cause constriction of coronary blood vessels and result in decreased myocardial oxygen supply. For those who suffer from angina when inhaling cold air (75), discomfort can be reduced or alleviated by wearing a face mask to warm the inspired air. The incidence of cardiovascular accidents is high among middle-aged men who perform hard work that involves an isometric component in a cold environment. The increase in myocardial oxygen consumption due to the increased heart rate, coupled with the substantial rise in blood pressure prompted by isometric work, makes snow shoveling a particularly dangerous activity for individuals at high risk.

Exercise in hot and humid weather may constitute an even greater hazard for the postcoronary exerciser. First, body temperature rises rapidly in response to exercise. This leads to a shunting of blood from the core to the periphery (skin) and causes excessive sweating. These mechanisms cause a reduction in effective circulating blood volume and a subsequent drop in blood pressure (76). Heart rate and myocardial oxygen consumption increase disproportionately to keep up with increasing metabolic demands. Men who are not acclimated to heat and who are exposed to temperatures greater than 24°C experience added heart rate increases of 1 beat/min/°C while exercising (Fig. 16) and 2–4 beats/min/°C with concomitant increased humidity (77). Finally, loss of sweat causes alterations in serum and cellular electrolytes (sodium and potassium), which can affect heart rhythm.

Specific suggestions for exercising in warm weather include the following:

· Maintain salt–water balance by drinking plenty of fluid (either water or a weak salt solution).
· Decrease exercise dosage at temperatures above 27°C and/or at 75% relative humidity. Under hyperthermic conditions, reduced speed or resistance will achieve the THR.
· Wear a light nylon running shirt (preferably mesh) and running shorts to facilitate cooling by evaporation. Rubberized clothing, often worn for "en-

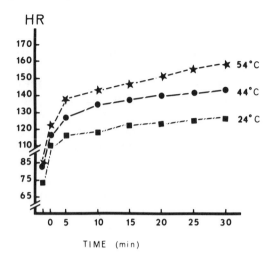

Figure 16. Influence of environmental temperature on heart rate responses at constant exercise work load. Heart rate increases approximately 1 beat/min for each degree Celsius increment in ambient temperature above 24°C. [Adapted from Pandolf et al. (77).]

hancement of weight loss," blocks sweat loss and deprives the body of its normal mechanism for cooling.

METABOLIC REQUIREMENTS IN ACTIVITY PRESCRIPTION

Exercise stress tests yield both diagnostic and functional information. The functional assessment is often based on the oxygen cost required to perform a given external work load. If not measured directly, the oxygen requirement can be obtained from published data by using the body weight of the individual and the treadmill speed and percentage grade or the bicycle ergometer resistance setting (6). When these parameters are defined, the external work load (if performed for 3 min or more) can be translated to an oxygen cost (corrected for body weight) that will not differ significantly from one individual to the next. For example, an individual at supine rest theoretically has an oxygen uptake of approximately 3.5 ml/kg bw/min. This metabolic requirement is defined as 1 met. The subject who negotiates a treadmill walk at 2 mph on a level grade has a mean oxygen requirement of 7.0 ml/kg/min or 2 mets.

The metabolic costs of many household, recreational, and occupational activities have been defined in terms of oxygen uptake (6). Consequently, activity prescription might also be made in terms of the metabolic equivalent (mets). This involves recommendation of activities that are sufficiently below the maximal metabolic rate achieved during exercise testing. For example, let us consider a subject who has a $\dot{V}O_2$ max of 28 ml/kg/min (8 mets) and associated highest heart rate of 170 beats/min. His recommended training intensities at average expenditure and peak expenditure during the training session are 16 and 22 ml/kg/min, with heart rates 120 and 144 beats/min, respectively. Table 4 in Chapter 9 provides a wide choice of activities for these energy levels: for average expenditure, walking at 3.0–3.5 mph, cycling at 8 mph, table tennis, dancing foxtrot, raking leaves, etc.; for peak expenditure, jogging at 4.5–5 mph, cycling at 11 mph, singles tennis, square dancing, etc. However, activities requiring expenditure of 8 mets or more would appear to be contraindicated, since presumably they would require maximal or supermaximal efforts. The concept is attractive and easy to understand, and it is frequently adopted as a training and activity prescription guide. However, there are several inherent limitations to the approach:

One shortcoming in prescribing exercise in terms of mets is the assumption that 1 met = 3.5 ml/kg/min. In our experience and in the experience of others (5) this underestimates the resting metabolic rate. Oxygen consumption during standing at rest is closer to 4.0 ml/kg/min, and this is probably a more appropriate value for 1 met. Multiples of this value would more nearly represent the actual work being undertaken when exercise is being performed in the upright position. Prescriptions for sitting and supine exercise should use the resting metabolic rates appropriate for them.

Another limitation is that met values of selected physical activities represent average energy expenditure levels, and these levels may vary considerably among individuals. The manner in which individuals participate in activity varies widely in terms of energy expenditure, ranging from the lackadaisical to the frenetic (6). Metabolic demands are also highly dependent on speed and efficiency (skill). Activities that are little affected by the skill of the performer include walking, jogging, and cycling. On the other hand, the experienced tennis player may expend an average of 5 mets during singles tennis, whereas the novice may be working at 7 mets. Table 4 in Chapter 9 lists singles tennis at 5–7 mets. Even one's competition during sports or recreational activity may alter the metabolic cost of the activity.

It cannot be assumed that all occupational work demanding oxygen consumption equal to that registered during leg exercise testing produces similar heart rate and systolic blood pressure responses (myocardial oxygen demand). Additional factors at work include the stresses of emotions, excitement, cognition, and climate (temperature and humidity), as well as activation of muscle groups not used during the exercise tests. For example, in our studies of surgeons we found that during an operation the average energy expenditure was low (1.5 mets/min); however, myocardial oxygen consumption as estimated from the HR × SBP product was equal to that of hard work in a steel mill (3–4 mets). Upper-extremity effort produces another disproportionate $M\dot{V}O_2/\dot{V}O_2$ response. Arm exercise performed at 70–85% maximal heart rate is equal to only 40–55% of $\dot{V}O_2$ max achieved during leg exercise. Thus, consideration of only oxygen consumption during work does not necessarily give an accurate estimate of cardiac demand.

Finally, the oxygen costs listed in Table 4 of Chapter 9 were derived from continuous steady-state work ($\geq$ 3 min), whereas the activities of daily life are predominantly intermittent rather than continuous. According to the table, a patient with a 5-met capacity should refrain from gardening (a requirement of 5–7 mets), since presumably it represents maximal or supermaximal effort. However, if the activity is performed intermittently (i.e., 2 min work, 1 min rest), the task can easily be accomplished at oxygen consumption levels well below

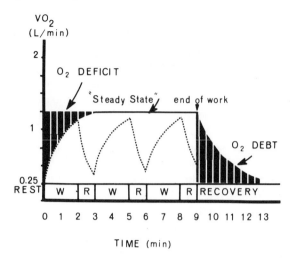

Figure 17. Oxygen uptake during intermittent effort that requires 1.25 liters of oxygen per minute during continuous effort. Oxygen consumption for the same activity performed intermittently [2 min of work (W) followed by 1 min of rest (R)] is shown by broken line. Oxygen consumption is lower during intermittent exercise than for continuous exercise because of partial repayment of oxygen debt during interspersed rest periods.

those estimated for the task (Fig. 17). Thus, by using the met concept, one may considerably underestimate the patient's capacity for physical work.

In summary, the met concept appears to have limited applicability in the recommendation of activities for cardiac patients. Heart rate response immediately after exertion will usually provide a better assessment of exertional demands than will metabolic equivalent tables.

REVISION OF EXERCISE PRESCRIPTION AND EVALUATION OF EXERCISE THERAPY

Fitness testing should be performed prior to the conditioning program and at intervals of 3–6 months during the conditioning program in order to assess the cardiac patient's response or lack of response to the exercise stimulus. Favorable cardiovascular adaptations to a physical conditioning program include decreased heart rate and systolic blood pressure at rest and at submaximal work loads, decreased myocardial oxygen requirements for comparable levels of submaximal work, increased working capacity, and decreased evidence of cardiac arrhythmias, especially premature ventricular contractions.

Periodic multistage exercise testing allows the exercise prescription to be appropriately modified. Recommendations may include increased, decreased, or unchanged exercise dosage, discontinuation of training, and/or recommendation for further diagnostic studies, coronary arteriography, and possibly revascularization surgery. Following reappraisal and medical or surgical intervention, the physician may return the patient to a reconditioning program.

Medication and dosage adjustments should be modified at the time of reevaluation. For example, conditioning bradycardia at rest and during submaximal work (thus decreasing cardiac work) may obviate or reduce the need for β-adrenergic blocking agents and/or nitrate drugs. Since progressive conditioning exercise may decrease the frequency of exercise-induced premature ventricular contractions (78), antiarrhythmic agents may possibly be decreased in dosage or even discontinued. Antihypertensive drugs may also need adjustment, since physical conditioning has been shown to have a beneficial effect on blood pressure, particularly in hypertensive individuals. Conversely, deterioration of cardiac status and performance may be compensated with appropriate increases in medication and/or dosage.

Finally, exercise testing with feedback of results provides an excellent way to motivate the individual to continue participation in the conditioning program. Exercise-induced reduction of body fat stores, increased cardiorespiratory reserves, and improved serum lipid profile are powerful motivators toward renewed enthusiasm and dedication.

FAILURE TO RESPOND TO TRAINING

It is helpful to be able to predict which patients will benefit from investing time and effort in a physical conditioning program. The primary determinants are the underlying disease process, the program design, and the patient's participation.

Underlying Disease Process

Patients who are unable to perform at 2 mets (equivalent to 2 mph at zero grade or 150–300 kpm/min) are considered to be ineligible for participation in exercise training programs. Patients who have poor rehabilitation potential often show reduced inotropic and/or chronotropic reserves, severe angina pectoris, ventricular dyskinesis and/or aneurysm, frequent early uniform (R on T) or multiform ventricular ectopic beats, or pronounced ST-T displacement during or after exercise. Despite demonstration of a significant correlation between aerobic capacity and infarct size, the latter has proved to be a poor predictor of the subject's ability to increase aerobic power with exercise training (79).

Our experience indicates that approximately 15% of myocardial infarction patients show minimal improvement or no improvement, despite faithful attendance and active participation in exercise programs. Angiograms have demonstrated severe involvement of the three major coronary arteries and 90% or more stenosis of two arteries (80). Thus the severity and/or progression of the underlying coronary disease represent major obstacles to improvement. In such patients, earlier consideration is now being given to surgical intervention. Coronary arteriograms are considered valuable in excluding patients unlikely to profit from a conditioning program (80).

Other Factors

Lack of improvement may be due to intercurrent illness or injury (e.g., concomitant disease, surgery, orthopedic complications), inadequate adherence to the exercise prescription, exercising below the threshold necessary for improvement, failure of supervision, or poor motivation. Improvement may be negated by the substantial reduction in aerobic capacity that results from as little as 1–3 weeks of inactivity (particularly bed rest due to illness or injury) (81).

Proscription of Practices That Modify Training Responses or Are Potentially Hazardous

Participants must be cautioned against certain practices that can counteract the benefits of exercise and are potentially dangerous. Some of the more important proscriptions follow.

Avoid ingestion of large meals, coffee, and other xanthine-containing beverages less than 2 hr before and within 1 hr after exercise. Large meals tend to divert a greater portion of the cardiac output to mesenteric vascular beds and produce marked shifts in serum electrolytes. Meals and xanthines can cause significant electrocardiographic changes, including arrhythmias and ischemic ST-T changes.

Abstain from alcohol prior to exercise and after exercise. Alcohol has a negative inotropic effect on the myocardium, and it possibly could produce temporary vasoconstriction (82).

Avoid wearing heavy clothes during sustained high levels of effort. Heart rate and blood pressure responses to steady-state exercise are consistently higher when one is wearing heavy clothing or rubberized sweat suits that interfere with heat loss than when wearing shorts (13). Thus at a given external work load the myocardial oxygen consumption becomes disproportionately high compared to the body's oxygen intake.

Avoid hot showers, saunas, and steam baths before and immediately after exercise. The added heat stress of a sauna or hot shower diverts blood to the periphery and may deprive the central circulation of returning blood. Consequences may include a rapid fall in blood pressure and/or serious cardiac arrhythmias. Sudden syncopal attacks when standing up to leave a sauna are not uncommon. Normal subjects and myocardial infarction patients have been shown to develop electrocardiographic evidence of myocardial ischemia and frequent ectopic beats on exposure to the intense heat of a sauna (83). Acute myocardial infarction and ventricular fibrillation have occurred during hot showers following normal responses to maximal exercise tests (84). Patients should be advised to refrain from saunas and steam baths and allow for adequate recovery from active exercise (at least 15 min) before taking a shower, preferably lukewarm.

Avoid spasmodic exercise efforts. Attempting to crowd all of one's exercise into 1 day per week may result in excessive fatigue and musculoskeletal and cardiovascular strain. Furthermore, an increase in the blood clotting mechanism may occur with sporadic high-level exercise bouts (85).

Avoid exercise during illness. Certain illnesses cause dehydration and reduction of blood volume, whereas others may predispose the individual to arrhythmias. Patients should be cautioned against exercise during illness or when unduly fatigued. Furthermore, the exercise dosage should be reduced following a period of inactivity due to illness or injury.

Tobacco should not be smoked, preferably not at any time, but particularly not before or after exercise. Smoking tobacco tends to negate the gains made by exercise training, and it imposes additional stresses on the cardiorespiratory system. Specific adverse effects include increased heart rate (15–20 beats/min) and peripheral resistance, increased cardiac work, increased circulating levels of noradrenaline, increased myocardial irritability, and increased formation of carboxyhemoglobin, which decreases (5–10%) the effective oxygen-carrying capacity of the blood.

Reduce the intensity of effort in extremes of temperature and humidity. The reasons for this proscription are discussed in a preceding section on environmental factors.

REFERENCES

1. Ford AB, Hellerstein HK: Work and heart disease. I. A physiologic study in the factory. *Circulation* 18:823, 1958

2. Ford AB, Hellerstein HK, Turell DJ: Work and heart disease. II. A physiologic study in a steel mill. *Circulation* 20:537, 1959

3. Hellerstein HK, Banerja JC, Biorck G, et al: Rehabilitation of Patients with Cardiovascular Diseases. *WHO Tech Rep Ser* 270, 1964

4. Jones NL, Campbell EJM, Edwards RT, et al: *Clinical Exercise Testing.* WB Saunders, Philadelphia, 1975

5. Sivarajan ES, Lerman J, Mansfield LW, et al: Progressive ambulation and treadmill testing of patients with acute myocardial infarction during hospitalization: A feasibility study. *Arch Phys Med Rehabil* 58:241, 1977

6. Hellerstein HK, Brock LL, Bruce RA, et al: *Exercise Testing and Training of Apparently Healthy Individuals: A Handbook for Physicians.* Committee on Exercise, American Heart Association, New York, 1972; *Exercise Testing and Training of Individuals with Heart Disease or at High Risk for Its Development. A Handbook for Physicians.* Committee on Exercise, American Heart Association, New York, 1975

7. Ellestad MH: *Stress Testing Principles and Practice.* FA Davis, Philadelphia, 1975

8. Naughton JP, Hellerstein HK (eds): *Exercise Testing and Exercise Training in Coronary Heart Disease.* Academic Press, New York, 1973

9. Bruce RA: Progress in Exercise Cardiology. In Ye PN, Goodwin JF (eds): *Progress in Cardiology.* Lea & Febiger, Philadelphia, 1974, p 113

10. Blomqvist CG: Clinical Exercise Physiology. In Wenger NK, Hellerstein HK (eds): *Rehabilitation of the Coronary Patient.* John Wiley, New York, 1978

11. Barnard RJ, Gardner GW, Diaco NV, et al: Cardiovascular response to sudden strenuous exercise—heart rate, blood pressure and ECG. *J Appl Physiol* 34:833, 1973

12. Shephard RJ, Allen C, Benade AJS, et al: The maximum oxygen intake. An international reference standard of cardiorespiratory fitness. *Bull WHO* 38:757, 1968

13. Hellerstein HK, Hirsch EZ, Ader R, et al: Principles of exercise prescription. Normals and cardiac subjects. In Naughton JP, Hellerstein HK (eds): *Exercise Testing and Exercise Training in Coronary Heart Disease.* Academic Press, New York, 1973, p 129

14. Fardy PS, Webb D, Hellerstein HK: Benefits of arm exercise in cardiac rehabilitation. *The Physician and Sports Medicine* Oct 1977, p 31

15. Bevegard S, Freyschuss U, Strandell T: Circulatory adaptation to arm and leg exercise in supine and sitting positions. *J Appl Physiol* 21:37, 1966

16. Secher N, Ruberg-Larsen H, Binkhorst RA, et al: Maximal oxygen uptake during arm cranking and combined arm plus leg exercise. *J Appl Physiol* 36:515, 1974

17. Bergh U, Kanstrup IL, Ekblom B: Maximal oxygen uptake during exercise with various combinations of arm and leg work. *J Appl Physiol* 41:191, 1976

18. Schwade J, Blomqvist CG, Shapiro W: A comparison of the response to arm and leg work in patients with ischemic heart disease. *Am Heart J* 94:203, 1977

19. Donald KW, Lind AR, McNicol GW, et al: Cardiovascular responses to sustained (static) contractions. *Circ Res* 20–21(Suppl 1):I-15, 1967

20. Elisberg EI: Heart rate response to the Valsalva maneuver as a test of circulatory integrity. *JAMA* 186:120, 1973

21. Levin AB: A simple test of cardiac function based upon the heart rate changes induced by the Valsalva maneuver. *Am J Cardiol* 18:90, 1966

22. Levison H, Cherniak RM: Ventilatory cost of exercise in chronic obstructive pulmonary disease. *J Appl Physiol* 25:21, 1968

23. Wenger NK, Hellerstein HK, Blackburn H, et al: Uncomplicated myocardial infarction: Current physician practice in patient management. *JAMA* 224:511, 1973

24. Ericsson M, Granath A, Ohlsen P, et al: Arrhythmias and symptoms during treadmill testing three weeks after myocardial infarction in 100 patients. *Br Heart J* 135:787, 1973

25. Hellerstein HK: Exercise therapy and coronary heart disease. Rehabilitation and secondary prevention. In de Haas JH, Hemker HC, Snellen HA (eds): *Ischaemic Heart Disease. Boerhaave Series for Postgraduate Medical Education.* University Press, Leiden, Holland, 1970, p 406

26. Bruce RA: Principles of exercise testing. In Naughton JP, Hellerstein HK (eds): *Exercise Testing and Exercise Training in Coronary Heart Disease.* Academic Press, New York, 1973, p 45

27. Kitamura K, Jorgensen CR, Taylor HL, et al: Hemodynamic correlates of myocardial oxygen consumption during upright exercise. *J Appl Physiol* 32:516, 1972

28. Nelson RR, Gobel FL, Jorgensen CR, et al: Hemodynamic predictors of myocardial oxygen consumption during static and dynamic exercise. *Circulation* 50:1179, 1974

29. Bruce RA, Fisher LD, Cooper MN, et al: Separation of effects of cardiovascular disease and age on ventricular function with maximal exercise. *Am J Cardiol* 34:757, 1974

30. Blomqvist G: The Frank lead exercise electrocardiogram. A quantitative study based on averaging technic and digital computer analysis. *Acta Med Scand [Suppl]* 178:1, 1965

31. Lester FM, Sheffield LT, Reeves JT: Electrocardiographic changes in clinically normal older men following near maximal and maximal exercise. *Circulation* 36:5, 1967

32. Sheffield LT, Holt JH, Lester FM, et al: On-line analysis of the exercise electrocardiogram. *Circulation* 40:935, 1969

33. Radke JE, Hellerstein HK, Salzman SH, et al: The quantitative effects of physical conditioning on the exercise electrocardiogram of subjects with arteriosclerotic heart disease and normal subjects. In Brunner D, Jokl E (eds): *Physical Activity and Aging.* S Karger, Basel, 1970, p 168

34. McHenry PL, Phillips JF, Knoebel SB: Correlation of computer-quantitated treadmill exercise electrocardiogram with arteriographic location of coronary artery disease. *Am J Cardiol* 30:747, 1972

35. Simoons ML, Hugenholtz PG: Estimation of the probability of exercise-induced ischemia by quantitative ECG analysis. *Circulation* 56:552, 1977

36. Erikssen J, Enge I, Forfang K, et al: False positive diagnostic tests and coronary arteriographic findings in 105 presumably healthy males. *Circulation* 54:371, 1976

37. McHenry PL, Fisch C: Clinical applications of the treadmill exercise test. *Mod Concepts Cardiovasc Dis* 46:21, 1977

38. Ellestad MH, Wan MKC: Predictive implication of stress testing: Follow-up of 2700 subjects after maximum treadmill stress testing. *Circulation* 51:363, 1975

39. Simonson E: *Differentiation Between Normal and Abnormal in Electrocardiography.* CV Mosby, St Louis, 1961

40. Rifkin RD, Hood WB Jr: Bayesian analysis of electrocardiographic exercise stress testing. *N Engl J Med* 297:681, 1977

41. McHenry PL, Morris SN, Kavalier M, et al: Comparative study of exercise-induced ventricular arrhythmias in normal subjects and patients with documented coronary artery disease. *Am J Cardiol* 37:609, 1976

42. Stoedefalke KG: Physical fitness programs for adults. *Am J Cardiol* 33:787, 1974

43. Åstrand PO, Rodahl K: *Textbook of Work Physiology.* McGraw-Hill, New York, 1970

44. Pollock ML: Quantification of endurance training programs. In Wilmore JH (ed): *Exercise and Sport Science Reviews, Vol 1.* Academic Press, New York, 1973, p 155

45. Shephard RJ: Intensity, duration and frequency of exercise as determinants of the response to a training regime. *Int Zeit Angew Physiol* 26:272, 1968

46. Karvonen MJ, Kentala E, Mustala O: The effects of training on heart rate. *Ann Med Exp Ferm* 35:307, 1957

47. Davies CTM, Knibbs AV: The training stimulus: The effects of intensity, duration and frequency of effort on maximum aerobic power output. *Int Zeit Angew Physiol* 29:299, 1971

48. Pollock ML, Broida J, Kendrick Z, et al: Effects of training two days per week at different intensities on middle-aged men. *Med Sci Sports* 4:192, 1972

49. Mead WF, Pyfer HR, Trombold JC, et al: Successful resuscitation of two near simultaneous cases of cardiac arrest with a review of fifteen cases occurring during supervised exercise. *Circulation* 53:187, 1976

50. Gualtiere WS, Zohman LR, Lopez RH, et al: Effects of physical training on cardiorespiratory capacity of patients with angina pectoris. Cited in Naughton JH, Hellerstein HK (eds): *Exercise Testing and Exercise Training in Coronary Heart Disease.* Academic Press, New York, 1973, p 166 (reference 26)

51. Siegel W, Blomqvist GB, Mitchell JH: Effects of a quantitated physical training program on middle-aged sedentary men. *Circulation* 41:19, 1970

52. Hollmann W, Venrath H: Experimentalle Untersuchungen zur Bedeutung eines Trainings unterhalf und oberhalb der Dauerbelastungsgrenze. In Korbs W, et al (eds): *Carl Diem Festschrift.* Frankfurt, a. M/Wein, 1962.

53. Dehn MM, Mullins CB: Physiologic effects and importance of exercise in patients with coronary artery disease. *Cardiovasc Med* 2 April 1977, p 365

54. Roskamm H: Optimum patterns of exercise for healthy adults. *Can Med Assoc J* 96:895, 1967

55. Pollock ML, Gettman LR, Milesis CA, et al: Effects of frequency and duration of training on attrition and incidence of injury. *Med Sci Sports* 9:31, 1977

56. Cumming GR: Variations in exercise and recovery stroke volumes. In: Proceedings 6th Annual Meeting, Canadian Association of Sports Science, Vancouver, October 1972. Williams & Wilkins, Baltimore, 1973

57. Hellerstein HK: Exercise therapy in coronary disease. *Bull NY Acad Med* 44:1028, 1968

58. Pollock ML, Dimmick J, Miller HS, et al: Effects of mode of training on cardiovascular function and body composition of adult men. *Med Sci Sports* 7:139, 1975

59. Holmer I, Åstrand PO: Swimming training and maximal oxygen uptake. *J Appl Physiol* 33:510, 1972

60. Baker JA: Comparison of rope skipping and jogging as methods of improving cardiovascular efficiency of college men. *Res Quart* 39:240, 1968

61. Currens J, White PD: Half a century of running. *N Engl J Med* 265:988, 1961

62. Costill DL: Metabolic response during distance running. *J Appl Physiol* 28:251, 1970

63. Bassler TJ: Marathon running and immunity to heart disease. *The Physician and Sports Medicine* 3:77, 1975

64. Hellerstein HK: Limitations of marathon running in the rehabilitation of coronary patients; anatomic and physiologic determinants. The marathon: physiological, medical, epidemiological and psychological studies. *Ann NY Acad Sci* 301:484, 1977

65. Green LH, Cohen SI, Kurland G: Fatal myocardial infarction in marathon running. *Ann Intern Med* 84:704, 1976

66. Ullyot J: The medical report. *Runner's World* 11 September, 1976, p 16

67. Fardy PS, Ilmarinen J: Evaluating the effects and feasibility of an at work stairclimbing intervention program for men. *Med Sci Sports* 7:91, 1975

68. Clausen JP, Trap-Jensen J, Lassen NA: The effects of training on the heart rate during arm and leg exercise. *Scand J Clin Lab Invest* 26:295, 1970

69. Clausen JP, Klausen K, Rasmussen B, et al: Central and peripheral circulatory changes after training of arms and legs. *Am J Physiol* 225:675, 1973

70. National Exercise and Heart Disease Project: Common protocol, 1975. Coordinating Center, George Washington Medical Center, Washington, DC

71. Belcastro AN, Bonen A: Lactic acid removal rates during controlled and uncontrolled recovery exercise. *J Appl Physiol* 39:932, 1975

72. Oldridge NB: What to look for in an exercise class leader. *The Physician and Sports Medicine* April 1977, p 85

73. Wilhelmsen L, Sanne H, Elmfeldt D, et al: A controlled trial of physical training after myocardial infarction: Effects on risk factors, nonfatal reinfarction, and death. *Prev Med* 4:491, 1975

74. Heinzelmann F, Bagley R: Response to physical activity programs and their effects on health behavior. *Public Health Rep* 85:905, 1970

75. Hattenhauer M, Neil WA: The effect of cold air inhalation on angina pectoris and myocardial oxygen supply. *Circulation* 51:1053, 1975

76. Rowell LB, Marz HJ, Bruce RA, et al: Reductions in cardiac output, central blood volume and stroke volume with thermal stress in normal men during exercise. *J Clin Invest* 45:1801, 1966

77. Pandolf KB, Cafarelli E, Noble BJ, et al: Hyperthermia: Effect on exercise prescription. *Arch Phys Med Rehabil* 56:524, 1975

78. Blackburn H, Taylor HL, Hamrell B, et al: Premature ventricular complexes induced by stress testing: Their frequency and response to physical conditioning. *Am J Cardiol* 31:441, 1973

79. Carter CL, Amundsen LR: Infarct size and exercise capacity after myocardial infarction. *J Appl Physiol Respir Environ Exercise Physiol* 42:782, 1977

80. Hellerstein HK: Anatomic factors influencing effects of exercise therapy of ASHD subjects. In Roskamm H, Reindell H (eds): *Das Chronisch Kranke Herz.* FK Schattauer Verlag, Stuttgart, 1973, p 513

81. Saltin B, Blomqvist G, Mitchell JH, et al: Response to exercise after bed rest and after training. A longitudinal study of adaptive changes in oxygen transport and body composition. *Circulation* 38(Suppl 7):1, 1968

82. Webb WR, Degerli IU: Ethyl alcohol and the cardiovascular system. *JAMA* 191:1055, 1965

83. Taggart P, Parkinson P, Carruthers M: Cardiac responses to thermal, physical, and emotional stress. *Br Med J* 3:71, 1972

84. Bruce RA, Hornsten TR, Blackmon JR: Myocardial infarction after normal responses to maximal exercise. *Circulation* 38:552, 1968

85. Burt JJ, Blyth CS, Rierson HA: The effect of exercise on the coagulation fibrinolysis. *J Sports Medicine* 4:213, 1964

9

Design and Implementation of Cardiac Conditioning Programs

William L. Haskell, Ph.D.

When a patient is discharged from the hospital following a myocardial infarction, a major concern is what physical activities can and should be performed. There will be numerous questions regarding job-related functions and leisure-time activities. The patient may want to know about undertaking an exercise program to develop cardiovascular capacity, to lose weight, or to regain muscle strength. Advising a patient to take it easy or to exercise moderately is no longer adequate. The patient needs specific information about activities that can be performed relatively safely, instructions on how to perform these activities, and advice about activities to be avoided. The physician should provide each patient with a concise exercise recommendation or prescription tailored to fit the patient's functional capacity, needs, and interests. The patient's interests, skills, and experience at various physical activities must be considered, as well as the accessibility of appropriate exercise equipment, facilities, and programs. Exercise recommendations should be formulated with the same care and precision used in prescribing other therapies. An overdose of exercise can produce new clinical manifestations of coronary atherosclerotic heart disease, including sudden cardiac death, whereas inappropriate activity restriction can result in cardiovascular deconditioning, psychologic trauma, and economic disability (Table 1).

The physical activity component of a comprehensive rehabilitation program must meet the patient's specific needs during each stage of recovery. For the patient discharged from the hospital after an uncomplicated myocardial infarction, an exercise plan can be organized into three stages:

· a posthospitalization convalescent period lasting from discharge to 8–20 weeks post infarction

Table 1. Contraindications to Exercise Training and Conditions Requiring Special Precautions[a]

Absolute contraindications
1. Congestive heart failure, uncontrolled
2. Recent myocardial infarction
3. Active myocarditis or pericarditis
4. Unstable angina pectoris
5. Recent systemic or pulmonary embolism
6. Acute infections
7. Thrombophlebitis
8. Ventricular tachycardia and other ventricular dysrhythmias
9. Severe ventricular outflow obstruction
10. Untreated severe systemic or pulmonary hypertension

Relative contraindications
1. Uncontrolled supraventricular dysrhythmias
2. Ventricular aneurysm
3. Moderate aortic stenosis
4. Uncontrolled metabolic disease (diabetes, thyrotoxicosis, myxedema)
5. Marked cardiac enlargement
6. Severe anemia
7. Overt psychoneurotic disturbance requiring therapy
8. Neuromuscular or musculoskeletal disorder that would prevent activity

Conditions requiring special consideration and/or precautions
1. Conduction disturbance
   a. Complete atrioventricular block
   b. Left bundle branch block
   c. Wolff-Parkinson-White syndrome
2. Fixed-rate cardiac pacemaker
3. Certain medication
   a. Digitalis
   b. β-adrenergic blocking agents and drugs of related action
4. Angina pectoris
5. Marked obesity

[a]Adapted from Fox SM, Naughton JP, Haskell WL: Physical activity and the prevention of coronary heart disease. *Ann Clin Res* 3:404, 1971.

· physical reconditioning activities that begin at the end of convalescence and continue until appropriate functional capacity is achieved
· activity maintenance, which lasts indefinitely

Systematic physical activity for each stage of recovery should be prescribed by a knowledgeable physician after a careful evaluation and should be supervised and monitored by the physician or by well-trained allied health personnel. The precise steps in the evaluation, supervision, and monitoring will depend on the patient's clinical and functional status. As recovery progresses, the specific activities performed and the immediate objectives of the exercise plan will change, but the general principles of exercise evaluation, prescription, and training will remain the same.

The formulation of an exercise plan can be accomplished during a routine office visit, or the patient may be referred to a physician with special interest and expertise in exercise testing and training. Increasing numbers of medically supervised cardiac exercise programs are being set up in communities throughout the country. The American Heart Association listing of many of these facilities, a directory of cardiac rehabilitation units, can be obtained from any local heart association.

The guidelines and suggestions in this chapter will provide the general principles of design and implementation of physical activity programs for cardiac patients. An exact exercise plan for a particular patient must be determined by a physician. The interactions among the various circumstances that influence exercise programming for a specific patient require that each plan be individualized and that it be altered as the patient's status changes. The values given here for exercise conditioning responses of patients; the guidelines for intensity, frequency, and duration of the exercise program; and the instructions for program modification as a result of exercise conditioning should constitute a frame of reference and may not be applicable to all patients.

Whenever exercise is recommended for a cardiac patient, whether medically supervised or not, its guidelines should ensure that a relatively safe and effective plan is carried out. Adherence to these guidelines by the medical team and the patient makes it likely that exercise will be performed without major complications and with enhancement of cardiovascular functional capacity. However, as with other cardiovascular therapy, no absolute assurance of safety and benefit can be ascribed to exercise training for a specific patient.

PATIENT EVALUATION: BASIS OF AN INDIVIDUALIZED EXERCISE PLAN

A cardiac patient's exercise plan should be determined by objective assessment of clinical status, functional capacity, and exercise needs. What may be good for one patient may prove detrimental for the next. There are numerous medical conditions that are temporary contraindications to an increase in physical activity, and these can be determined only by cardiovascular evaluation, including multilevel exercise testing. Some common contraindications to increased physical activity and some conditions that require that exercise conditioning be closely monitored and supervised are discussed in Chapter 8. Exercise tolerance indicates the exercise intensity at which the patient becomes fatigued and does not wish to continue or at which clinical contraindications to further exercise occur. Medical evaluation and exercise testing procedures for exercise prescription were described in Chapter 8.

In addition to making a medical evaluation, the physician must determine, by questionnaire or interview, the patient's exercise needs, interests, abilities, and previous habits. This information, combined with knowledge of the exercise equipment, facilities, and programs available to the patient, can be used to develop an individualized exercise plan, one that can be carried out with a minimum of inconvenience, that the patient has the skill to perform, and that might be found enjoyable or at least not unpleasant. These considerations are important if the patient is to make successful long-term changes in exercise habits.

EXERCISE CHARACTERISTICS

The individualized exercise plan should be characterized according to type, intensity, duration, and frequency of exercise (see Chapter 8). Appropriate activities should be selected, and guidelines should be prepared regarding how, when, where, and under what conditions these activities are to be performed. Precautions regarding when not to exercise should also be included.

The selection of physical activities and the description of how they are to be performed by the cardiac patient must take into consideration both safety and conditioning effectiveness. Patient safety relates primarily to the myocardial oxygen demands made by the activity. Conditioning effectiveness requires that exercise stress of adequate intensity, duration, and frequency be exerted on the cardiovascular and metabolic systems, particularly sustained increases in cardiac output and in energy expenditure by a large skeletal muscle mass. Thus the exercise design should be such that during peak exercise the myocardial oxygen demand will remain within the oxygen supply limitations while producing a sustained increase in oxygen delivery to exercising muscles.

Type of Exercise

Exercises that increase metabolic, cardiovascular, and respiratory function are necessary to achieve the desired adaptation in functional capacity (6). The activities selected should involve rhythmic low-resistance contractions of large muscle masses of the legs and trunk that are performed aerobically. These activities can include walking, jogging, stationary and regular cycling, swimming, bench stepping, certain continuous rhythmic calisthenics and selected active sports or games, self-care activities, household chores, and occupational tasks.

The physician and the patient should select activities that are pleasurable and that do not produce discomfort. Emphasis should be placed on active recreational games and on ways to use commonplace opportunities for exercise, such as walking, climbing stairs, and gardening.

For exercise prescription, activities can be classified according to the difficulty involved in regulating their intensity. Activities whose exercise intensities can be easily prescribed by the physician and maintained by the patient include walking, jogging, and cycling. A constant work-rate can be maintained, and the interindividual variability of energy cost at any given velocity is small. Activities in which work-rate is easily maintained but that have wide interindividual variation in energy cost at a given work load often involve particular skills. For example, swimming with a given stroke at a specified velocity may have an energy cost three or four times greater for an inefficient swimmer than for an efficient swimmer; this difference may occur even if they have the same exercise capacity. The third type of exercise includes activities in which exercise intensity varies greatly and is sporadic in nature (e.g., dancing, most sports and games, and mountain climbing or hiking).

Thus walking, cycling, and bench stepping are useful activities during the early phases of rehabilitation when precise control of effort is necessary to ensure that patients do not exceed their exercise tolerance. These activities continue to be useful during all phases of a cardiac exercise program because, in addition to the element of control, they enable the patient to expend the most energy per unit time and readily see improvements, plateaus, or recidivism in performance.

If activities in the exercise plan involve a significant amount of arm work, a lower exercise intensity, as determined by energy cost, will be required to achieve the prescribed target heart rate. Dynamic arm work produces higher heart rate and blood pressure responses than leg work, thus creating greater myocardial oxygen demand (as expressed by HR × SBP product) for the same amount of external work as measured in physical (watts, kilogram meters per minute) or metabolic (kilocalories, mets) terms. Patients who plan to return to occupational or leisure activities requiring moderate or heavy arm exercise should include arm training in the exercise program to achieve maximal benefit. An increase in arm-work functional capacity requires that arms be used during training. Arm cranking using a modified stationary bicycle, low-resistance rowing, shoulder wheels, and selected calisthenics can be used for arm training (6).

Coronary patients should be informed about the difference in myocardial oxygen demand between isometric or high-resistance exercise and low-resistance or dynamic exercise. With isometric contraction the heart rate and particularly the blood pressure rise rapidly and disproportionately to the low metabolic demand for the activity (see Chapter 7). Since the magnitude of cardiovascular response to isometric exercise is related to the percentage of maximal contraction rather than to the absolute magnitude of contraction (pounds), the myocardial stress produced by isometric contraction of a small weak muscle can be similar to or even greater than that produced by contraction of a larger and stronger muscle. Patients who have undergone prolonged inactivity and have lost muscle strength achieve substantial increases in heart rate and blood pressure with isometric exercises of relatively low intensity, especially arm exercise. Activities that produce sustained isometric contraction include defecation, micturition, carrying objects from one place to another, and maintaining unusual postures, such as holding the arms above the head to paint a wall or ceiling, or carrying weights at chest height rather than at a lower level. Activities requiring high-resistance effort, such as near-maximal weight lifting, do not improve cardiovascular function and should not be included in a beginning activity program. Patients should be instructed not to perform the Valsalva maneuver or close the glottis for prolonged periods during exercise. To counteract this tendency, patients should be encouraged to practice rhythmic breathing during exercise.

Exercise Intensity

The ability of the patient to maintain an appropriate exercise intensity is the key to a safe and effective exercise program (6). The exercise must be of sufficient intensity to produce favorable cardiovascular and metabolic changes, but not so strenuous as to produce detrimental side effects. Some major adverse effects of overexertion are listed in Table 2.

The basic guidelines for prescribing exercise intensity are that the exercise intensity (work of the heart) during training be less than that safely achieved at the most recent exercise test and that the exercise intensity reach 60–80% of the

Table 2. Manifestations of Excessive Effort During or Following Exercise Training[a]

During exercise and immediately thereafter:
Anginal discomfort above level 2 on scale of 1–4
Increased frequency of dysrhythmias
Inappropriate bradycardia
Inappropriate tachycardia for effort
Ataxia, light headedness, confusion
Nausea, vomiting
Leg pain (claudication)
Pallor, cyanosis
Dyspnea persisting for more than 10 min
Delayed:
Prolonged fatigue
Unusual insomnia
Weight gain due to fluid retention
Persistent tachycardia (heart rate should be below 100–110 beats/min by 6 min after exercise)

[a]Appearances of these signs and symptoms in cardiac patients during or following exercise training indicate that the exercise intensity in subsequent sessions should be reduced.

patient's functional capacity. The concept of exercise prescription based on exercise test results was described in Chapter 8.

The patient should be instructed to begin exercise slowly, gradually building up to an intensity below that achieved at the most recent exercise test. The easiest and most accurate way for the physician to prescribe exercise intensity and for the patient to regulate exercise intensity is to use the target heart rate concept, as discussed in Chapter 8. The patient is instructed to exercise until reaching a given range of heart rate, as determined by prior response in an exercise test. If the patient did not exhibit signs or symptoms that required termination of the exercise test, then the initial prescription for exercise intensity can be to reach a heart rate that is 70–85% of the heart rate achieved at the end of the exercise test. Figure 1 provides a method for rapid calculation of this heart rate range. However, if the occurrence of a sign or symptom required that the exercise test be terminated, then the prescribed exercise intensity should be such as to elicit a peak heart rate no higher than 85% of that at which the sign or symptom occurred. Application of this approach also depends on the nature and severity of the abnormality that occurred during the exercise test; for example, if a serious arrhythmia such as ventricular tachycardia occurred, no exercise should be recommended until the arrhythmia has been adequately treated and it has been found that the arrhythmia has not recurred during subsequent exercise testing.

A slightly different approach to selection of the target heart rate for training is the Karvonen method, in which the intensity of training is based on a percentage of the chronotropic reserve. As discussed in Chapter 8, the Karvonen formula has limited application unless reliable heart rates at rest and at peak effort are

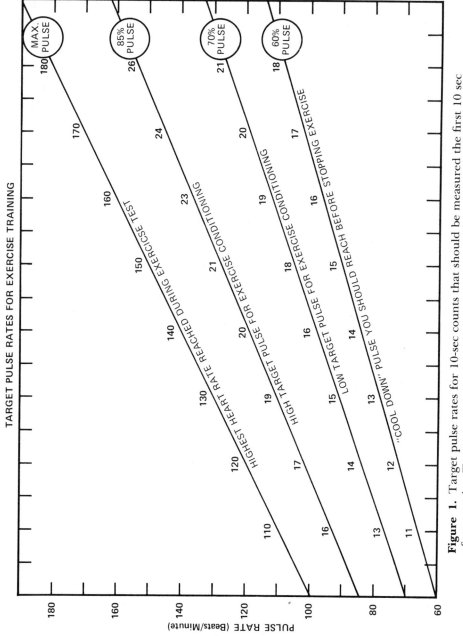

Figure 1. Target pulse rates for 10-sec counts that should be measured the first 10 sec after exercise. To convert the count to beats per minute, multiply by 6. To determine a patient's target pulse rate range, identify the highest heart rate safely achieved during the most recent exercise test on the top line (maximum pulse line); then locate the corresponding values on the 85% and 70% lines directly below. These two values represent the limits of target rate range for exercise conditioning.

209

obtained. Determination of target heart rate based on a percentage of heart rate during the exercise test is similar to determination by the Karvonen method (Table 3).

For cardiac patients, a target heart rate range is preferable to a single target heart rate value. The lower limit of this range is the level the patient should sustain for most of the activity session, whereas the upper limit of the range should not be exceeded at any time. This approach provides more flexibility for the patient and allows for intermittent as well as continuous activity, during which high levels of activity are interspersed with low levels. Sixty percent of peak exercise test heart rate could be used as the lower value and 80% as the higher value (Table 3).

Exercise Duration

The duration of exercise required for improvement in cardiovascular function is inversely related to the intensity of exercise, expressed as a percentage of the patient's working capacity. The higher the intensity (relative to capacity) the shorter the duration needed to elicit improvement. At an exercise intensity of 60–80% of aerobic capacity, a duration of 15–20 min will produce substantial objective and subjective effects. Activity at a lower intensity will require a longer duration to produce changes of a similar magnitude. Many patients cannot exercise for more than a few minutes before they become "too tired" to continue, or they experience leg fatigue or angina pectoris. This may be a result of the deconditioning produced by prolonged bed rest or inactivity, or it may be due to myocardial dysfunction or ischemia. These patients respond best to a program of intermittent activity, e.g., exercising at a target level for a few minutes, recovering by performing light activity for a short period of time (30 sec to several minutes), and then exercising at the target level once again; this procedure is repeated until target-level exercise has been performed for a total of 12–20 min. For patients requiring this type of training, the exercise session may last for 30–60 min. As capacity increases, the duration of the intermittent rest periods can be reduced until patients can perform exercise at the target level for the entire conditioning phase of the exercise session.

Exercise Frequency

Exercise should be performed on a regular basis to obtain sustained benefit. This is especially true for the patient with limited exercise capacity whose exercise sessions are of limited intensity and duration. Depending on the prescribed intensity and duration, exercise should be performed at least three times weekly on nonsuccessive days or preferably daily during early convalescence or when exercise intensity and total energy expenditure are low.

For the patient whose prescription is walking at slow or moderate speed, it may be best to walk several times daily rather than once. Reducing the exercise duration and increasing its frequency allows the patient to perform more exercise each day with less fatigue and soreness. Also, with short periods of exercise several times daily, the patient who misses one session still gets some exercise and has not "gone off the program." The patient who admits to "going off the

Table 3. Training Heart Rates[a]

| Peak Exercise Test Heart Rate | Percentage method | | Resting Heart Rate (beats/min) | | | | | | | | | | | | | | |
| | | | 50 | | | 60 | | | 70 | | | 80 | | | 90 | | |
	70%	85%	60%	70%	80%	60%	70%	80%	60%	70%	80%	60%	70%	80%	60%	70%	80%
110	77	94	86	92	98	90	95	100	94	98	102	98	101	104	102	104	106
120	84	102	92	99	106	96	102	108	100	105	110	104	108	112	108	111	114
130	91	111	98	106	114	102	109	116	106	112	118	110	115	120	114	118	122
140	98	119	104	113	122	108	116	124	112	119	126	116	122	128	120	125	130
150	105	128	110	120	130	114	123	132	118	126	134	122	129	136	126	132	138
160	112	136	116	127	138	120	130	140	124	133	142	128	136	144	132	139	146
170	119	145	122	134	146	126	137	148	130	140	150	134	143	152	138	145	154
180	126	153	128	141	154	132	144	156	136	147	158	140	150	160	144	157	162
190	133	162	134	148	162	138	151	164	142	154	166	146	157	168	150	160	170
200	140	170	140	155	170	144	158	172	148	161	174	152	164	176	156	167	178

[a]Training heart rate values calculated from percentage of peak test heart rate for different resting and peak exercise heart rates (Karvonen method). Training heart rate equals the difference between the peak heart rate and the resting heart rate times the given percentage (60%, 70%, or 80%) plus the resting heart rate.

program" is less likely to return to full participation than is the patient who performs some exercise, even though it is less than optimal.

UNSUPERVISED VERSUS MEDICALLY SUPERVISED EXERCISE

A critical decision in developing an exercise plan for the cardiac patient is whether the exercise is to be done with or without medical supervision. When possible, coronary atherosclerotic disease (CAD) patients and individuals at high risk of developing clinical manifestations of CAD should, at least initially, exercise under medical supervision. Medical supervision is defined as having in attendance at all exercise sessions one or more health professionals who can provide exercise instruction, who can identify medical contraindications to exercise, and who can perform cardiopulmonary resuscitation, including electrical defibrillation.

Experience in numerous cardiac exercise programs has demonstrated the value of experienced medical supervisors for exercise guidance, for motivation, and for emergency care of cardiovascular complications of exercise, especially cardiac arrest. Thus, for the patient exercising without direct supervision, the physician must assume more responsibility in explaining the exercise prescription and assuring that the patient knows exactly what to do and what to expect, as well as ensuring compliance.

Twenty-two medically supervised outpatient cardiac exercise programs in the United States and Canada were recently surveyed in regard to major cardiovascular complications in participants during exercise. All programs required exercise testing prior to participation, and all had on-site medical supervision. A major cardiovascular complication was defined as one requiring hospitalization. As of June 1975, with 748,133 person-hours of participation, there were 37 nonfatal and 10 fatal cardiovascular complications. Nonfatal complications included 24 cardiac arrests, 2 myocardial infarctions, and 11 other complications, including paroxysmal atrial tachycardia (3 cases), atrial fibrillation, ventricular bigeminy (2 cases), hypoglycemic reaction, and Stokes-Adams syncope with asystole. Fatal complications included 6 cardiac arrests, 2 cases of pulmonary embolism, 1 case of pulmonary edema, and 1 case of shock. The event rate (person-hours of participation divided by total nonfatal and fatal events) was one major cardiovascular complication per 16,556 person-hours of participation. The range was from one event per 4600 person-hours in one program to one event per 25,000 person-hours in another program. Twenty-four of 30 cardiac arrest patients were successfully resuscitated, a higher percentage than usual, even with expert resuscitation capability immediately available.

Medically supervised exercise programs attract only a small percentage of eligible cardiac patients. It appears that substantially fewer than 20,000 cardiac patients join medically supervised exercise programs each year. All others either do not exercise or exercise without medical supervision. Many patients who exercise to improve cardiovascular function without medical supervision do so either because supervision is not available or because they or their physicians do not believe supervision is necessary. Other cardiac patients who could exercise do not do so because they or their physicians do not believe exercise is of benefit, because they are not sufficiently motivated to participate, or because programs considered appropriate by the physician or the patient are not available due to geographic, financial, or logistical reasons.

UNSUPERVISED EXERCISE DURING CONVALESCENCE

Since numerous postinfarction patients participate in physical activity programs that are not medically supervised, those who design and conduct such programs should ensure that they are as safe and effective as possible. Whether long-term beneficial effects of exercise counteract any immediate increased risk of sudden death associated with exercise remains unknown.

The design and implementation of cardiac exercise programs that are not medically supervised will be presented in three sections. The first will deal with low-level physical activity during early convalescence, from the time of hospital discharge until 8–20 weeks following an uncomplicated myocardial infarction. The second will consider guidelines for selected cardiac patients performing higher-intensity conditioning programs following convalescence. The third will be concerned with patient participation in selected active games or sports.

Exercise During Early Convalescence

Patients are usually considered eligible to participate in medically supervised outpatient exercise programs at 8–12 weeks following infarction; this delay is recommended by those who believe that most patients do not have the capacity to participate in conditioning programs in the early weeks following hospitalization, whereas others are concerned that the myocardium is still healing or that patients cannot exercise at sufficient intensity and duration without excessive fatigue to warrant commuting from home to such a program. There are exceptions to this approach, e.g., the cardiac exercise programs conducted at the Dallas Cardiac Rehabilitation Institute in Dallas, Texas, and at Rancho Los Amigos Hospital in Downey, California. Some programs provide medically supervised ambulatory exercise programs as early as 4 weeks after infarction or after coronary bypass surgery.

When medically supervised exercise is not available or is not feasible, the patient with an uncomplicated course following hospitalization should be provided a plan for unsupervised low-level activity. This plan, tailored to the individual's capacity, should encompass walking or low-intensity stationary bicycle riding, easy calisthenics, light household chores or recreational activities, and for patients who have returned to work, low-level job-related tasks. High-intensity exercise, high-resistance activities, and competitive situations should be avoided.

There are two primary goals during this phase:

· to increase the frequency, duration, and intensity of activity gradually so that by 8–12 weeks after infarction the level of exertion reached is commensurate with that required by the job to which the patient is to return
· to provide psychologic support for the patient and family with the prospect of successful long-term recovery

Table 4. Approximate Energy Requirements of Selected Activities

Category	Self-care or Home	Occupational	Recreational[a]	Physical Conditioning
Very light <3 mets <10 ml/kg/min <4 kcal	Washing, shaving, dressing Desk work, writing Washing dishes Driving auto	Sitting (clerical, assembling) Standing (store clerk, bartender) Driving truck[a] Crane operator[a]	Shuffleboard Horseshoes Bait casting Billiards Archery[a] Golf (cart)	Walking (level @ 2 mph) Stationary bicycle (very low resistance) Very light calisthenics
Light 3–5 mets 11–18 ml/kg/min 4–6 kcal	Cleaning windows Raking leaves Weeding Power lawn mowing Waxing floors (slowly) Painting Carrying objects (15–30 lb)	Stocking shelves (light objects)[b] Light welding Light carpentry[b] Machine assembly Auto repair Paper hanging[b]	Dancing (social and square) Golf (walking) Sailing Horseback riding Volleyball (6 man) Tennis (doubles)	Walking (3–4 mph) Level bicycling (6–8 mph) Light calisthenics
Moderate 5–7 mets 18–25 ml/kg/min 6–8 kcal	Easy digging in garden Level hand lawn mowing Climbing stairs (slowly) Carrying objects (30–60 lb)[b]	Carpentry (exterior home building)[b] Shoveling dirt[b] Pneumatic tools[b]	Badminton (competitive) Tennis (singles) Snow skiing (downhill) Light backpacking Basketball Football Skating (ice and roller) Horseback riding (gallop)	Walking (4.5–5 mph) Bicycling (9–10 mph) Swimming (breast stroke)

Heavy 7–9 mets 25–32 ml/kg/min 8–10 kcal	Sawing wood[b] Heavy shoveling[b] Climbing stairs (moderate speed) Carrying objects (60–90 lb)[b]	Tending furnace[b] Digging ditches[b] Pick and shovel[b]	Canoeing[b] Mountain climbing[b] Fencing Paddleball Touch football	Jog (5 mph) Swim (crawl stroke) Rowing machine Heavy calisthenics Bicycling (12 mph)
Very heavy >9 mets >32 ml/kg/min >10 kcal	Carrying loads upstairs[b] Carrying objects (>90 lb)[b] Climbing stairs (quickly) Shoveling heavy snow[b] Shoveling 10/min (16 lb)	Lumber jack[b] Heavy laborer[b]	Handball Squash Ski touring over hills[b] Vigorous basketball	Running (≥6 mph) Bicycle (≥13 mph or up steep hill) Rope jumping

[a]May cause added psychologic stress that will increase work load on the heart.
[b]May produce disproportionate myocardial demands because of use of arms or isometric exercise.

215

If return to work is not a consideration or if the patient's job requires a peak energy expenditure greater than 6–8 mets, the activity level during this time should reach that necessary for complete self-care and for the performance of selected leisure-time activities, including sexual activity. The exercise plan should include the following:

· information regarding the exercise to be performed
· instruction in how to perform the exercise
· instruction in monitoring responses to exercise and indications to terminate exercise

Ideally, a written prescription should contain specific information on exercise implementation.

If a low-level exercise test has been performed either before or after hospital discharge, the patient can be given an exercise prescription based on the target heart rate concept described in Chapter 8. Experience in the Stanford Cardiac Rehabilitation Program has demonstrated that low-level treadmill exercise testing within 1 week after hospital discharge of uncomplicated postinfarction patients is safe and valuable in determining the appropriate activity level for these patients. If no contraindications to exercise are present, patients are given a target heart rate range 15–30 beats/min below the peak rate achieved during the test. For example, a patient who reaches a peak heart rate of 130 beats/min will be assigned a target range of 100–115 beats/min.

For the patient who has not had an exercise test, exercise recommendation should be based on clinical judgment, considering cardiovascular status, duration of convalescence, previous exercise habits, and age. Such patients should be given a conservative exercise plan in which the intensity of exercise is low and the duration and frequency are increased. Activities should produce an increase in heart rate of no more than 30–40 beats/min above resting rate, or not above 110–120 beats/min, an energy requirement of 4–6 mets.

The activities to be recommended are dynamic exercises using large muscle groups, e.g., walking, slow stair climbing, stationary bicycle riding at low resistance, regular bicycle riding on reasonably flat terrain, easy swimming in water at moderate temperature, light household chores (not heavy lifting, carrying, or pulling or pushing), light calisthenics, and light occupational tasks. The energy requirements of various household, occupational, recreational, and conditioning activities are listed in Table 4. Activities of the proper type, but of too high an intensity for patients soon after myocardial infarction, include jogging, running, hiking in hills or mountains, and most active sports and games such as basketball, handball, squash, and singles tennis. Inappropriate activities include any high-resistance or isometric exercises such as heavy lifting or water skiing. Because their intensities are readily controlled, walking, stationary bicycle riding, and low-level bench stepping are useful conditioning activities during early rehabilitation. A combined program of walking and stationary bicycle riding or bench stepping can be used for all ambulatory patients. Walking can be performed when environmental conditions (weather, daylight, terrain, etc.) permit, and bicycle riding or bench stepping can be used when it is necessary or advisable to exercise indoors. The same target heart rate method is used for each of these activities.

When medical supervision of exercise during convalescence is not feasible, control of exercise intensity can be improved by the use of a portable heart rate monitor. Based on the patient's exercise test response, high and low heart rate indicators can be set on the monitor. An electrocardiographic signal is obtained from a bipolar chest lead, and the monitor uses the electrocardiographic signal to determine the patient's heart rate. Signals of different tones inform the patient when heart rate is too high, too low, and within the prescribed range of target heart rate. More sophisticated monitors not only trigger an alarm when the heart rate is too high or too low but also trigger an alarm when premature ventricular contractions increase above a preset number, transmitting the electrocardiographic signal via telephone for recording and evaluation in the physician's office. We have used these units successfully to control exercise intensity during physical training and occupational activities of early postinfarction patients, especially patients prone to exertional arrhythmias.

During early convalescence, many patients are anxious about exercising; thus the physician's instructions must be specific (Table 5) and must include the following:

· exercise type, intensity, duration (distance), and frequency; i.e., walk 1 mile over flat terrain in approximately 24 min (2.5 mph) twice each day, once in the morning and once in the evening
· how to check exercise pulse rate, what target pulse rate range is, and what to do if the pulse is above or below the target range while exercising; e.g., if the pulse rate is consistently below target rate, the patient should increase the exercise intensity slightly and recheck the pulse rate; if it is not close to target rate, further adjustment and rechecking should be carried out until the pulse is close to target rate; conversely, if the pulse rate is higher than target rate, the patient should slow down and recheck the pulse rate until it is within target range
· what to avoid, e.g., too much exercise too soon, exercise too soon after a heavy meal or after alcohol consumption, exercise during extremely hot or humid times of day or during very cold weather, hot showers, cold showers, steam baths, and saunas after exercise
· what to wear to maintain body temperature as close to normal as possible (warm clothing in winter and light clothing in warm weather); how to protect feet while walking on hard surfaces (shoes should have firm thick soles, good arch supports, padded heels, and soft pliable tops); good shoes can help to prevent the orthopedic problems of feet, ankles, and knees frequently experienced by sedentary adults during the early phase of an exercise program
· indications of overexertion and how to respond to them; Table 6 lists exercise-related symptoms, their causes, and remedial actions; all patients should be familiar with this information

Exercise Following Early Convalescence

By 8–20 weeks after infarction the patient who has been performing low-level exercise on a reasonably regular basis may be ready for additional physical activities of higher intensity. A multistage exercise test should be performed at

Table 5. Exercise Prescription Form

TO: Exercise Specialist/Physical Educator
RE: Exercise Prescription & Exercise Test Summary
FOR: _____ AGE: ___ OCCUPATION: _____
FROM: _____ DATE: _____ TELEPHONE: _____
Rx EXERCISE DOSAGE: Recommended (circle one)
Frequency (sessions/week)   2   3   4   5   6   7
Duration (min/session)   Specify (   )
   A. Continuous (   )   5–10   10–20   20–30   30–40
   B. Intermittent (work–rest) (   ) _____
Intensity   (% × peak heart rate)   65   70   75   80   85   × ____ = ____
Type of activities _____
Recreational preferences _____
SUMMARY—EXERCISE TEST: Conducted on _____
Highest stage of exercise
   mph   _____
   % grade _____   Estimated $\dot{V}O_2$ max (ml/kg/min) _____
   kpm/min _____   Estimated mets _____
Signs and symptoms _____
Peak HR _____   SBP _____   DBP _____
ECG changes _____
Reason for terminating the test _____
Medications _____

CAUTIONS: Reduce exercise dosage in case of severe environmental stress (temperature and/or humidity), recent overindulgence in food or drink, emotional turmoil, anginal discomfort, increased frequency of arrhythmias, inappropriate tachycardia or bradycardia, pallor or cyanosis, persistent dyspnea, prolonged fatigue, intercurrent illness, orthopedic injury, cerebral dysfunction (i.e., dizziness), recent minor surgery, other recent changes in clinical status and/or physical appearance.

DEFERRAL OF TRAINING: Discontinue exercise training with orthopedic problems aggravated by activity, marked progression of cardiac illness (i.e., severe arrhythmia), development of new systemic disease, major surgery, psychiatric decompensation, acute alcoholism. Advise patient to contact referring physician.

REFILL: Next evaluation _____

that time to evaluate the patient's exercise capacity. The results of this test, combined with medical history and examination data, will provide the information necessary to update the exercise plan. If the intensity of exercise is to be increased to the level of jogging or running, the patient should enter a medically supervised program (see following section).

The exercise plan for the patient not in a supervised program should restrict the intensity to 60–70% (Karvonen method) of capacity and should emphasize longer exercise sessions (30–60 min) and increased exercise frequency (four to five times per week instead of three to four). The warm-up period at the beginning of each exercise session should be lengthened (10 min), as should the cool-down period (5–10 min) at the end. To ensure accurate control of exercise intensity, brisk walking, intermittent walking and jogging, continuous jogging, stationary bicycle riding, or regular bicycle riding should be used as the primary activities. Slow- or moderate-speed stair climbing, bench stepping, and walking over hilly terrain are activities within the capacity of many patients that can be added to their exercise plans. Vigorous or competitive sports and games such as handball and singles tennis should be delayed until the patient's exercise capacity has been increased and the patient has been cleared by a multistage exercise test. Isometric or high-resistance activities should not be prescribed.

The same considerations in prescribing unsupervised exercise during the early convalescence phase still apply. As cardiovascular capacity improves, the patient should learn to recognize the early signs of overexertion, chronic fatigue, and orthopedic problems outlined in Tables 5 and 6. The patient should know when to slow down, when to stop, and when not to exercise.

As exercise capacity increases with training, a decision must be made regarding the level of exercise capacity to be achieved. The patient's capacity for exercise will vary with the severity of disease, age, sex, previous exercise habits, and heredity. A general guide is that to achieve and maintain benefits from exercise, the patient should exercise regularly (three to five times per week) for approximately 30 min per session at 60–80% of functional capacity. Exercise capacity can be maintained by regular participation at the lower limits of this recommendation.

As the heart attack recedes further into the patient's past, there may be a tendency to revert to a preillness life-style. If a sedentary life-style was the norm prior to the attack, the patient may need frequent encouragement to remain motivated to continue exercising. Such encouragement can be provided by the physician when the patient is reevaluated and is found to be progressing well. Some patients need reinforcement to continue exercising regularly; others need guidance to avoid overexercising. Competitively oriented patients have to understand the potential dangers of overexertion and accept the desirability of exercising within the levels determined by their exercise tests.

Participation in Sports and Games

Cardiac patients frequently request a physician's advice regarding participation in active sports, games, and leisure-time activities. Such questions are difficult to answer categorically because of the substantial intraindividual and interindividual variations in total body energy requirement and myocardial oxygen demand of many such activities. These variations are due to a number of factors: the intermittent nature of the intensity required by many of these activities; differences in skill and proficiency among the participants; variations in competitiveness and aggressiveness among the participants; changes in the ambient environment (temperature, humidity, wind velocity, and altitude); variations in the amounts of upper-body exercise and isometric exercise performed; differences in the amounts of excitement, thrill, and danger associated with the activity.

A multitude of activities can present such problems: competitive sports and games (handball, squash, tennis, badminton, volleyball, basketball); activities requiring isometric contraction or isotonic contraction against high resistance

Table 6. Exercise Warnings and What to Do About Them[a]

	Symptom	Cause	Remedy
STOP — SEE A PHYSICIAN BEFORE RESUMING	1. Abnormal heart action; e.g.: pulse becoming irregular; fluttering, jumping, or palpitations in chest or throat; sudden burst of rapid heartbeats; sudden very slow pulse when a moment before it had been on target (immediate or delayed)	Extrasystoles (extra heartbeats), dropped heartbeats, or other disorders of cardiac rhythm. This may or may not be dangerous and should be checked by your physician.	Consult physician before resuming exercise program. Medication may be provided to temporarily eliminate the problem and allow you to safely resume your exercise program, or you may have a completely harmless cardiac rhythm disorder.
	2. Pain or pressure in the center of the chest or in the left arm or throat precipitated by exercise or following exercise (immediate or delayed)	Possible heart pain	Consult physician before resuming exercise program
	3. Dizziness, light-headedness, sudden incoordination, confusion, cold sweat, glassy stare, pallor, blueness or fainting (immediate)	Insufficient blood to the brain	Do not try to cool down. Stop exercise and lie down with feet elevated, or put head down between legs until symptoms pass. Later consult physician before next exercise session.

Table 6. (Continued)

	Symptom	Cause	Remedy
REMEDIES THAT MAY BE SELF-ADMINISTERED	4. Persistent rapid heart action near the target level even 8–10 min after the exercise was stopped (immediate)	Exercise is probably too vigorous	Keep heart rate at lower end of target zone or below. Increase the vigor of exercise more slowly. If these measures do not control the excessively high recovery heart rate, consult physician.
	5. Flare-up of arthritic condition or gout that usually occurs in hips, knees, ankles, or big toe (weight-bearing joints) (immediate or delayed)	Trauma to joints, which are particularly vulnerable	If you are familiar with how to quiet these flare-ups of your prior joint condition, use your usual remedies. Rest and do not resume exercise program until the condition subsides. Then resume the exercise at a lower level with protective footwear on softer surfaces, or select other exercises that will put less strain on the impaired joints, e.g., swimming will be better for people with arthritis of the hips, since it can be done mostly with the arms. If this is new arthritis, or if there is no response to usual remedies, see physician.

221

Table 6. (Continued)

	Symptom	Cause	Remedy
	6. Nausea or vomiting after exercise (immediate)	Usually not enough oxygen to the intestine. You are either exercising too vigorously or cooling down too quickly.	Exercise less vigorously, and be sure to take a more gradual and longer cool-down.
	7. Extreme breathlessness lasting more than 10 min after stopping exercise (immediate)	Exercise is too taxing to your cardiovascular system or lungs	Stay at the lower end of your target range. If symptoms persist, do even less than target level. Be sure that while you are exercising you are not too breathless to talk to a companion.
	8. Prolonged fatigue even 24 hr later (delayed)	Exercise is too vigorous	Stay at lower end of target range or below. Increase level more gradually.
	9. Shin splints (pain on the front or sides of lower leg) (delayed)	Inflammation of the fascia connecting the leg bones, or muscle tears where muscles of the lower leg connect to the bones	Use shoes with thicker soles. Work out on turf, which is easier on your legs.
CAN BE REMEDIED WITHOUT MEDICAL CONSULTATION	10. Insomnia that was not present prior to the exercise program (delayed)	Exercise is too vigorous	Stay at lower end of target range or below. Increase intensity of exercise gradually.
	11. Pain in the calf muscles that occurs on heavy exercise but not at rest (immediate)	May be caused by muscle cramps due to lack of use of these muscles, or exercising on hard surfaces. May also be due to poor circulation to the legs (claudication)	Use shoes with thicker soles; cool down adequately. Muscle cramps should clear up after a few sessions. If muscle cramps do not subside, circulation is probably faulty. Try another type of exercise, e.g., bicycling instead of jogging in order to use different muscles.
	12. Side stitch (sticking under the ribs while exercising) (immediate)	Diaphragm spasm; the diaphragm is the large muscle that separates the chest from the abdomen	Lean forward while sitting, attempting to push the abdominal organs up against the diaphragm
	13. Charley horse or muscle-bound feeling (immediate or delayed)	Muscles are deconditioned and unaccustomed to exercise	Take hot bath and usual headache remedy. Next exercise should be less strenuous.

^aAdapted from Zohman LR: *Beyond Diet: Exercise Your Way to Fitness and Heart Health.* CPC International, New York, 1974, p 24.

222

(water skiing, weight lifting, weight training); activities with components of speed, excitement, and danger (snowmobiling, motorcycling, downhill skiing).

Before participating in sports or games, patients should be encouraged to participate in a systematic reconditioning program. Postinfarction patients should not participate in high-intensity games or recreational activities until 24–36 weeks after infarction, and then only after clearance by their physicians.

Because of the difficulty in estimating the total body energy requirement or myocardial oxygen demand for a specific patient performing such activities, advice regarding participation should be conservative. Activities requiring sustained isometric activity (more than 10–15 sec) or high resistance should not be recommended. Clearance for participation in vigorous sports and games should include a maximal or symptom-limited multistage exercise test during which the work load achieved has an estimated energy requirement substantially higher than that listed for the planned activity and during which the patient does not develop signs or symptoms contraindicating unmonitored exercise of that intensity (see Table 4).

If the activity being considered has a major component of arm or upper-body activity, an exercise test involving arm work is appropriate (see Chapter 7). Monitoring the patient during simulation of the activity in the clinic or office, or use of a Holter-type electrocardiogram recorder to monitor the patient during actual performance of the activity, can provide objective information about the appropriateness of many activities.

Patients cleared for participation in active games or sports should be cautioned to avoid extremes of environmental conditions, e.g., they should not play tennis or hike on hot, sunny, or humid days, and they should not ski on the coldest days or ski at resorts at the higher altitudes. Extremes in water temperature should be avoided when participating in water sports. Also, the cardiovascular demands of a given activity can be reduced; e.g., by playing doubles instead of singles tennis, badminton, or paddleball; by avoiding highly competitive opponents or situations; by planning frequent rest periods; by carrying loads in a backpack rather than with the arms when hiking.

OUTPATIENT MEDICALLY SUPERVISED EXERCISE PROGRAMS

Because of the increased risk of cardiovascular complications during high-level physical activities such as jogging, running, and active games and sports, these activities should, at least initially, be performed under medical supervision when possible. On occasion, the increased myocardial work load of exercise may precipitate cardiac arrest. Appropriate medical supervision may enable successful management of this problem without detrimental complications.

Several hundred medically supervised ambulatory cardiac exercise programs currently exist in the United States. The programs vary in design and implementation, but there is substantial similarity. As various procedures have been found to be of value in one program, they frequently have been incorporated into other programs.

The design and implementation of an effectively supervised ambulatory cardiac exercise program are summarized in the remainder of this section.

General Organization

Most successful long-term cardiac exercise programs have a multidisciplinary staff working at least part time with the program. Patients are referred by community physicians, and program personnel evaluate the exercise capacity of each patient. The exercise program usually is conducted in a community gymnasium. Individual activity is guided by the patient's heart rate response to exercise. Programs are medically supervised, and participation is on a fee-for-service basis.

Personnel

The staff should consist of a medical director with training in internal medicine and/or cardiology and experience in exercise testing and exercise training (additional physicians may be needed in larger programs), one or more cardiovascular nurses, and a physical director to serve as an exercise leader. Additional personnel may be needed, depending on the size of the program and the nature of the support provided by the sponsoring agency (YMCA, university, hospital, etc.). Attempts to conduct cardiac exercise programs without a medical director but with community physicians evaluating patients and assuming supervisory responsibility for the exercise program have not been successful. One physician should take primary responsibility for the medical aspects of the program.

The exercise leadership in most supervised group programs is provided by a physical educator or a staff member trained in exercise physiology. The exercise leader teaches the patients to exercise properly, leads them through their exercises, and makes observations and comments during the exercise session. In conjunction with the medical supervisor, the exercise leader is responsible for seeing that patients exercise properly and within their capacity. The exercise leader must have knowledge of functional anatomy, exercise physiology, behavioral psychology, group dynamics, and cardiopulmonary emergency procedures. The exercise leader is important in assuring that the patient understands the exercise regimen and in motivating the patient to continue participation.

Appropriate medical supervision requires either a physician or an experienced cardiovascular nurse acting under the direction of a physician. Maximal safety and long-term participation are enhanced by the attendance of a physician, although economic realities may favor the nurse. A recent survey of major cardiovascular complications during outpatient cardiac exercise programs suggests that in programs using nurses instead of physicians there are no differences in major medical complications and that complications, including cardiac arrest, are appropriately managed. Suggested qualifications for each member of the cardiac exercise team have been published by the American College of Sports Medicine (1).

Facilities

Cardiac exercise programs have functioned successfully in facilities owned by YMCAs, YMHAs, community centers, schools, and hospitals. These facilities usually include at least a gymnasium, locker room, and showers. In some cases outdoor exercise areas, running tracks, and swimming pools have been used effectively. Increasing numbers of programs have renovated facilities such as offices and storage space into areas where stationary exercise equipment can be used for medically supervised exercise. If only stationary equipment such as bicycles, treadmills, and rowing machines are used, an exercise program can be conducted in a reasonably small space; rooms no larger than 20 feet by 20 feet have been found acceptable for programs with limited numbers of participants. The total number of participants such a facility can accommodate will depend on scheduling. An example of this approach is the Cardiac and Pulmonary Rehabilitation Center operated by AMSCO/REHAB of Mechanicsburg, Pennsylvania.

Patient Referral and Recruitment

Patients should be accepted only on referral of their personal physicians. The patient and physician must understand that the medical care of the patient remains with the physician and that the exercise program should be considered an adjunct to health care, similar to an outpatient physical therapy clinic. Some patients referred to exercise programs by community physicians decide to change physicians and may request an exercise program physician to assume this role; acceptance will endanger future referrals from that patient's physician and others. For individuals who wish to enter the program but who do not have personal physicians, referral to physicians other than the program physicians is appropriate.

Most cardiac exercise programs have found it necessary to conduct intensive educational and promotional programs for the first several years in order to recruit adequate numbers of patients. Such promotion initially should be directed to community physicians, but information provided to the general public can be a valuable recruitment procedure. The latter should take place only after community physicians have been informed about the program by personal contacts, letters, brochures, newsletters, and presentations at hospital staff meetings, local medical society meetings, and heart association meetings.

One approach to obtaining greater participation by the local medical community is to establish a medical advisory committee for the program. Included should be interested physicians or allied health professionals representing various segments of the health care delivery system for cardiac patients (private physicians, hospital staff in coronary care units, heart associations, etc.).

Patient Evaluation

When a patient is referred to an exercise program, a summary of the patient's medical history should be provided to the program physician, including current medical status, medications, recent laboratory evaluations including chest x-ray, blood chemistry values, coronary angiography (if available), and resting, ambulatory, and exercise electrocardiograms. This information is essential if the program physician is to determine the patient's eligibility for exercise.

In most cases the medical director or a physician associate will obtain an interim medical history and resting 12-lead electrocardiogram and will perform a cardiovascular examination. If it is not medically contraindicated, the patient should perform a multistage exercise test on either a motor-driven treadmill or a stationary bicycle ergometer to determine eligibility for participation in an exercise program and to establish the initial exercise intensity (see Chapter 8 for details of exercise testing and prescription). At times, patients will have had the exercise test performed by their primary care physicians. A summary of the initial and subsequent evaluations should be sent to the referring physician.

Program Orientation Session

After being cleared for participation, the patient should be scheduled for an individual or small group orientation session. This should include an explanation of the purpose and operation of the program, discussion of each patient's exercise tolerance and the factors that limit capacity (angina, fatigue, etc.), an explanation of how exercise capacity is used to develop an individualized exercise plan, instructions on the do's and don'ts of exercise, and an explanation of administrative details. Potential participants should sign an informed consent form for exercise as treatment (see Appendix 1, pp. 230–231). A well-planned coronary risk factor education program that is acceptable to the referring physician and is conducted in conjunction with the exercise program can substantially enhance the benefit of the program to the patient and family. Participation in a group exercise program appears to increase the likelihood that other coronary risk factors such as obesity, elevated lipids, and cigarette smoking can be favorably modified if systematic attention is given by the program staff.

Exercise Sessions

Patients should attempt to attend at least three exercise sessions per week; some programs encourage patients to participate in additional sessions. Each session should last approximately 1 hr, including time for changing clothes, a warm-up period, conditioning activity, tapering off, and a lukewarm shower. The actual time on the exercise floor is about 45 min. The time of day does not seem to be important in regard to the conditioning effectiveness or safety, but sessions must be scheduled to be reasonably convenient for the patient. Early morning (7:00–8:30 A.M.) and early evening (4:30–6:30 P.M.) are the most popular times; noontime sessions seem to result in sporadic attendance.

Each exercise session should have a warm-up period, conditioning activities, and a tapering-off or cool-down period. Some programs also include a game or recreational period after the conditioning activities to help promote attendance, whereas others use modified games as conditioning activities.

Warm-up
The primary purposes of the warm-up period are to increase the readiness of the joints for more vigorous activity and to slowly increase respiratory, cardiovascular, and metabolic rates. Warm-up periods usually begin with low-level calisthenics performed in the supine or sitting position. Stretching activities performed at a slow tempo in a horizontal plane should be emphasized (see Appendix 2, pp. 231–241). Following stretching and a few light resistance activities, the warm-up should be completed with brisk walking or easy jogging, depending on the capacity of the patient. A warm-up period usually lasts 6–15 min.

Conditioning Activities

The conditioning period is usually scheduled for approximately 30 min. It should be dominated by endurance activities such as walking, jogging, running, stationary bicycle riding, swimming, and in some cases modified games or sports. Walking and jogging are used most frequently because their intensity can be controlled easily, they require limited skill, and they can be performed using a diversity of facilities.

The intensity at which patients exercise can be controlled effectively if patients monitor their own heart rates and modify the intensity to achieve the target heart rate determined by a prior multistage exercise test.

Patients should be instructed to measure pulse rate by palpation at the carotid, brachial, or radial artery. Most patients learn this procedure quickly and can obtain accurate pulse rates immediately after exercise. Heart rate should be monitored frequently during the conditioning period. New patients, patients with low exercise capacity, and patients returning to class after an absence of a week or more should check the pulse rate every few minutes, whereas experienced patients with reasonably good exercise tolerance should check at least every 5–10 min. Pulse rate should be determined for the first 10 sec immediately following exercise. If monitored for a longer time (15–30 sec), the rate will have slowed significantly from the exercise rate, and an inaccurately low rate will be obtained. Attempting to count for a shorter time, such as 5–6 sec, is difficult and results in errors. While counting the pulse rate the patient should not stand still but should walk slowly or in place (or pedal slowly at no resistance if on a stationary bicycle) to protect against postexercise hypotension resulting from blood pooling in the dilated vessels in the legs. If heart rate is below the target range, the patient can slightly increase exercise intensity; if heart rate is above the target range, the patient can slow down. Keeping the heart rate at or below target level is one of the best ways of ensuring patient safety.

Patients with low exercise capacity tend to tolerate more exercise per session, and heart rate can be monitored more effectively if exercise is performed intermittently, i.e., with higher-level activity that elicits the target heart rate for a short period, followed by low-level exercise or rest for a short period. As exercise tolerance increases, the duration of the higher-level exercise periods can be increased and the duration of the low-level periods or rest periods decreased.

Cool-down Period

The cool-down or tapering-off session usually lasts 5–10 min and includes easy jogging, walking, and light calisthenics. This tapering off of exercise intensity, instead of suddenly stopping, is designed to reduce postexercise hypotension, and the time can be used to observe patients in the medically supervised exercise area for a short period after peak exercise intensity. Since cardiovascular complications of cardiac exercise programs often occur at this time, it is important that the staff be alert. The patient should continue to walk slowly until heart rate returns to near the preexercise level (see Fig. 1).

Safety Procedures

The primary purposes of medically supervised exercise for cardiac patients are prevention or reduction of cardiovascular complications and appropriate treat-

Table 7. Indications for Temporarily Deferring or Reducing
Intensity of Physical Activity Conditioning Program

Progression of cardiac disease: increasing angina, new or increasing
    PVCs
Intercurrent illness: febrile, gastrointestinal, injury
Orthopedic problem aggravated by activity
Cerebral dysfunction: dizziness, vertigo
Emotional turmoil: anxiety, frustration, or anger
Sodium retention: edema, weight gain
Substantial dehydration
Environmental factors
    Weather: excessive heat or cold, humidity, or wind
    Air pollution: smog, carbon monoxide
Overindulgence
    Large, heavy meal within 2 hr
    Coffee, tea, coke (xanthines and other stimulating beverages)
    Alcoholic hangover
Drugs: decongestants, bronchodilators, atropine, weight reducers
    (anorectics)

ment of complications that occur. Successful prevention of complications must
include the following:

· selection criteria to exclude inappropriate patients
· periodic reevaluation to identify patients who do not respond to exercise or
  whose disease manifestations have progressed since the previous evaluation
  (Table 7)
· medical supervision during each exercise session to ensure that patients exercise within prescribed limits and to detect recent changes in disease status
· conservative target heart rate values for patients with ventricular arrhythmias
  or exertional angina
· regular communication with the patient's private physician regarding health
  status or changes in medication
· specific instructions to patients regarding signs or symptoms that preclude
  participation in the exercise program (unusual fatigue, anxiety, changing cardiovascular symptoms, especially increasing angina or arrhythmias)
· reasonably small class size, ideally 30 patients or less
· sign-in and sign-out procedures to ensure regular participation and to aid in
  reducing exercise intensity if a patient has missed several consecutive sessions

Even with the best of precautions, major cardiovascular events may occur. The
most frequent serious complication appears to be sudden cardiac arrest. The
chances of successful resuscitation are increased if the following precautions are
taken:

· all members of the program staff are well trained and certified in emergency
  cardiac care, including cardiopulmonary resuscitation procedures (CPR)

Table 8. Emergency Equipment and Drugs for Cardiac Exercise Program[a]

Equipment	Drugs
1. Defibrillator (portable synchronized direct current preferable)	1. Morphine or meperidine
2. Oxygenator (intermittent positive-pressure capability)	2. Nitroglycerin tablets and amyl nitrite pearls
3. Airways, oral and endotracheal	3. Catecholamines Aramine Epinephrine 1/10,000 i.v. Norepinephrine i.v. Isoproterenol i.v.
4. Bag-valve-mask hand respirator (Hope non-rebreathing bag)	
5. Syringes and needles	4. Antiarrhythmics Lidocaine i.v. Procainamide i.v. Propranolol i.v./oral
6. Intravenous sets	
7. Intravenous stand	5. Atropine sulfate
8. Adhesive tape	6. Digoxin, Cedilanid
9. Laryngoscope (desirable)	7. Sodium bicarbonate solution
	8. Dextrose, 5% in water
	9. Furosemide (Lasix) i.v.
	10. Edrophonium (Tensilon)

[a]Adapted from Committee on Exercise, American Heart Association: *Exercise Testing and Training of Apparently Healthy Individuals: A Handbook for Physicians.* American Heart Association, 1972, p 22.

· they have frequently practiced CPR as a team and all members know their assignments

· they have the appropriate emergency equipment and supplies that have been maintained properly (Table 8)

· the telephone number of the emergency transportation service is readily available and arrangements have already been made with the transportation service regarding the location of the facility

SUMMARY

Most postinfarction patients should be provided individualized exercise instructions at the time of discharge from the hospital. Ideally, these instructions should be based on objective evaluation of the patient's functional capacity, as well as assessment of clinical status. The instructions must be specific and are best provided in writing. They should describe the following procedures: type, intensity, duration, and frequency of exercise; how the patient can check exercise intensity by monitoring pulse rate and symptoms; when to reduce intensity, stop exercising, or report symptoms to the physician. During early posthospital convalescence, low-intensity dynamic exercises performed daily or several times per day are recommended.

As time passes and capacity increases, higher-intensity dynamic exercises can be performed less often, but still at least three times per week on nonconsecutive days. Isometric or high-resistance exercises should be avoided by cardiac patients because of the pressure work load they impose on the myocardium. When feasible, cardiac patients who undertake exercise programs of higher intensity (jogging, running, swimming, etc.) should do so initially in a medically supervised program to provide closer supervision, instruction, motivation, and cardiopulmonary resuscitation capabilities. Before postinfarction patients return to active games or sports, they should participate in a regular program of physical activity for 3–6 months and then be cleared by successful performance of a multistage exercise test.

REFERENCES

1. *Guidelines for Graded Exercise Testing and Exercise Prescription.* American College of Sports Medicine. Lea & Febiger, Philadelphia, 1975, p 116

2. Morse RL (ed): *Exercise and the Heart: Guidelines for Exercise Programs.* Charles C Thomas, Springfield, Ill, 1972, p 265

3. Zohman LR, Tobis JS: *Cardiac Rehabilitation.* Grune & Stratton, New York, 1970, p 248

4. Kasch FW, Boyer JL: *Adult Fitness: Principles and Practices.* All American Productions and Publications, Greeley, Colo, 1968, p 147

5. Fletcher GF, Cantwell JD: *Exercise in the Management of Coronary Heart Disease: A Guide for the Practicing Physician.* Charles C Thomas, Springfield, Ill, 1971, p 57

6. Hellerstein HK, Franklin BA: Exercise testing and prescription. In Wenger NK, Hellerstein HK (eds): *Rehabilitation of the Coronary Patient.* John Wiley, New York, 1978, chapter 8

APPENDIX 1: INFORMED CONSENT FOR EXERCISE AS TREATMENT

I desire to engage voluntarily in an exercise treatment program in order to improve my cardiovascular function. This program has been recommended to me by my physician, Dr. —————.

Before I enter such a program I will have a clinical evaluation including a medical history and/or physical examination that includes but is not limited to measurement of heart rate and blood pressure and EKG at rest and with effort. The purpose of this evaluation is to detect any condition that would indicate that I should not engage in an exercise program.

The program will follow an exercise prescription prepared by Dr. ————— and will be carefully followed by the supervisor of the treatment program. The amount of exercise will be regulated on the basis of my tolerance.

Before starting the program I will be instructed as to the signs and symptoms that will alert me to modify my activities. I will also be observed by the supervisor of the exercises who will also be alert to changes that would suggest that I modify my exercise.

The activities are designed to place a graduated increased work load on the circulation and thereby to improve its function. The reaction of the cardiovascular system to such activities cannot be predicted with complete accuracy. There is the risk of certain changes occurring during or following the exercise. These changes include abnormalities of blood pressure, increased irregular or ineffective heart rate, and in rare instances "heart attacks" or "cardiac arrest."

Every effort will be made to avoid such events by the preliminary medical examination and by observation during the exercise. Emergency equipment and trained personnel are available to deal with and minimize the dangers of untoward events should they occur.

I have read the foregoing and I understand it. Any questions that have arisen or occurred to me have been answered to my satisfaction.

Signed _____
                                                                                    Patient

_____   _____
Date   *Witness*

_____
Physician Supervising Test

APPENDIX 2: WARM-UP AND DEVELOPMENTAL EXERCISES

Warm-up Exercises

Begin your warm-up exercises at Level I. Plan to spend 4 weeks at each level. During this time, progress from the lowest number of repetitions to the highest within that level. After 4 weeks, proceed to the next level. Once you have reached the highest number of repetitions in Level III, continue it as part of your maintenance program.

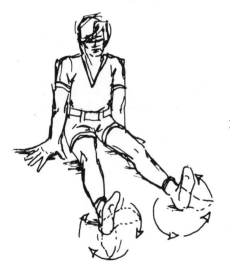

1. ANKLE ROLLS
Starting Position: Sitting position on floor with hands on floor alongside hips.
Action: Count 1: Rotate ankles in 360° circle, clockwise, using full range of motion. Count 2: Reverse and repeat in counterclockwise direction.
Level: I   3–5
                 II   6–8
                 III 9–12

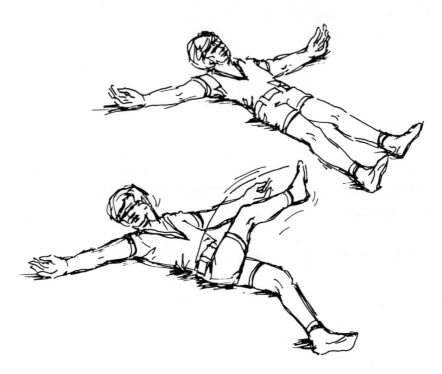

2. OPPOSITE LEG OVER

Starting Position: Lie on back with arms outstretched to side at shoulder level, palms up.

Action: Count 1: Carefully kick the right foot to left hand (exhale). Count 2: Return to starting position. Count 3: Carefully kick the left foot to the right hand (exhale). Count 4: Return to starting position.

Level: I   3–5
            II   6–8
            III 9–12

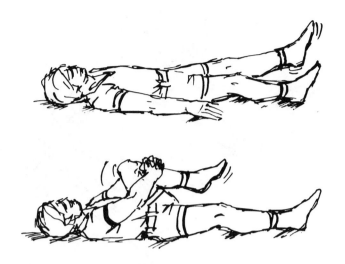

3. LEG RAISE AND BEND

Starting Position: Lie on back, legs extended, feet together, arms at sides.

Action: Count 1: Raise extended left leg about 10 inches off the floor. Count 2: Bend knee and bring knee toward chest as far as possible, using abdominal, hip, and leg muscles; then clasp knee with both hands and pull slowly toward chest. Count 3: Return to Count 1 position. Count 4: Return to starting position. Counts 5, 6, 7, and 8: Repeat with right leg.

Level: I   1–4
           II   5–8
          III   9–12

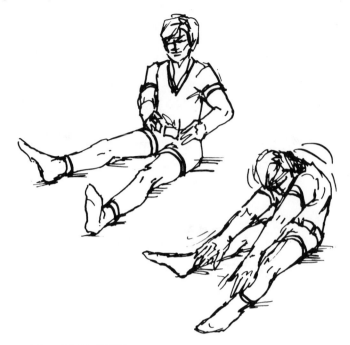

4. SITTING FORWARD BEND
Starting Position: Sit erect, legs straight, feet shoulder-width apart, hands on waist.
Action: Count 1: Bend trunk forward and down, and attempt to touch lower legs or toes with fingers, keeping legs straight. Count 2: Return to starting position. Do slowly, stretching and relaxing at intervals rather than in rhythm.
Level: I   2–4
            II   5–8
            III   9–10

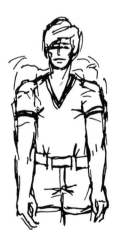

5. SHOULDER SHRUG
Starting Position: Stand relaxed with arms hanging down at sides.
Action: Shrug shoulders high into the neck, then relax and stretch shoulder down. Rotate shoulders in rearward direction and then in forward direction.
Level: I, II, and III   5–10

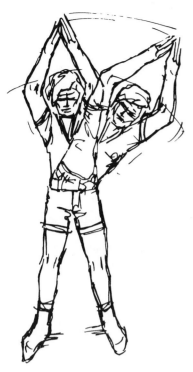

6. SIDE BODY BEND

Starting Position: Stand with feet shoulder-width apart, hands extended overhead, fingertips touching.

Action: Count 1: Bend trunk slowly sideward to left as far as possible, keeping hands together and arms straight (don't bend elbows). Count 2: Return to starting position. Counts 3 and 4: Repeat to the right.

Level:　　I　　2–5

　　　　　　II　　6–9

　　　　　　III　10–12

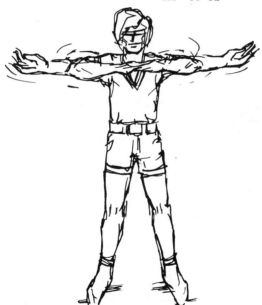

7. CHEST AND SHOULDER STRETCH

Starting Position: Stand erect, bend arms in front of chest, with fingertips touching and elbows at shoulder height.

Action: Counts 1, 2, and 3: Pull elbows back as far as possible, keeping arms at shoulder height. Return to starting position each time. Count 4: Swing arms outward and sideward, at shoulder height, palms up. Return to starting position. This is bouncy, rhythmic action, counting "one-and-two-and-three-and-four."

Level:　　I　　3–6

　　　　　　II　　7–10

　　　　　　III　11–15

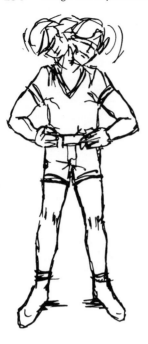

8. HEAD ROTATION
Starting Position: Stand erect, feet shoulder-width apart, hands on hips.
Action: Count 1: Slowly rotate the head in an arc from left to right. Count 2: Slowly rotate head in the opposite direction. Use slow, smooth motion; close eyes to help avoid losing balance or getting dizzy.
Level: I   2–4
      II   5–8
      III   9–10

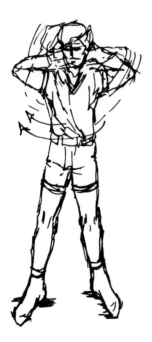

9. TRUNK ROTATION
Starting Position: Stand erect, feet shoulder-width apart, fingers interlocked behind head.
Action: Count 1: Rotate trunk to right, keeping feet flat on floor. Count 2: Return to starting position. Count 3: Rotate trunk to left. Keep feet flat on floor. Count 4: Return to starting position.
Level: I   2–4
      II   5–8
      III   9–10

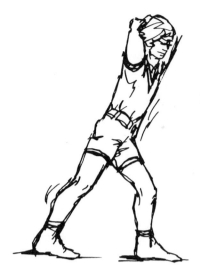

10. CALF STRETCHER

Starting Position: Place one foot ahead of the other about 24 inches in a stride position with the forward knee flexed and rear leg extended. Place hands behind head.

Action: Lean trunk forward carefully until a continuous stretch occurs to the rear calf; hold for 8–12 sec. Change leg positions and repeat. Remember to breathe freely.

Level: I   2–4 each leg
            II   4–6 each leg
            III 4–6 each leg

Developmental Exercises

Begin your developmental exercises at Level I. Plan to spend 4 weeks at each level. During this time, progress from the lowest number of repetitions to the highest within that level. After 4 weeks, proceed to the next level. Once you have reached the highest number of repetitions in Level III, continue it as a part of your maintenance program.

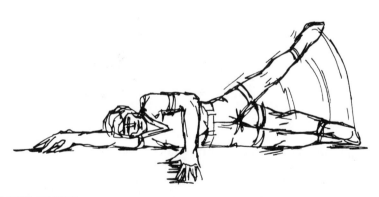

1. SIDE LEG RAISES

Starting Position: Right side of body on floor, head resting on right arm.

Action: Count 1: Lift leg sideways off floor to approximately 45°. Count 2: Return to starting position. Do the desired number of repetitions with the left leg and then turn over; lie on left side and exercise the right leg.

Level: I   3–6
            II   7–10
            III 11–15

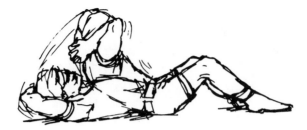

2a. HEAD AND SHOULDER CURL

Starting Position: Lie on back, legs bent at knees so that feet are together and flat on the floor. Clasp hands behind neck (hold that way throughout).

Action: Count 1: Tighten abdominal muscles and lift head and shoulders so that shoulders are about 10 inches or 45° off the floor. Hold this position 2–4 sec. Count 2: Return slowly to starting position, keeping abdominal muscles tight until shoulders and head rest on floor. Relax. The head should lead in a "curling" motion, chin tucked to chest, with back rounded, not arched.

Level: I   2–8

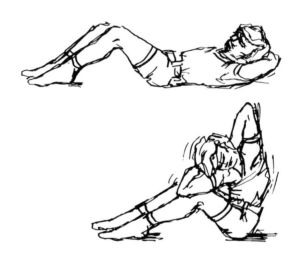

2b. BENT-KNEE SIT-UP

Starting Position: Lie on back, legs bent at knees so that feet are together and flat on the floor. Clasp hands behind neck (hold that way throughout).

Action: Count 1: Tighten abdominal muscles and sit up so that back is approximately perpendicular to the floor. Count 2: Return slowly to starting position, keeping abdominal muscles tight until shoulders and head rest on floor. Relax. The head should lead in a "curling" motion, chin tucked to chest, back rounded, not arched. When returning, "uncurl" back down.

Level: II   2–10
          III   11–20

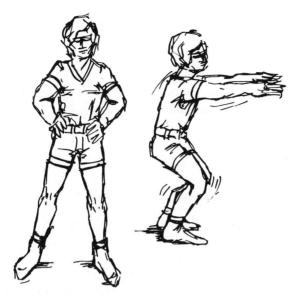

3. HALF KNEE BENDS

Starting Position: Stand erect, feet shoulder-width apart, hands on hips.

Action: Count 1: Bend knees halfway while extending arms forward, palms down. Keep heels on floor. Count 2: Return to starting position.

Level: I   2–5
II   6–9
III 10–15

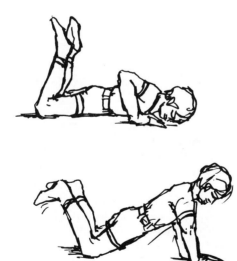

4a. KNEE PUSH-UP

Starting Position: Lie on floor, face down, legs together, knees bent with feet raised off floor, hands on floor under shoulders, palms down.

Action: Count 1: Push upper body off floor until arms are fully extended and body forms straight line from head to knees. Count 2: Return to starting position.

Level: I   3–10

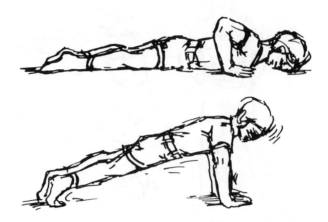

4b. REGULAR PUSH-UP
Starting Position: Lie on floor, face down, legs extended, hands on floor under shoulders, palms down.
Action: Count 1: Push body off floor until arms are fully extended and body and legs form straight line from head to heels. Count 2: Return to starting position.
Level: II   2–8
            III   9–20

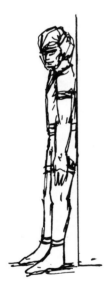

5. WALL PRESS
Starting Position: Stand erect, head not bent forward or backward, back against wall, heels about 3 inches away from wall.
Action: Count 1: Pull in the abdominal muscles and press the small of the back tightly against the wall. Hold for 4 sec. Count 2: Relax and return to starting position. Keep entire back in contact with wall on Count 1, and do not tilt head backward.
Level: I   2–5
            II   6–8
            III   9–10

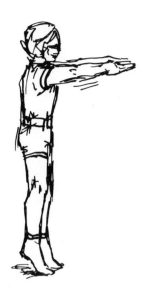

6. DIVER'S STANCE

Starting Position: Stand erect, feet slightly apart, arms at sides.

Action: Rise on toes and bring arms upward and forward so that they extend parallel with the floor, palms down. When this position is attained, close eyes and hold balance. Head should be straight, and body should be held firmly throughout.

Level: I   5 sec
II   6–10 sec
III   11–15 sec

10

Psychologic Aspects of Rehabilitation After Myocardial Infarction

Thomas P. Hackett, M.D.

Ned H. Cassem, M.D.

The psychologic symptoms encountered in individuals recovering from myocardial infarction (MI) are largely centered around two states of mind: depression and anxiety. They are interwoven as closely as warp and woof. Anxiety is a state resembling fear. The sufferer is apprehensive and hyperalert, and there are signs of heightened autonomic (sympathetic nervous system) activity. In the coronary disease patient the main reason for continued anxiety is the threat of sudden death; other worries, such as one's ability to remain employed and to function successfully as spouse, parent, and citizen, can augment this fear of death and contribute to anxiety. Depression is defined as a state of sadness due to a loss. Following MI, one almost invariably feels as though one has lost a part of oneself; usually it is a valued part—strength, energy, independence. During the first month of convalescence, depression is abetted by a subjective sense of depletion, weakness, and easy fatigue. The result is post-MI depression, about which Paul Dudley White (1) said, "It is of importance to realize that the heart may recover more rapidly than the depressed mental state which is so often a complication."

Although there are many individual psychologic problems that may be experienced during coronary rehabilitation (e.g., loss of libido, decreased potency, insomnia, irritability, inattentiveness), these problems, and others as well, have their roots in underlying depression. Many physicians who are unaware of the manifestations of depression or unfamiliar with its importance in coronary convalescence remain blind to its presence while treating its individual symptoms

Work prepared under contracts PHS 43-67-1443 and HE-13781 from the National Institutes of Health, Public Health Service, U.S. Department of Health, Education and Welfare.

243

in vain. For example, a 38-year-old commercial fisherman who had sustained MI and who went through hospitalization and convalescence without complication found himself unable to return to work on his father's trawler. Although he had been assigned a position requiring only a minimum of heavy exertion, he experienced extreme weakness and dyspnea as soon as he set foot aboard the vessel. His baffled physician continued to take serial electrocardiograms, along with Masters 2-step exercise tests, and to examine his blood chemistries. When these efforts failed to unearth the source of the problem, he was referred to a cardiologist; after a brief examination, the cardiologist sent him on to a psychiatric consultant. It turned out that his weakness was but one of a galaxy of symptoms that had come in the wake of MI: early morning awakening, difficulty in maintaining erections, markedly increased appetite, and a tendency to fall asleep every time he sat down. Although at first he denied fear or depression, closer questioning brought out his concern that death was just around the corner. He believed that his weakness and shortness of breath were signs that his cardiac condition was far worse than his doctors had told him. Once he began to talk, a stream of fears and concerns poured out—all related to his conviction that he had only months to live. Even a short time at sea took him away from his wife and children, with whom he desperately wanted to spend his remaining days. When this information was out, the psychiatrist was able to confront the patient's fears directly with explanations and reassurance and to guide the family doctor toward an understanding of the patient's concerns. A series of counseling sessions, along with dietary precautions, proper tranquilization, and bedtime sedation, served to restore him to his full measure of health.

Even under the best of circumstances there can be difficulties in recognizing and diagnosing depression. To begin with, it must be clearly understood that depression is a normal response to having an infarction. It is rare to find an individual who does not experience some degree of desolation, sadness, or resentment in the weeks after sustaining an infarction. However, it need not, and often does not, come to the doctor's attention. Typically, when first admitted with the symptoms of MI, the patient is frightened, worried about the diagnosis, and concerned about the immediate future. Once in the coronary care unit (CCU), after receiving a sedative and expert medical attention, the patient tends to relax. The patient's worries are centered on the immediate future, the next few days, not the more distant horizon of months. As the condition becomes stabilized and the patient begins to feel better, there is also a great deal of support provided by nurses and doctors. Anxiety usually is obvious only when the patient first comes to the CCU; by the second day it will decrease considerably (2,3). This diminished anxiety is a function of the defense of denial (as will be discussed presently) and of the effectiveness of tranquilizers and reassurance. However, depression seldom makes its appearance before the third day, and then it declines only slowly. If, during this period, the doctor asks "Are you depressed?" the patient may deny it. Instead of admitting depression, patients often say that they are concerned about what will happen to their jobs and how they will manage to change their living habits. Some patients mention the fear of shortened life span, but the usual response will have to do with more prosaic concerns. It is unlikely that tears or other signs of anguish will accompany the response. After such an encounter the physician frequently is impressed by how well the patient is bearing up, but the patient may or may not be holding up well. In many cases the underlying disturbance, if present, does not surface until after discharge from the hospital.

The depression that begins in the CCU often becomes manifest when the patient returns home. There are many reasons to account for this, but one seems to stand out from the rest. While hospitalized, the patient seldom has the chance to move about in an ordinary fashion. Unless the hospital is fortunate enough to have a physical conditioning program, the patient's movements are restricted to a hospital room, or perhaps a walk up and down a corridor. In such circumstances there is little opportunity to develop normal fatigue. As a consequence, when the range of activity increases on returning home, the patient quickly experiences the twin symptoms of weakness and easy tiring. Although these occur because of newly expanded activities, the patient is apt to misinterpret them as evidence of cardiac decline. The pleasure of recovery and the joy of returning to the family vanish in the first 48 hr. Often they are replaced by what the patient perceives to be a future in which life will be measured by limitations and restrictions. The hope of returning to full health that was engendered by the hospital experience is shattered and replaced by despair. We have used the term *homecoming depression* to describe this response (4).

Most patients are able to weather the discouragement of the early weeks at home without major disruption of their own lives or the lives of their families. However, there is little doubt in the mind of any physician who has treated post-MI patients that early convalescence at home is a time fraught with difficulty. Aside from being depressed, the patient is apt to feel unprotected and vulnerable after the close scrutiny and care provided in the hospital. Furthermore, the severe restrictions placed on smoking, eating, and the use of alcohol are discouraging. Then, too, there are questions about sexual, social, and physical activities that cause worry. All of these add up to a situation that tends to work against peace of mind. One patient summarized his mental state: "No smokes, no booze, low salt, low fat, low energy, low sex or no sex—I feel like a cardiologic capon."

When does homecoming depression become pathologic? In understanding any depression it is helpful to use grief as a model. When a loved one dies, the bereaved experiences a feeling of emptiness and loss. The depth of this reaction usually has a direct relationship to the closeness of the tie. Parents mourn the loss of children long and bitterly. Grieving is accompanied by physical symptoms such as anorexia, insomnia, weakness, constipation, agitation, physical depletion, and loss of interest in usual pleasures. Mourning is most acute during the first 3 months following the loss. During the fourth month the individual may begin to take interest again in certain aspects of life, regaining appetite and the ability to sleep. Generally, after a year has passed the process of mourning has ended, although the sense of loss may still be keenly felt. By that time the person usually has returned to the company of friends and society and is able to work effectively and enjoy life. Grieving is said to be pathologic when it does not end within certain broadly defined time limits ranging from 3 months to 1 year. These limits are, of course, arbitrary and can vary, depending on the relationship between the survivor and the deceased.

The same type of time scale can be applied in coronary heart disease. Following an uncomplicated first MI, the patient should be able to resume involvement in work, in society, and in the home within 3 months of leaving the hospital. In more complicated cases there seems to be a direct relationship between the severity of the cardiac condition and the extent of depression. In this sense the cardiac patient's response has parallels with the observation that the depth of grieving is a function of the depth of the severed relationship. When depression in the post-MI patient really is related to severe cardiac impairment, there is little that can be done from the psychologic standpoint; however, that is not the type of patient about which this chapter is written. There are many patients who become cardiac cripples without the necessary credentials; despite uncomplicated recovery and maximum physiologic return of the myocardium, the members of this group continue being depressed and fearful. They do not return to work and do little to attempt renewal of their former ways of life. They suffer from the syndrome of "unwarranted invalidism." There are hundreds of thousands of them in this country, and their cost to the nation in lost time, compensation, and settlement is enormous. The financial dimension is measured in billions; the toll in human suffering is incalculable.

In our studies and in the studies of others we have noticed a considerable difference between the effects of uncomplicated MI on blue-collar workers and the effects of uncomplicated MI on white-collar executives (5,6). Blue-collar patients appear to know less about the illness. They may not want to learn about the condition; they may have trouble understanding explanations; or it may be simply that medical caretakers do not take enough time to teach them what they should know. One fact is apparent: blue-collar patients do not ask as many questions as their white-collar counterparts. Their resulting lack of knowledge often sets the stage for anxiety, uncertainty, and a sense of helplessness. A simple example will demonstrate this. We routinely ask convalescent MI patients to draw an outline of the heart showing where the trouble was, how large an area it covered, and what the lesion looked like. Generally, white-collar patients do a reasonably good job of describing the infarction, although few have any idea of its size. They also know about the process of repair. Blue-collar patients, in contrast, can describe the damage done, but they have little or no idea of how the scar tissue fills in the defect. Many of them imagine that a hole has been punched out of the heart wall forming a permanent leak in the pumping system. It is not difficult to understand why persons who harbor such a notion are inclined to regard themselves as cripples. Lack of information is undoubtedly one of the reasons why unwarranted invalidism is more widespread among the laboring class.

The speed and ease of recovery from MI are also related to job security. The executive can generally expect to have the same job waiting when the time comes to return. This is not true for the factory worker or laborer. Not only do unfair personnel practices discriminate against the blue-collar coronary patient, but labor union contracts also frequently impose shortsighted and unrealistic regulations. It is difficult to design a program for physical rehabilitation when a harsh world offers so little incentive for improvement. Fortunately, many of these bylaws are undergoing change, but they still must be taken into account in the management of coronary convalescence.

At this point the reader might well ask what the MI patient does have going for him. Is everyone destined to get depressed in the same way during the course of recovery? Although we share Hellerstein's conviction that depression is "virtually universal in the period following onset of infarction," there are wide individual variations in its depth and duration (7). Some people are better at adjusting to adversity than others. An important clue to the way in which a patient will respond to MI can be obtained by learning how the patient dealt with stress in the past (e.g., death or sickness of family members, financial reversals, induction into the armed service and combat). Answers to these questions can help predict the patient's capacity to cope with MI.

Earlier in this discussion mention was made of the defense of denial. Denial is a defense mechanism defined as conscious or unconscious repudiation of all or part of the available meaning of an event to allay anxiety or other unpleasant emotions. Denial is the most commonly used defense in coronary heart disease. It is a normal method of handling stress. For example, when we enter an airplane at the start of a trip, we usually avoid thinking about hijackings, midair collisions, engine failures, and fogged-in landing strips. Instead, we focus on the forthcoming cocktail and meal and arrival at our destination. Thus we deny or push aside the fearful aspects of air travel while occupying ourselves with the pleasant advantages of being aloft. Similarly, the cardiac patient in the CCU denies the serious, life-threatening aspect of the illness and focuses on the monitor and other aspects of intensive care as benevolent life rafts. In this way the patient can avoid facing the fact that the need for them signifies a high state of personal danger. The person who denies is able to replace worry and morbid preoccupation with positive plans and more tranquil thoughts. The successful denier is the nonworrier. Such is the following example. A 56-year-old architect who had recently suffered an anterior MI impressed the examiner as being unusually complacent and unperturbed in the face of his illness. He explained his peace of mind by stating that he was "indestructible." A Texan by birth and inclination, he identified with President Lyndon B. Johnson, who had also sustained an MI and survived. Furthermore, both his father and a paternal uncle had done well following heart attacks, and the patient firmly believed he shared their immunity to harm. There was no reason to doubt that his confidence and composure were anything but genuine. Without denying the heart attack itself, this man denied all of its threatening aspects and accentuated the potential for survival.

Not all people who attempt to deny are equally successful. Some individuals simply do not worry or do not appear to suffer unduly from the threat of death. There are others who keep fear at a greater distance. Some put on a convincing front, but secretly suffer anguish. Others appear to have no ability whatever to control or stifle their worries. Most of us fall somewhere between these extremes. Denial, or the conscious ability to reduce worry, may reduce mortality and morbidity in coronary heart disease. Studies have shown that patients who are able to deny worry have a better chance of surviving hospitalization for MI. Furthermore, such patients tend to return to normal sexual activity and to work sooner than individuals who are unable to reduce fear through denial. It is important for the physician to understand that denial plays a critical role in recovery; more than anyone else, the physician can institute, bolster, and maintain denial. Denial does not mean lying with optimism in the face of grim reality;

rather, it means pointing out the positive by emphasizing the patient's strengths rather than dwelling on the threat to health. The following case illustrates how a physician can reassure by using denial. A 47-year-old nightclub comedian had difficulty staying in bed his first day in the CCU. Although his pain had abated, he complained of uneasiness and "inner tensions." His doctor, sensing that he was alarmed at suddenly finding himself for the first time in an intensive care setting, said, "Some people don't like the restraint of being hooked to the monitor. You get used to it. The fact is you couldn't be in a safer place. While your heart is healing, it needs to be watched closely. It is like setting down cement. Wet or 'green' cement has to be roped off so people won't step on it and make a mark. You have scar tissue rapidly filling in the bruised area in your heart. Soon it will be as firm and sound as set concrete, but until then we will watch it closely with this monitor. While you're attached to it, nothing can happen to you that we can't take care of." The patient was considerably heartened by this explanation that dealt entirely with the positive aspects of healing while avoiding (denial) the negative. Later, when the patient expressed doubt about ever being able to perform before an audience again, his physician pointed out the examples of Peter Sellers and Pearl Bailey, both of whom had sustained severe MIs and had returned to the stage. Had the patient questioned specifically about risks such as reinfarction, arrest, and arrhythmias, he would have been answered honestly, but in as reassuring a way as the circumstances warranted.

What are the best tactics to use in managing the convalescent MI patient? We have listed the following steps, some of which may not be possible because of limitations of time and staff and restrictions imposed by the severity of the illness. However, any one of these points would be helpful to the patient.

CLEARING UP MISCONCEPTIONS THROUGH EDUCATION

Every disease is surrounded by long-established myths that tend to resist all attempts to rout them. MI is no exception. Because it is both common and lethal, it has accumulated more than its share of folklore. The most frequently encountered myths are the following:

· Even mild exercise is dangerous.
· Sexual intercourse should never be attempted, because following MI one is "over the hill."
· Repeated infarction or sudden death is more likely to occur at sexual orgasm.
· Driving must be avoided.
· The arms must not be suddenly raised above the head, especially the left arm.
· The patient is apt to die at the same age as a parent who had heart disease.
· Recurrence is apt to take place around the anniversary of the first infarction.
· The heart is more vulnerable to repeat infarction and sudden death while the patient sleeps.

Patients rarely, if ever, volunteer these beliefs and ask the physician's opinion about them. Consequently, the physician must bring them up in order to determine if the patient entertains any such ideas. Those cited are more common in blue-collar populations, but they occur across all strata of society. Queries about sex are more commonly made by the educated. Patients from lower socio-economic backgrounds are often too embarrassed to speak of sex.

The best time to clarify these misconceptions and impart the facts is just before the patient leaves the hospital. It is important to set aside half an hour or more to chat with the patient and spouse. Point by point the doctor should discuss medications, activities, diet, and various restrictions, as well as the tendency of the family to overprotect and baby the patient. This education can be reinforced by other health care personnel.

With the couple alone, advice should be given about sexual performance. Good articles are available on this topic (8). Liberal use should also be made of the excellent pamphlets and booklets offered by the American Heart Association.

ANTICIPATION

The first portion of this chapter provided a description of post-MI depression. The patient should be warned about the sense of tiredness and easy fatigue that may be experienced on arriving home. It should be made clear that this does not indicate a failing heart; it is a natural response to 2 or 3 weeks of inactivity. Even young athletes who are kept at bed rest for only a few days are out of condition for days thereafter. It should also be made clear that anxiety may occur as the patient's range of activities is expanded, especially in regard to returning to work or doing anything that has produced social stress in the past. Simple anticipation can do a great deal to reduce anguish.

MEDICATION

It is important to consider the use of psychotropic drugs during convalescence. Recurrent anxiety is best handled by trying to determine its cause and by offering explanations and reassurances when these are in order. Tranquilizers should be used in conjunction with counseling. They are often valuable in maintaining equanimity. It should be emphasized that one's state of mind is important to one's physical health. For patients who are chronically anxious, tranquilizers should be accorded the same importance as diuretics, digitalis, and other cardiac drugs. The benzodiazepines are tranquilizers that are safe for cardiac patients. Generally, the dosage schedule is as follows: diazepam (Valium) 2–5 mg, chlordiazepoxide (Librium) 5–10 mg, or oxazepam (Serax) 15 mg, three or four times a day. Since some patients, especially men from lower socio-economic strata, consider it unmanly to take pills continually, the physician should stress the importance of following a regular regimen and should emphasize that the use of tranquilizers no more casts aspersion on manhood than does taking a drink of alcohol (and it is far more beneficial than alcohol).

Use of tricyclic antidepressants is contraindicated because of associated disturbances in heart rate and rhythm. They, along with the phenothiazines, have been implicated in sudden deaths. Similarly, it is unsafe to use the monoamine oxidase inhibitors during convalescence from MI because of the danger of hypertensive crisis when tyramine-containing food is ingested.

Insomnia, particularly during the first month at home, should be treated with a hypnotic. The most convenient method of achieving this is to double the dose of the benzodiazepine given for daytime sedation. Flurazepam (Dalmane) is a popular hypnotic, largely because it does not suppress REM sleep. The usual adult dosage is 30 mg at bedtime.

ACTIVITY AND PHYSICAL CONDITIONING

Most of the patients we have seen, particularly those in the blue-collar category, have stated that inactivity is the most frustrating aspect of convalescence. Most did not have hobbies to pursue, nor were they content to watch television all day long. On the other hand, often they were afraid to move about very much, particularly during inclement weather and when moving about involved exertion. As a consequence, our advice for the physician or the cardiac nurse is to outline a program of activity on a day-to-day basis. Working with both patient and spouse, a trained nurse can draw up a course of activities compatible with the patient's cardiac status just before discharge.

As a result of three decades of effort in evaluating cardiac work in various facilities across the country, there are now lists available that tell how strenuous the common daily activities are. These lists quantify the energy spent in self-care, vocational activities, housework, and recreational activities. Quantification is in terms of metabolic equivalents, called mets (1 met or metabolic unit is the energy expenditure per kilogram of body weight per minute for an average subject sitting quietly in a chair, which is approximately 1.4 K Cal/min or 3.5–4 ml of oxygen per kilogram per minute).

The best means of preventing depression from developing or of arresting the growth of depression that has begun is a program of physical conditioning. Far too few hospitals have fully accepted the importance of the concept of physical conditioning, and even fewer have seen fit to finance units to put the concept into practice. But in hospitals where this has been done, tangible gains have been made. Anxiety and depression are less troublesome, it is reported, when patients are actively engaged in physical conditioning. Aside from the physiologic benefit, these activities give the patient a sense of participating in the recovery process, rather than being the passive recipient of care. Confidence in performance is restored as patients see their potential for various activities expand. Physical conditioning can help fill the long days of recovery and can provide a welcome do as relief from the many don'ts of convalescence (don't smoke, don't eat too much, don't hurry, don't worry). For most human beings, physical activity is an important part of living and being alive; when the patient is deprived of it, self-esteem declines, and living becomes a hollow experience.

Following uncomplicated MI, average men of middle age in supervised programs are capable of performing at a level of 8–9 mets. This level encompasses running at 5.5 mph, cycling at 13 mph, skiing at 4 mph, noncompetitive squash and handball, and vigorous basketball. If less than ordinary activity produces symptoms in the post-MI period, then the patient's capacity is closer to 4 mets. Even though such a patient's performance is clearly impaired, the following activities should be possible: swimming breast stroke at 20 yards/min, cycling at 5.5 mph, walking up a 5% incline at 3 mph, table tennis, golf, badminton, doubles tennis, and raking leaves. These are quantitative capacities, carefully computed; prescribing them is far more precise than making statements such as "Use your own judgment" or "Do it in moderation." We believe it is much better to explain the concept of mets and provide a booklet listing all the values for common activities, as well as values for those activities that are particularly applicable to the patient's life-style. The Colorado Heart Association has printed this information for patients in its program.

Supervised exercise programs are becoming increasingly available for post-MI patients throughout the country. Many patients, of course, will not want to be so active on a regular basis, but knowing that referral to such a program is possible at some future date (ordinarily not before 2–3 months after infarction) can provide reassurance that they are not considered invalids by their physicians.

It may be of help to point out to the recently infarcted patient who is still in the hospital that five runners from Toronto who had sustained MI completed a recent year's Boston marathon. This will come as a surprise to most patients; it illustrates quite vividly that levels of activity may be obtainable that had not been thought possible.

CLUB ACTIVITIES

There have been reports from a variety of sources that group meetings of post-MI patients, managed by a cardiac nurse clinician, can be an excellent means of exchanging information and discussing mutual experiences (9). Most of these groups assemble while patients are hospitalized and continue for 3–4 months after discharge. They may be run by a physician or a nurse clinician who instructs the patients on what they should and should not do in various situations. The leader may answer questions and encourage patients to share their experiences with each other. Since this group concept has not yet been tested on a sufficiently large scale under controlled conditions, its value remains to be demonstrated scientifically. However, individuals who have participated in these groups enthusiastically endorse them. In our experience this has been a valuable method of educational therapy.

TELEPHONE FOLLOW-UP

The procedure of having a nurse telephone the patient and family on a weekly basis for 2 months after discharge to ask if there is anything about which advice is needed has been greatly appreciated by our patient population. Numerous issues can arise about which the patient would not ordinarily feel justified in bothering the physician. (Can I walk my dog? He's an elderly dalmatian.) The patient is faced with a problem that needs an answer, however trifling. This is especially true in conditioning programs where activity is stressed; often the patient is unsure about how far to go. Fears concerning sexual activity comprise a considerable proportion of telephone queries.

TRANSCENDENTAL MEDITATION, HYPNOSIS, AND RELAXATION TECHNIQUES

Transcendental meditation (TM) has received considerable attention in recent years, but there has been no sizable controlled study of its usefulness in coronary convalescence. The same holds true for hypnosis and muscular relaxation. However, responsible investigators put great store in spending one or two periods each day practicing some form of relaxation technique. Autohypnosis has long been recognized as a useful tool in a variety of conditions, but it is limited by the fact that not everyone is a good hypnotic subject. TM and relaxation techniques such as those advocated by Jacobson are more useful for the general population. It seems to us that these relaxation techniques have a strong attraction for certain individuals but, like jogging, have limited appeal for the majority.

PSYCHOTHERAPY

Short- or long-term psychotherapy is indicated only when post-MI depression is protracted or when the individual is besieged by chronic anxiety spells or the physical concomitants of either of these two states. Persistent loss of libido, impotence, anorexia, insomnia, hypersomnia, and hypochondriacal complaints (all or any of which may occur or persist in the wake of MI) might well be evaluated by a psychiatrist and might require psychotherapy. However, we do not advocate psychotherapy routinely for the post-MI patient in depression unless the depression compromises marriage, job, or happiness for an extended period (3 months).

SUMMARY

Anxiety and depression are the major psychologic hurdles in cardiac rehabilitation. Each can result in unwarranted invalidism, which extracts a huge toll in money and anguish. By means of a few simple interventions, the most important of which are education and activity, the morbidity of the rehabilitative process can be considerably reduced.

REFERENCES

1. White PD: *Heart Disease.* Macmillan, New York, 1951
2. Hackett TP, Cassem NH, Wishnie HA: The coronary care unit: An appraisal of its psychological hazards. *N Engl J Med* 279:1365, 1968

3. Cassem NH, Hackett TP: The psychiatric consultation in the coronary care unit. *Ann Intern Med* 75:9, 1971

4. Wishnie HA, Hackett TP, Cassem NH: Psychological hazards of convalescence following myocardial infarction. *JAMA* 215:1292, 1971

5. Hackett TP, Cassem NH: White collar and blue collar responses to heart attack. *J. Psychosom Res* 20:85, 1976

6. Croog SH, Levine S, Lurie, Z: The heart patient and the recovery process. *Soc Sci Med* 2:111, 1968

7. Hellerstein HK: Rehabilitation of the post-infarction patient. *Hosp Pract* 7:45, 1972

8. Hellerstein HK, Friedman EH: Sexual activity in the post-coronary patient. *Arch Intern Med* 125:987, 1970

9. Bilodeau CB, Hackett TP: Issues raised in a group setting by patients recovering from myocardial infarction. *Am J Psychiatry* 128:73, 1971

11

Social Aspects of Rehabilitation After Myocardial Infarction: A Selective Review

Sydney H. Croog, Ph.D.

A universal feature of rehabilitation of cardiac patients is that it takes place in social contexts. Further, the participants (the patients and those who provide care and support) are also influenced in many ways by social factors in their immediate situations and in their backgrounds. These varied social influences may, taken as a whole, serve either to enhance or to impede the processes of rehabilitation and recovery. In the latter case, social influences may constitute barriers sufficient to endanger the health and long-term welfare of patients.

In this chapter some of the principal social influences on recovery and rehabilitation will be reviewed briefly. The main emphasis will be on barriers and problems with which the physician may be concerned in patient management and in rehabilitation planning. These include elements in the physician–patient relationship, work situations, family relationships, and availability and use of rehabilitation services. The focus will be primarily on rehabilitation in the period after discharge from the hospital following treatment for the acute episode of coronary disease.

DATA AND GOALS

One inevitable influence in any review of social factors in cardiac rehabilitation must be the character and adequacy of currently available data. Many sophisti-

Preparation of these materials has been supported in part by Social Security Administration grant 10-P-57537, "Health Services Use and Life Problems in Chronic Disease," and by USPHS grant HS-00268, "Social Factors in the Recovery of Heart Patients." Some illustrative materials have been used previously in research reports and in manuscript prepared in connection with the National Heart and Lung Institute Task Force on Cardiovascular Rehabilitation. U.S. Government Printing Office, DHEW publication (NIH) 75-750, December, 1974.

255

cated clinical reports have dealt with such matters as the physician–patient relationship, the role of the family, the effects of interpersonal relationships in the work situation, and the influences of the sociocultural context as a whole. Numerous writers have suggested ways in which such matters should or can be considered in rehabilitation management. However, there have been few studies specifically concerned with the social and psychologic influences on rehabilitation, as compared with the large volume of research on the etiology and epidemiology of heart disease (1). Aside from scarcity of data on general trends and relationships, few studies have illustrated the variability in the effects of these factors within social subgroups, whether differentiated in terms of social class, sex, age, region, rural–urban, race, or other key traits.

Another matter of importance is the relationship of cardiac rehabilitation as a system to the nature of the society as a whole. The larger society and its health care system influence the physician–patient relationship, the use of services, and family relationships (2,3). The health care system reflects the society in which it exists, varying in such elements as political organization, economic system, values and beliefs regarding health care, level of bureaucratic organization in government, conceptions of the rights of individuals in the society, and other features. However, the current literature fails to provide a basis for detailed comparisons of rehabilitation outcomes for cardiac patients living in diverse societies, such as China, Germany, Great Britain, India, Japan, New Zealand, Scandinavia, and the United States.

Numerous materials, however, provide at least indirect evidence and preliminary data relevant to issues in this chapter. For example, we can refer to studies in other areas, such as those that deal with adherence to medical advice in illnesses other than heart disease. Some discussion is based in part on specialized studies in cardiac rehabilitation that only peripherally relate to social aspects but that are useful nonetheless. I have also drawn from our long-term longitudinal study of heart patients in Boston (4–7). This review will focus on a series of relevant factors in the complex processes of rehabilitation, with emphasis on raising questions and offering tentative interpretations.

PHYSICIAN–PATIENT COMMUNICATION AND ADHERENCE

During hospitalization and after being discharged, the cardiac patient comes into contact with a variety of health professionals and hospital personnel. Although care and rehabilitation of the coronary patient include the efforts of many health professionals, in addition to the efforts of the patient, the primary physician is a key person. The elements of the physician–patient relationship have been analyzed often, and numerous psychologic and sociologic reviews are available (8,9). Two concerns will be discussed as they relate to cardiac rehabilitation: patient adherence to the medical regimen and the problem of physician–patient communication (including associated social and psychologic barriers).

Adherence

A continuing problem in cardiac rehabilitation is patient adherence to the medical regimen. Although few controlled studies have dealt with eventual outcomes of patients classified by differing levels of adherence, it seems clear that adherence to the physician's advice affects the course and success of rehabilitation. The factors that promote or impede adherence among cardiac patients may best be understood as sharing common characteristics with factors that influence adherence in patients with other chronic illnesses.

Seen in these terms, numerous reports dealing with research, clinical experiences, and case studies become relevant (8,9). The many reviews present a picture of adherence as a multifaceted phenomenon that cannot be explained with simple models. Rather, a number of operant factors must be considered, including patterns of communication, the character of the message, the complexity of the instruction, the personalities of the participants, the relativity and severity of the threat perceived, etc. Such research has helped to rule out relatively unimportant factors and has directed attention to more critical variables. For example, Becker and Maiman (9) recently reported that "in general, studies show that compliance is not consistently related to sex, intelligence, education, or marital status."

In our study of cardiac patients, several principal findings related to their adherence (4). It appeared that physicians had an optimal opportunity to influence patients. A year after hospitalization for a first myocardial infarction, for example, a pattern of continuity of relationship with the physician and confidence in the physician was evident. Over 90% of patients had seen their physicians during the year, and virtually all indicated they would continue with the same physician. Although advice to patients covered many subjects, physicians reported a high level of general adherence by their own criteria, with about 70% of physicians rating patient adherence as good or better. Adherence by patient ratings was highest during the first year in specific matters that required clear action, such as taking medication, changing jobs, and the like.

A key factor in coronary atherosclerotic heart disease, smoking, was clearly modified in response to physician advice. Although the literature shows few instances of long-term modification of smoking behavior, such change was found in our study. Seventy-five percent of the men studied had smoked over a pack of cigarettes per day prior to myocardial infarction; 42% had smoked two packs of cigarettes or more, an amount several times higher than that encountered in males of comparable age at that time in the general population. After discharge from the hospital, the proportion of smokers dropped drastically and was maintained 1 year later. At the year's end, 58% classified themselves as nonsmokers, and the proportion smoking one pack or more declined to 23%. Only 6% still smoked two packs or more.

At present we are studying the same men 7–8 years later. Preliminary data from the survivors shows that, after this long period, smoking is still at the lower level of the postinfarction year. In fact, the rate of consumption is not significantly different from that of other men of the same age in the general population.

The basis for such change cannot be ascribed entirely to the advice that most smokers received from their physicians. However, the power of this influence, as reported by patients, was of great importance. It is significant that a long-term behavioral change occurred, supported by continued reinforcement from the physician. Even in the case of a difficult behavior to change, smoking, this population achieved an outcome favorable for reduction of a coronary risk factor.

Physician–Patient Communication

In the physician–patient relationship, factors that limit or impede communication are important barriers to rehabilitation of the cardiac patient (5,10). Although communication is a two-way process, one avenue has received greater attention than the other in the medical literature: How can the physician communicate best with the patient? The counterpart (the problems of communicating to the physician the patient's problems, needs, and goals as they relate to rehabilitation) has received less emphasis. Physicians must recognize the importance of both sides of communication.

For example, in the treatment of cardiac patients the possibility of development of iatrogenic illness is well known. Inadequate or misinterpreted information about the illness may provoke anxieties in patients and may hamper their ability to resume normal activities. Although the message may be perfectly clear to the physician, the patient may become anxious because of what the patient believes the physician said and because of what the physician failed to say.

Restrictions that physicians place on patients may also constitute symbolic communications, conveying unintended messages. Reduction or deprivation of smoking, drinking, physical activity, and sexual activity may mean more than simple restriction. For example, to the male patient they may signify a symbolic loss of manhood and of personal competence, confirming his concern that illness has transformed him into an aging cardiac cripple, an incomplete man.

Another potential problem for cardiac patients is the lack of adequate guidance from their physicians in regard to management of life-style. This may stem from ambiguous advice or no information at all about avoidance of stress, sexual performance, and the symptoms that are danger signals and those that are not.

In our study of cardiac patients, at 1 month after discharge from the hospital about one-third continued to have questions about which they desired further information from their physicians (4). Although both patients and physicians reported that these topics were discussed, patients still felt inadequately informed. They cited such matters as the future course of their disease, acceptable levels of activity, causes of the illness, and factors that might bring on recurrences. Ironically, many of these issues could well have been handled by persons acting as educators on behalf of physicians, such as coronary care unit nurses, visiting nurses, and other health professionals.

Social and Psychologic Barriers

There is increasing evidence that the barriers to communication may be greater when physicians and patients have different social and cultural backgrounds. The difficulties of communication between physicians and patients with marked cultural or language gulfs are well known. One example is the difficulty patients experience in communicating to physicians their own goals and conceptions of rehabilitation. Whereas the physician may provide guidance attuned to a classic medical model, this may sometimes take place without adequate communication concerning the patient's own goals and needs in rehabilitation. The life patterns and values of persons from differing social classes, races, and ethnic groups help account for heterogeneity among patients in regard to both short-term and long-term goals for rehabilitation (5).

The frustrations of physicians who are not adequately understood by their patients are shared by those patients who feel that they have not had the time for discussion or who do not have verbal skills to inform their physicians about their hopes and needs in rehabilitation. As part of modern American folklore there has emerged the picture of the frustrated and anxious patient lamenting that the really important issues have not been discussed with the doctor. Together with variables that influence the quality and content of communication, recent data on time limitations are pertinent. One study of cardiologists showed that the average time the patient spends with the physician ranges from 6 to 12 min (11). Moreover, when the physician has a large office caseload (25–50 patients per day) it is probable that time restrictions limit the patient's opportunity to explore problems and receive counseling and teaching from the physician.

Recent reports have suggested that small teaching groups of postcoronary patients led by a nurse, a physician, or another health professional have reduced the anxiety and depression experienced during rehabilitation (12,13). These groups are not to be confused with psychotherapy groups. Heart Clubs are organized while patients are still in the hospital, and they meet at scheduled intervals for weeks or months. The primary purpose is educational. Patients exchange experiences and question the group leader about their concerns, and they are given information appropriate to their stages of recovery. This appears to be a practical and economical method of improving the exchange of information and enhancing the education of the postcoronary patient.

FAMILY ROLES AND REHABILITATION

Changes in Power Relationships and Authority

One potential source of problems lies in the changes in family roles brought about by illness. When illness afflicts the husband, major reorganization in responsibilities, activities, and authority may be necessary. As the wife and children undertake new roles, the husband may be placed in a subordinate position. This situation can raise two types of problems. In one instance, the husband accepts his passive role and takes a place in the family as a permanent cardiac cripple. Such an individual may have had longstanding conflicts with his wife in regard to dominance. The illness finally provides the means whereby he accepts being overprotected, cared for, and having decisions made on his behalf. In the other situation, the husband fights back, while wife and children struggle with him for dominance and justify their efforts as being for his own good. Thus the illness may trigger new arrangements of power and control within the family. The struggle may continue, altering in form and intensity as the patient regains his health, as new illness occurs, or as new situations arise within the family.

Goals and Life-style

The influence of family goals and life-style on the course of rehabilitation may also be significant. Whether recognized or not, a family may have psychologic and social needs whose fulfillment is linked to its style of life and position in the community. The illness and the possible continuation of the patient's disability alter that way of life, not only for the patient but also for the other members of the family. The economic impact may include the need to restrict funds, to change residence, or to limit future planning for the education of children and for other major expenditures. Because of the reduction in the style of life and changes in plans, the patient may feel guilty for handicapping the lives of others. Aggression and resentment, expressed or latent, often appear among family members and cause problems for others. Some patients deal with this situation by denial of the illness and by continuing a stressful, pressured life-style in order to maintain the customary pattern of the whole family.

Marital Conflicts and Illness

In addition to rearrangement of roles and changes in the power structure of the family, marital conflicts may affect rehabilitation. The occurrence of illness may exacerbate preexisting interpersonal conflicts and disagreements. Irritability, anxiety, and depression in the patient, often eliciting negative responses from the spouse, are not uncommon in families where severe illness strikes. Thus the patient must cope not only with the physical problems of the illness but also with the emotional tensions of the marriage.

Is marital conflict a significant factor affecting the course of cardiac rehabilitation? No accurate survey is available. However, the high divorce rate in the United States is one partial indication that many marriages are unstable, as is the high incidence of legal separations, desertions, and marital discord. It seems inevitable that the high incidence of marital conflict in the nation may be an important factor affecting the recovery course of large numbers of patients.

Some indication of the character of family relationships within which rehabilitation takes place appeared in our study of 345 men discharged from the hospital after a first myocardial infarction. All patients were presented a list of items dealing with common concepts about the etiology of coronary heart disease; they were asked to designate those that they believed to be important in their own case. Among married men, one-fifth reported that problems with their wives were important causes. Twenty-five percent of men with children indicated that "upsetting problems with their children" were important (4).

Lacking other evidence, we cannot judge whether the patients' beliefs about the illness reflected the general emotional tone of the relationships in the family or in the marriage. It is possible that they do. However, regardless of the level of emotional tension between patient and family, the holding of such beliefs has many implications, both for the men who held these convictions privately and for those who expressed them to their wives and children. The assumption by the practitioner that the family is always a source of support during rehabilitation may be less justified after subtle inquiries are made into the actual home situation.

Variability and Change in Family Patterns

Although some general descriptions can be developed that sum up the multiple principal effects of the family on the course of rehabilitation, it may be useful also to note some sources of variation. Thus the contexts within which family factors operate may differ in terms of social class, level of cohesiveness or togetherness in the family, number of family members, and situations involving widowhood, divorce, and separation. Ethnic traditions, race, and cultural beliefs may be important. The effects induced by social change, such as the influence of the women's liberation movement, remain to be assessed. These numerous traits can be classified in terms of major common characteristics. When sufficient empirical data become available, it will be possible to outline the primary patterns and processes within family structures as they influence the course of rehabilitation.

Quasi-Family Aid and Support

Whereas it is recognized that the spouse and the family influence the course of rehabilitation, the potential influences of quasi-family members or surrogate family are less frequently cited. For example, the cardiac patient may have stronger and closer associations with neighbors and friends than with relatives and in-laws.

In our study, some assistance from friends during the first year after hospitalization was noted by 85% of the cardiac patients; 40% rated their friends as being as helpful as parents, siblings, and in-laws (6). Neighbors were also cited by 66% as being helpful. Similar assistance was reported by patients of differing social status and education. These quasi-family sources provide services, moral support, and even financial assistance, and they can be important factors in rehabilitation.

The strength and supportive power of the family, the power of love between husband and wife, and the positive assistance of children and members of the extended family as factors in recovery from illness are all well known and need no reemphasis. Yet, the true meaning and implications of relationships within the family are often difficult to discern. It is easy for the hurried physician to accept at face value superficial descriptions that are given in office interviews by patients and spouses. The physician may not take the time to acquire information that would facilitate recognition of the more subtle processes and signs in the family that influence rehabilitation.

WORK SITUATIONS AND RELATIONSHIPS

Physical Stresses and Employer Attitudes

One of the main criteria used in assessing the success of rehabilitation is the return of the patient to work. Return to work relates to such matters as physical capacity, emotional state, social role, financial independence, and other factors. However, in the work situation, a number of elements act as barriers to rehabilitation. For example, the physical stresses of work may constitute a problem, especially for the blue-collar worker whose life may be endangered by tasks requiring high levels of energy expenditure.

Attitudes of employers may play a role, as reflected in their reluctance to hire cardiac patients or their refusal to place them in responsible positions. One of our cardiac patients summed up the problem with these words: "My heart condition has limited my chances with the company. There are jobs which carry more responsibilities and more pressure. The company, knowing of my heart attack, does not give me the consideration I would have received if I were well."

Furthermore, limited opportunities for changing to less demanding jobs may present difficulties for some wage earners, particularly those in blue-collar categories. Thus the difficulty of obtaining reentry into employment after the acute phases of cardiac illness may be a barrier to return to normal life.

Relationships With Fellow Employees

Another relevant rehabilitation factor concerns standards and requirements of social situations at work. To maintain the image of competence in the eyes of fellow workers, the cardiac patient may be led to overexert. In cases where teamwork is necessary, the cardiac patient who tries to avoid overexertion may be accused of malingering or may be resented by fellow workers for not doing the job properly. The question of maintaining status among fellow workers or acting to protect health can constitute a difficult choice. For some, the job may be perceived as a barrier to personal welfare and safety, a place of frustrated ambitions, of reminders of incapacity and inadequacy.

Work and Physician Decisions

Physician decisions may constitute a barrier to return to work. A physician may be reluctant to permit patients to return to full activity, despite their ability to do so. The physician may be fearful that too bold an approach may result in deaths, which would reflect on the quality of his professional care, his reputation and his means of earning a livelihood. The net effect on the patient may be delayed rehabilitation. On the other hand, overeager endorsement by the physician of the patient's ability to return to the former job may also become an obstacle to long-range vocational rehabilitation; the patient may be fired or downgraded because of inability to perform at the required level.

Work as a Cause of Heart Attack: Beliefs and Their Implications

Among the common patient conceptions about the "causes of heart attacks," the belief that work stresses are of etiologic importance is widespread. Many workers are aware that courts have made liberal interpretations about work stress being causative in making awards under workmen's compensation laws and in related cases. The belief was readily reflected in our study (4). Among the factors that patients thought were important in the etiology of their illness, "emotional tension at work" and "physical stress at work" were among the most frequently cited. Eighty-six percent rated one or both of these factors as important in etiology.

Given such misconceptions (which have no basis in epidemiologic studies), going to work each day may engender a sense of concern or danger. Furthermore, many employers, knowing of these beliefs and perhaps sharing them, may act in ways that further handicap cardiac employees. This discrimination may occur in subtle ways, with patients being eased into inappropriate retirement and situations of financial dependency. Such instances are common, despite the findings of work classification clinics that 80–90% of cardiac patients can return to work in a variety of jobs with safe performance.

Blue-Collar, White-Collar, and Women Workers

Our study illustrates some of the more common problems relating to work (4). Heart attacks influenced the employability of blue-collar workers more than that of white-collar men. The blue-collar men were out of work for longer periods than the white-collar men. Five months after uncomplicated myocardial infarction, only 19% of the executive-professional group were not at work, whereas almost 60% of the semiskilled and unskilled were still unemployed. Moreover, 25% of the latter were still unemployed at 1 year after hospital admission, as compared with 2% unemployed among the executive-professional group.

The necessity of changing jobs, making adjustments in tasks at work, obtaining part-time employment, etc., also fell most heavily on the blue-collar group. The effects of job changes on seniority under union rules, eligibility for pensions, and capacity to hold a job while working at reduced performance brought insecurity to the blue-collar workers in particular, although they affected white-collar employees as well. Such data would be more negative had they been collected during a period of economic recession and high unemployment.

Social changes during World War II and in the decades that followed included larger numbers of women entering the work force. Although the incidence of coronary disease is lower among premenopausal women than among men of comparable age, the incidences become similar with advancing age. What are the work prospects of women who develop heart disease while employed? Their prospects regarding future employment, making changes in their jobs, and other aspects related to work tend to be even more precarious than those for men under conditions of full national employment.

During economic recession the occupational outlook for the female cardiac patient is even more insecure. Although only limited data are available, it appears that she faces particularly difficult problems of employability and tenure. She may share this situation with other cardiac patients, who even before their illnesses were typically among the last to be hired and the first to be fired; these include members of certain racial or ethnic minority groups, the less skilled and less well educated, and individuals with prior unstable employment records.

INSTITUTIONS, AGENCIES, AND SERVICES
FOR CARDIAC REHABILITATION

In the United States at present numerous hospitals, institutions, agencies, and services contribute directly and indirectly to the rehabilitation of cardiac patients. Among these are programs specifically directed to the cardiac patient: physical reconditioning; therapy for psychologic problems; job counseling, training, and placement; resocialization services to combat dependency and withdrawal. To carry out the functions associated with these types of rehabilitation activities, a broad range of services and programs exists. These include exercise testing and training programs, antismoking clubs, heart clubs, group therapy programs, weight reduction clubs, work evaluation units, services for patient education, vocational counseling, and services of other community organizations such as the Visiting Nurses Association, etc.

The general pattern of use of rehabilitative services and agencies can present barriers that hamper or impede rehabilitation. Several brief illustrations can be cited.

Use of Cardiac Rehabilitation Services

What are the pattern and extent of use of rehabilitation services following discharge from the hospital after the acute phase of the illness? Unfortunately, data are not available that would permit detailed conclusions, but there are some indications of extent of use (14). Some perspective on the magnitude of the problem can be obtained from the finding that over 600,000 people are discharged from hospitals each year after treatment for acute coronary incidents. According to a Social Security Administration report, it is estimated that 4.4 million persons had disabling cardiovascular conditions in 1966 (15). About 6% of these received formal rehabilitation services from clinics, physicians, and public agencies such as vocational rehabilitation units.

Describing the State-Federal Vocational Rehabilitation Program in 1972, Commissioner Reedy (16) stated: "We estimate we are serving 20,000 cardiac patients and rehabilitate 7,400 per year." He described this number of cardiac clients on the case rolls as being "relatively low." In our study, 70% of cardiac patients had no contact with any rehabilitation agency or service other than their hospitals and physicians during the first year after their initial myocardial infarction (6). The majority of the patients who used a service were in contact with unemployment offices and the Veterans Administration.

Availability and Barriers to Access

There is wide variation among areas of the country in regard to availability of cardiac rehabilitation services and facilities. Differences exist between regions, between states, and between rural and urban areas, as well as on the basis of other criteria. The immediate barrier may be geographic, with services being sparse in that location. In areas where services exist, another problem is unequal access for various segments of the cardiac patient population. The impediments to access are many: nonreferral by physicians, patients' lack of knowledge of availability, inability to pay for services, as well as barriers associated with race, socioeconomic status, etc. Whether the barriers to access are geographic, economic, social, or psychologic, the net result is that many patients with definite needs do not receive rehabilitation services.

Limited data on the distribution of services are available through a directory of cardiac rehabilitation units published by the American Heart Association (17). As recently as 1975–1976, the directory listed 148 rehabilitation units, located in 35 states. In the remaining 15 states, no cardiac rehabilitation unit was cited. Furthermore about 60% of units were located in 6 states. It appears that large segments of the cardiac population in the United States do not have cardiac rehabilitation services in their areas.

The key to use of rehabilitation services is the physician as the primary source of referral. In the absence of such guidance, the cardiac patient must make contacts and find his way through the maze of organizations and facilities. A view of the current situation was presented by the Task Force on Arteriosclerosis (18):

> At present there is no systematic approach to the rehabilitation of the patient after myocardial infarction either from a psychological or physical point of view. Medical and nursing curricula generally contain little on this aspect of myocardial infarction and often provide inadequate information concerning available techniques and community services.

Effectiveness of Services and Programs

Another problem concerns the effectiveness of various types of rehabilitation procedures or programs. Few systematic data are available (19,20) to indicate how well patients with similar problems respond to differing modes of rehabilitation. For example, the efficacy of exercise training programs still needs evaluation regarding long-term physiologic and psychologic effects (19–22). Other components of rehabilitation intervention require similar evaluation. The development of more sensitive measures and better evaluation methods will aid in improving current services and in planning for more effective new ones.

There are many unresolved questions about the desirability and effectiveness of assigning nurses rehabilitative tasks generally performed by physicians, such as education and counseling of patients. Will the additional responsibilities interfere with medical care and hamper the clinical progress of cardiac patients or perhaps cause other problems? Questions concerning whether current or proposed procedures will benefit the patient's recovery and rehabilitation may be resolved by appropriately designed scientific studies.

An even more provocative question relates to the effects of use and nonuse of rehabilitation services. Few comparisons have been made between patients for whom no services were provided and those who received various services. Indeed, for many patients no rehabilitative intervention or assistance may constitute the most beneficial therapeutic program. The lack of data on how to classify patients by needs and by potential to benefit from specific services constitutes an impediment to the planning of economical cardiac rehabilitation programs.

Internal Organization of Institutions and Agencies

Organizational arrangements within and among institutions and agencies can constitute a barrier to effective rehabilitation. Although many institutions, agencies, and programs perform their tasks efficiently and effectively, many health care professionals can identify some that are hampered by their internal organization. Common problems in large complex organizations include bureaucratic procedures, red tape, personnel turnover, poor motivation and morale, conflicts between occupational groups, rivalries among professionals, and inefficient administration. When these organizational arrangements hamper effective delivery of services, they impede cardiac rehabilitation.

Routine administrative policies and the quality of performance by workers in the institution may have consequences that are not intentional. For example, the transfer of a patient from the coronary care unit to another area of the hospital may be stressful, as the patient may feel alone and vulnerable away from the protection of the coronary care unit (23). Routine restrictive policies on visiting may create feelings of isolation and emotional deprivation so severe as to call the policies into question. Contradictory advice from various personnel about illness and prognosis can generate feelings of uncertainty and depression in patients.

Some customary operational aspects of hospitals, rehabilitation agencies, and other services may create difficulties for patients. The high turnover of personnel in health and social service agencies may interfere with continuity of care and supportive relationships with patients. Frequently a patient will experience a setback in psychologic and social readjustment to illness if an individual with whom rapport has been developed suddenly leaves. Once again the patient's circumstances and feelings must be explained to a new worker. When this occurs repeatedly, the patient must bear added discomforts and the inevitable delays (24).

There is ample evidence that the beliefs and values of the society outside the hospital or rehabilitation agency influence decisions and performance within such agencies (25,26). The cardiac patient may feel alienated, depressed, helpless, or angry if he believes the staff responds adversely to him because of his color, ethnic origin, religion, or class status. Whether these reactions influence physical process in cardiac disease is not known, but this type of experience can adversely affect rehabilitation. It can discourage some patients from returning for further beneficial services.

SUMMARY

This chapter has centered on some aspects of the social and psychologic factors that influence the course and quality of rehabilitation. Several subjects were selected to illustrate major barriers and problems in patient management, rehabilitation planning, physician–patient relationships, family relationships, work situations, roles of rehabilitation agencies, the role of the individual, and the effects of the larger societal context in which rehabilitation takes place. The emphasis has been on barriers and problems, as these illustrate both the challenges to patient and physician and the normal processes and structures currently operative.

Given the complexity of the social and psychologic variables influencing cardiac rehabilitation, what is the appropriate course for the practicing clinician? Three classes of problems involve different approaches. First, in rehabilitation planning and management, many social or psychologic traits exist that are beyond the sphere of responsibility or influence of the physician. These include the patient's social class, ethnic or racial origins, family history, past beliefs and values, etc.; all may influence the patient's behavior and course during rehabilitation. The appropriate physician role is to recognize the relevance of these elements and to develop information about them when necessary to understand the patient and accordingly guide rehabilitation.

A second category of social factors can be influenced or controlled: adherence of the patient to the medical regimen; the quality of communication between physician and patient; the framing of key decisions such as job changes, retirement, and referrals to appropriate agencies or services dealing with the physical, social, and emotional aspects of rehabilitation. A third class of problems consists of social factors that do not directly involve a particular patient but that may influence rehabilitation of many patients. There are various means by which the physician can promote the interests of the patient: by supporting the establishment of cardiac rehabilitation services in the community where needed; by encouraging appropriate patterns of referral among colleagues; by supporting the dissemination of rehabilitation information to the lay public, to employers, and to patients; by advising legislators in the preparation of laws on behalf of comprehensive rehabilitation for cardiac patients.

A common theme in this chapter has been the variability of barriers and the ways in which they affect subsegments of the cardiac population according to age, sex, race, ethnic origin, social class, urban–rural locale, etc. The manner in which the various factors operate in differing contexts and in various subpopulations remains to be investigated. Whereas clinical judgment, common sense, and logic may serve as initial guides, optimal development of more comprehensive rehabilitation programs for individual patients and for populations of cardiac patients requires additional specific information based on well-designed scientific studies. The social science aspects of cardiac rehabilitation have received less attention than other areas of cardiovascular research. It is hoped that the present review will be succeeded in future years by discussions supported by an extensive research literature, one that deals directly with the multifactorial elements in the social and psychologic aspects of cardiac rehabilitation.

REFERENCES

1. Jenkins CD: Psychologic and social precursors of coronary disease. *N Engl J Med* 284:244, 307, 1971

2. Hellerstein H: Reconditioning and the prevention of heart disease: Report of a study trip to West Germany, *Modern Medicine* 32:266, 1964

3. WHO: Evaluation of Rehabilitation Programmes for Patients with Myocardial Infarction: Report of a WHO Working Group, Prague, 4–7 October, 1971. EURO 8206(6)

4. Croog SH, Levine S: *The Heart Patient Recovers: Social and Psychological Factors.* Human Sciences Press, New York, 1977

5. Croog SH, Levine S: Social status and subjective perceptions of 250 men after myocardial infarction. *Public Health Rep* 84:989, 1969

6. Croog SH, Lipson A, Levine S: Help patterns in severe illness: The roles of kin network, non-family resources, and institutions. *Journal of Marriage and the Family* 34:32, 1972

7. Croog SH, Shapiro DS, Levine S: Denial in male heart patients. An empirical study. *Psychosom Med* 33:385, 1971

8. Marston M: Compliance with medical regimens: A review of the literature. *Nurs Res* 19:312, 1970

9. Becker MH, Maiman LA: Sociobehavioral determinants of compliance with health and medical care recommendations. *Med Care* 13:10, 1975

10. Francis V, Korsch BM, Morris MJ: Gaps in doctor-patient communication: Patients' response to medical advice. *N Engl J Med* 280:535, 1969

11. *New York Times*, February 14, 1974, p 24

12. Bilodeau CB, Hackett TP: Issues raised in a group setting by patients recovering from myocardial infarction. *Am J Psychiatry* 128:73, 1971

13. Rahe R, Tuffli CF, Suchor RJ, et al: Group therapy in the outpatient management of post-myocardial infarction patients. *Psychiatry in Medicine* 4:77, 1973

14. Smith RT, Lilienfeld A: The Social Security Disability Program: An Evaluation Study. DHEW publication SSA 72-1180, Research Report 39, 1971

15. Treitel R: Rehabilitation of the Disabled. Social Security Survey of the Disabled: 1966. Social Security Administration, Office of Research and Statistics, Report 12, September, 1970

16. Reedy C: The state-federal vocational rehabilitation program in cardiac rehabilitation. In Naughton J, Hellerstein H (eds): *Exercise Testing and Exercise Training in Coronary Heart Disease.* Academic Press, New York, 1973, p xvii

17. American Heart Association: Directory. Cardiac Rehabilitation Units, 1975–76. January 1976

18. National Heart and Lung Institute: Report by Task Force on Arteriosclerosis. DHEW publication (NIH) 72-137, Vol 1, June 1971, p. 67

19. Blackburn H: Disadvantages of intensive exercise therapy after myocardial infarction. In Ingelfinger F, et al (eds): *Controversy in Internal Medicine II.* WB Saunders, Philadelphia, 1974, p 162

20. Fisher S: Unmet needs in psychological evaluation of intervention programs. In Naughton J, Hellerstein H (eds): *Exercise Testing and Exercise Training in Coronary Heart Disease.* Academic Press, New York, 1973, p 289

21. Hackett TP, Cassem NH: Psychological adaptation to convalescence in myocardial infarction patients. In Naughton J, Hellerstein H (eds): *Exercise Testing and Exercise Training in Coronary Heart Disease.* Academic Press, New York, 1973, p 253

22. Heinzelmann F: Social and psychological factors that influence the effectiveness of exercise programs. In Naughton J, Hellerstein H (eds): *Exercise Testing and Exercise Training in Coronary Heart Disease.* Academic Press, New York, 1973, p 275

23. Klein RF, Kliner VA, Zipes DP, et al: Transfer from a CCU: Some adverse responses. *Arch Intern Med* 122:104, 1968

24. Safilios-Rothschild C: *The Sociology and Social Psychology of Disability and Rehabilitation.* Random House, New York, 1970

25. Duff RS, Hollingshead AB: *Sickness and Society.* Harper & Row, New York, 1968

26. Croog SH, Ver Steeg D: The hospital as a social system. In Freeman HE, Levine S, Reeder LG (eds): *Handbook of Medical Sociology.* Prentice-Hall, Englewood Cliffs, NJ, 1972, p 274

12
Legal Aspects of Rehabilitation After Myocardial Infarction

Elliot L. Sagall, M.D.

The physician directing the rehabilitation program for a myocardial infarction (MI) patient must recognize that practical realities often make legal and socioeconomic factors rather than medical factors the ultimate determinants of achievement of the primary goal of returning the post-MI patient to gainful employment.

The physician must also recognize that under current laws many benefits frequently are available to MI patients during periods of disability and that whether or not the patient obtains these benefits often influences the rehabilitation potential. Furthermore, it must be realized that the physician has a particular duty not to impose obstacles to the patient who is applying for benefits to which the patient is legally entitled either by reason of a statute or under the terms of an insurance policy.

Finally, inasmuch as many aspects of medical advice peculiar to MI rehabilitation programs, even though not involving the prescription of medication or the performance of surgery, do constitute medical treatment in the eyes of the law, the physician and the other health care team members involved in the program must recognize that they become legally liable and may become involved in malpractice litigation should untoward reactions stem from such advice. Their responsibility is the same as with other more obvious forms of medical and surgical treatments, and the same legal principles apply.

DISABILITY BENEFITS AND REHABILITATION

Under most current disability pension statutes and private insurance contracts, the benefits provided for disabled persons usually are considerably greater when the disability is due to an "accident" or "injury" than when it is due to an "illness" or "disease." Therefore, the legal or insurance distinction whether an acute MI resulted from accident or from illness not infrequently becomes a key issue; if

269

disputed, the decision ultimately must be resolved by the administrative agency or other legal tribunal assigned jurisdiction over the claim.

For the post-MI patient, disability pension considerations often are of prime importance in the rehabilitation program. On the one hand, when financial benefits are being received that will ensure economic survival for the patient and family during the period of incapacity, the patient may be willing to accept a protracted, medically advisable job retraining program; but without such a source of income, the patient may be forced by economic concerns to reject a medically advisable rehabilitation program in favor of a premature return to medically inadvisable work. On the other hand, the freedom from economic worry afforded the cardiac patient by disability pension benefits, particularly when the tax-free component is considered, often acts as an effective deterrent to the prime incentive to return to work, thereby precluding the success of any rehabilitation program that has as its primary objective the goal of returning the patient to gainful employment.

Finally, although it is commonly denied, employer awareness that a candidate for reemployment or for new employment is receiving disability benefits or has pending a claim for such benefits, particularly under workers' compensation, often motivates the employer against hiring a recovered MI patient. Such employer reluctance to offer positions to MI patients most often stems from fear that the employer's insurance premiums (workers' compensation, group life insurance, and group medical expense insurance) will sharply increase should subsequent disabilities occur as a result of unpreventable progression of existing disease.

Although ultimate determination of eligibility for statutory, contractual, or common law benefits rests with legal authorities, prosecution of a disputed claim requires that the claimant present expert medical opinion in support of the claim before the insurance company, the Workmen's Compensation board, or other administrative agency. This means that the physician who is directing the rehabilitation of a post-MI patient may be called on for expert opinions on the various medicolegal issues emanating from the patient's cardiac disorder. Accordingly, the physician has an obligation to the patient to maintain adequate records detailing the history obtained, the findings of physical examinations, and the results of electrocardiographic, laboratory, x-ray, and other medical studies documenting the diagnosis and the disability. The physician also should be prepared to provide written reports or oral testimony outlining findings and opinions on key medicolegal elements, e.g., diagnosis, extent and duration of impairment and disability, possible or probable causal connection of the cardiac disorder and disability to an accident or to work. In this regard, the physician will find involvement in the legal process much less frustrating and much more meaningful if an attempt is made to acquire some familiarity with the purposes, principles, mechanisms, and administrative procedures involved.

WORKERS' COMPENSATION AND OTHER INSURANCE BENEFITS

It is in the area of workers' compensation that most of the medicolegal problems involving cardiology arise. In all 50 states and in various federal and territorial jurisdictions, workers' compensation protection is afforded to most employees for injuries "arising out of" and occurring "during the course of" their employment. Many employees not covered by state workers' compensation acts are covered by similar legislation such as the federal Longshoremen's and Harbor Workers' Compensation Act, the federal Employers' Liability Act, the federal employers' compensation system, and for maritime workers, the Jones Act.

Workers' compensation coverage is based on the fundamental social principle that financial expenses stemming from work-induced injury should be assumed by the employer as an expense of doing business, not assessed on the worker or on public welfare or charitable institutions. Without exception, the various state and federal workers' compensation acts establish a right to the benefits prescribed within the act without regard to fault. The key determinant of compensability is that the injury, disability, disorder, or death "arise out of" and occur "during the course of" the employment; it is not a matter of who was at fault. Under this formula, compensation benefits have generally been extended to cover occupationally related cardiac disability and death along with other more easily defined "injuries," and state by state there has been a recent trend to more liberal definitions of "compensable" heart disorders. Thus, currently, many acute cardiac episodes, particularly acute MI, occurring "on the job" or in close temporal relationship to work hours are accepted legally as compensable injuries and provide the victim and family with weekly compensation payments and coverage of associated medical expenses.

In some states, recovery for work-connected cardiac attacks has been considerably narrowed by restrictive clauses incorporated into the governing statutes that limit compensation for disability or death only to conditions caused by "accident" or due to "unusual strain" of work effort. For many years, adherence to these concepts excluded many heart attack victims from compensation benefits. However, within recent years there has been a trend toward removing these restrictions under expanding legal concepts that the cardiac attack itself, since it is unpredictable as to when and where it will occur, constitutes "an accident." Similarly, the legal requirement of "unusual strain" is being eroded on a state-by-state basis. Thus workers' compensation is becoming available to larger numbers of persons who sustain MI or other sudden cardiac dysfunctions while in the course of their employment, even when performing so-called "usual work," provided that such work can be indicted as a "proximate precipitating" or "triggering" cause of the attack.

For the physician it is particularly important to recognize that in workers' compensation determinations there is universal acceptance of the common law concept that prior infirmity is no bar to receiving benefits. Compensation is due if it can be shown that employment aggravated a preexisting heart disorder or pathology to bring about injury, disability, or death sooner than ordinarily would have been expected during the natural history of the underlying disease. The fact that the disability or death occurred only because the worker was previously afflicted with heart disease does not, in the eyes of the law, relieve the employer of legal responsibility for the consequences of work-precipitated or work-hastened disability or death.

In heart cases, the agents or elements most generally accepted by compensation authorities as competent causes of cardiac disability and death are the following:

- physical effort (usual or unusual, depending on the jurisdiction where the claim originates)
- traumatic injury to the chest (nonpenetrating as well as penetrating)
- alleged work-connected psychologic tensions, such as sudden and severe psychologic upset resulting from heated arguments, emotionally disturbing discussions, or frights, as well as mounting mental stress or strain such as might be imposed by quotas, deadlines, and business reverses
- exposures to potentially harmful work environments, such as extremes of heat and cold
- inhalation or ingestion of toxic chemical agents that might produce cardiac disability by interfering with the oxygen-carrying capacity of the blood (e.g., carbon monoxide) or directly have a toxic effect on the myocardium
- accidental electric shocks
- adverse cardiac responses to therapy primarily directed to the treatment of any industrial injury, such as an adverse cardiac reaction to medication, surgery, or rehabilitative exercises.

Prolonged mental tensions and psychologic "pressures" alleged to be inherent in or derived from hazardous and demanding jobs generally have not been accepted by compensation authorities as legally acceptable causes of heart disease or hasteners of acute MI.

In order to prepare for the possibility of giving testimony or opinion regarding causation, it is important that the rehabilitation physician inquire into the circumstances preceding and surrounding the onset of the patient's MI, particularly in regard to work activities, with special inquiry regarding those elements that might fall into the category of "proximate precipitating" or "triggering" causes. It is also important that the physician ascertain whether or not the patient is contemplating legal action under the covering workers' compensation act or similar statutes or is already receiving compensation; such questions are of practical significance in determining if the rehabilitated MI patient can return to gainful employment.

For certain categories of public employment, some state legislatures have made available preferential retirement and death benefits of which the physician should be aware. These laws, the so-called heart laws, generally cover uniformed policemen and firemen, prison guards, and other specifically named employment groups; they provide benefits for disability or death due to heart disease or hypertension. For these specifically named groups, the question of a causal relationship between the disabling cardiac disorder or hypertension and the employment has, for all practical purposes, been eliminated by inclusion in the law of a clause stating that in the absence of substantial evidence to the contrary it is to be presumed that the employee's heart disease or hypertension emanated from the "hazards" of the employment. Therefore, generally, it need be established, usually by testimony of the attending physician, only that the employee does in fact suffer from heart disease or from high blood pressure; it is not necessary to establish a causal connection between the heart condition and the employment—a much more difficult task.

The disability insurance program instituted by the Social Security Act is at the present time the largest source of disability income for disabled persons in the United States. The Social Security Administration's insurance program currently covers almost 90% of persons in this country who work for a living, and it includes many dependents and survivors. Monthly cash benefits are available to eligible individuals when family earnings are cut off by severe disability or by old age (62–65 years of age and over).

A disability benefit program has been administered by the Social Security Administration since 1954. Originally, disability benefits were limited by "freezing" a worker's earnings at the time of commencement of the "disability," so that the amount of prescribed retirement and survivor benefits received was governed by the income of the worker at the time when disability began. Subsequent legislative amendments to the program have greatly extended coverage and benefits. Presently, cash benefits are available when current definitions of disability are met, namely, an "inability to engage in a substantial activity by reason of any determinable physical or mental ailment or impairment which can be expected to result in death or which has lasted or can be expected to last for a continuous period of not less than twelve months."

Disability benefits under the Social Security Act do not commence until after a waiting period of five full calendar months of disability. Disability income payments are terminated when the beneficiary recovers from the disability or returns to substantial work despite any impairment. A number of provisions have specifically been added to the act to encourage the rehabilitation of a disabled person, particularly one who attempts a return to work even though not fully recovered from the impairment sustained.

Benefits for disability under the Social Security Administration's insurance program are provided independent of income status. Eligibility is dependent solely on the patient's degree of disability according to the criteria defined in the law. However, disability benefits are not paid in addition to other Social Security benefits, and they may be reduced if the beneficiary is receiving workers' compensation simultaneously.

In the private sector of our economy, many disabled MI patients are entitled to financial payments of varying amounts and for varying periods of time as defined in insurance contracts, privately purchased or provided as fringe benefits by their employers. However, most such policies exclude benefits when the disability, injury, or death results from work and is covered by workers' compensation.

The physician in charge of the rehabilitation of the MI patient may be called on to provide medical reports supporting the patient's claim for insurance benefits, which will involve determinations such as the following:

· whether the insurer should accept an acute MI demonstrated to have been precipitated by some identified incident as an "accident" rather than an "illness" when the policy provides extra benefits for "accidental injury"

- whether a preexisting coronary atherosclerotic condition excludes MI as an "accident" when the policy restricts accidental benefits for disabilities due "solely and exclusively to accidental injury"
- whether a second or third episode of acute MI in the same individual constitutes a "new" illness and a "new" period of disability under the terms of an insuring contract with deductible features
- whether the degree and duration of disability resulting from the MI are "reasonable"
- whether the policyholder, in fact, voided the policy by misrepresenting the existence of heart disease in the original application for insurance coverage

EMPLOYER HIRING ATTITUDES

Return of the post-MI patient to gainful employment, except in cases of self-employment, ultimately depends on the attitudes of prospective employers regarding the hiring of known cardiac patients. From a practical point of view, it is well recognized that opinion in the labor market toward employment of persons with known heart disease is influenced to a greater degree by legal and insurance considerations than by medical considerations (1). Thus prospective employers often are motivated largely by concern over increased compensation and other liability premium costs by reason of alleged exacerbation or aggravation of a known preexisting condition; the medical condition of the applicant is of little concern. To a lesser extent, prospective employers may be reluctant to hire known cardiac patients because of concern about excessive illness absenteeism, as well as worry about increased legal liability should the employee's job be such that sudden physical incapacity from a cardiac cause might result in increased risk of injury to others.

In some cases, state and federal regulations, such as those applying to drivers in interstate commerce or drivers of school buses or passenger buses, may prevent return of rehabilitated MI patients to their former employment because of laws specifically excluding known cardiac patients from such employment.

In most instances, an employee seeking to return to a former job after recovery from acute MI, even when armed with medical clearance for such employment by the attending physician, has little or no recourse should the employer refuse reinstatement. However, in situations where labor contracts govern the return of medically disabled workers to their jobs and their seniority rights, an employer may be required under the terms of a contract to substantiate a refusal to hire by presenting supportive medical opinion from a company physician or from an impartial medical examiner. Often, should there be conflict between the opinions expressed by the employee's physician and the physician examining the patient on behalf of the employer, the dispute may be subject to resolution by the opinion of a third examining physician acceptable to both parties or mandated by binding arbitration.

In some instances union contracts may act as deterrents to proper work placement of rehabilitated cardiac patients. For example, some management–union agreements, particularly in the motor transport, stevedore, and construction fields, require that employers hire new employees only from union-provided employment pools. Selection of workers under these circumstances frequently is influenced primarily by seniority rights. Often this results in hiring practices that reserve the easier and physically less taxing jobs for those workers who have acquired the most seniority, thereby tending to prevent placement of the recovered MI patient in a job whose requirements are within the physical limitations imposed by the cardiac disorder.

MEDICAL MALPRACTICE CONSIDERATIONS

The risk of the physician being subjected to suit for professional negligence should the patient suffer an untoward result from the therapy prescribed or from failure of the physician to prescribe certain therapy is an inescapable fact in professional life today. Under current legal concepts, the physician directing a program to rehabilitate the MI patient is liable, in the eyes of the law, to the same extent as for other medical treatments and diagnostic procedures should harm result to the patient or should an untoward reaction occur during the course of testings or treatment or from advice given or from failure to properly advise.

In all instances where professional negligence is charged, the law assigns the plaintiff the burden of proving certain items. In a legal action based on alleged professional negligence, the plaintiff must establish the following points:

· that the defendant physician owed the patient a duty to conform to a particular standard of medical care
· that the defendant physician was derelict in that the physician's conduct breached this duty by not being in conformity with the recognized standard of medical care
· that the plaintiff suffered harm (damage)
· that the harm or damage suffered by the plaintiff was directly and proximately caused by the negligent conduct of the defendant physician

Failure of the plaintiff to establish each and every one of these items will in most jurisdictions and under most circumstances result in dismissal of the suit. In some jurisdictions, the plaintiff also must establish that the plaintiff's own conduct did not negligently contribute to the harm alleged ("contributory negligence").

Should the patient suffer harm, the physician may be liable, separately or additionally, to several legal actions besides the one charging negligence (tort):

· charges that the patient did not give valid consent to a prescribed diagnostic test or treatment by reason of lack of sufficient information having been imparted by the physician to enable the patient to give "informed consent"
· actions based on alleged breach of contract should a particular result or cure promised and thereby "guaranteed" by the treating physician not be achieved
· actions based on the expanding legal doctrine of "strict liability," involving the concept that the patient is entitled to certain treatments by law, independent of currently recognized and accepted standards of medical care, so that failure

to provide such treatment (or testing) renders the physician legally liable for any harmful consequences.*

Malpractice actions in these latter areas are increasing in number for two reasons: in some of these actions the governing statute permits the bringing of a suit that would otherwise be barred by statute of limitations were the action only in tort; in these types of legal actions the plaintiff's burden of proof is eased because the plaintiff usually is not required to produce supportive medical opinion to substantiate the claim. Thus the legal issue in dispute in actions that are not actions in tort primarily concerns whether the physician did or did not say what the patient alleges the physician did or did not say. Demonstration of negligence generally is not at issue.

EXERCISE TESTING

Exercise stress testing is widely employed as a guide to graded exercise prescription in medically recommended physical fitness programs for both cardiac and noncardiac patients. When performed under the supervision of a physician or by a physician's order, an exercise test, in the eyes of the law, constitutes a medical procedure that renders the prescribing or supervising physician liable to those legal obligations attendant on all medical procedures and treatments.

Although admittedly they are relatively uncommon, untoward reactions to exercise stress tests have been reported in both medical and lay literature (e.g., ischemia leading to MI, serious ventricular rhythm disorders, and even death) in sufficient numbers that physicians employing or recommending exercise testing can be expected by the law to be alert to the potential danger of vigorous exercise. Accordingly, should a serious consequence result to a patient from an exercise stress test or during a medically prescribed exercise physical fitness program, there will be a solid legal basis for a malpractice action against the physician if one or more of the following points can be established:

· improper ordering of an exercise stress test in the face of generally recognized contraindications to its performance
· improper performance of the test
· failure to provide adequate monitoring during the test
· failure to detect promptly and to heed promptly signs heralding impending catastrophe or serious reaction
· continuation of the exercise in the face of a response that should have called for immediate cessation of the exercise
· performance of the test or exercise under circumstances such that maximal

*This legal philosophy is illustrated in a recent decision of the Supreme Court of the state of Washington, which in *Helling* v. *Carey and Laughlin* ruled (March 14, 1974) that failure of the defendant ophthalmologists to make a routine test for glaucoma in a 26-year-old female patient under observation for contact lenses constituted negligent professional conduct as a matter of law, despite testimony from medical experts for both plaintiff and defendant that such testing in patients under 40 years of age is not a regular practice or standard treatment even for ophthalmologists. One of the reasons given for the court's finding was that by law patients under the age of 40 years are entitled to the same standards of treatment as those over that age.

resuscitative equipment and trained personnel thoroughly familiar with its use
were not on hand

· failure to impart to the patient sufficient information concerning the potential
risks and hazards of the test to enable the patient to give "informed consent"

To minimize the potential for malpractice charges, the physician who employs
exercise testing in a post-MI program or who recommends graded exercise must
make sure that a thorough pretest screening examination is performed to bring
to light those conditions generally recognized as absolute or relative contraindications to exercise stress testing or vigorous exercise programs. These include
MI that occurred less than 8–12 weeks previously, severe aortic stenosis, persistent
congestive heart failure, increasing or unstable angina pectoris, untreated or
uncontrolled atrial fibrillation, high degrees of atrioventricular block, significant
ventricular irritability such as runs of three or more consecutive ectopic beats,
uncontrolled hypertension, dissecting aneurysm, active myocarditis, acute infec-
tious disease, recent pulmonary or systemic embolization, marked anemia, severe orthopedic or neurologic impairments interfering with exercise, and uncontrolled metabolic disorders such as diabetes, thyrotoxicosis, or myxedema. The
physician who permits or conducts an exercise test in the face of a recognized
absolute or relative contraindication has the onus of explaining why such a test
was ordered and performed; furthermore, the physician takes on medical and
legal responsibility to ensure that the exercising of such a high-risk patient be
performed only under direct supervision of a physician, only with constant
electrocardiographic monitoring, only in a facility equipped with properly functioning resuscitative equipment, and only with individuals on hand who have
been adequately trained in resuscitation.

Symptoms and signs generally recognized as requiring immediate termination
of an exercise test include the following: development of significant chest pain or
other anginal equivalents; fainting or a feeling of faintness; severe dyspnea;
excessive fatigue; leg claudication; sudden pallor or other changes in skin color;
development of cold, moist, or clammy skin; profuse or sudden sweating; signs
of cerebral vascular insufficiency such as staggering, confusion, or head nod-
ding; undue changes in blood pressure (rise or fall); paroxysmal cardiac rhythm
disorders, particularly runs of three or more consecutive ventricular ectopic
beats, ventricular tachycardia, or fibrillation; onset of atrioventricular heart
block or other serious conduction disturbances; appearance of ST-T ischemic
alterations greater than 3–4 mm (.3–.4 mV). The development of any of these calls
for immediate termination of exercise. The patient should then be allowed to rest
in a comfortable position, usually supine, and should be carefully observed, with
prompt institution of cardiopulmonary resuscitation if appropriate and with other
therapeutic procedures administered as needed.

To guard against charges of lack of informed consent, the physician prescribing or supervising an exercise test should make certain that prior to its performance the patient is told in sufficient detail the reasons for performing the test
and is given an explanation of what the test procedure will entail and the risks
and hazards that might be encountered, including the risk of acute MI or
fatality. Unless the physician has given the patient this information, a court may
later rule that the consent of the patient was not legally valid because it was not
"informed consent," and that could make the physician liable for damages.

The consent forms proposed by the American Heart Association for exercise testing of patients with known heart disease (2) (Appendix, p. 280) can be used, or they can be adapted to secure written "informed consent" prior to exercise testing or entrance of patients into a myocardial rehabilitation program. However, it is important to appreciate that the signing of a consent form by a patient may not provide adequate defense should the patient later claim insufficient knowledge and insufficient appreciation of the procedure and its risks to have given informed consent, or should it be claimed that the patient did not know what was being signed. Thus, in further evidence that adequate pretesting information was imparted, the physician should make appropriate handwritten notations in the patient's office records or hospital records that the physician personally explained the procedure to the patient, as well as the reasons for its performance, the recognized risks and hazards, and the alternative procedures and their risks and hazards, and that the patient understood all of this before assenting to its performance.

EXERCISE PHYSICAL FITNESS PROGRAMS

Exercise as treatment has been widely recommended in graded amounts and with increasing levels of physical effort for the MI patient as an important component of the rehabilitation program, even (in one rehabilitation center) to the point of a progressive endurance running program leading to competition in the 26.2-mile Boston marathon some 1–4 years after MI (3,4).

As with exercise testing, medically prescribed physical fitness exercise programs, even under supervision, are not without danger. Sporadic reports of sudden death occurring while jogging (persons with and without known heart disease) and occasional reports of deaths of cardiac patients exercising at gymnasiums attest to such occurrences as foreseeable risks. Thus, for example, monitoring of exertional cardiac arrest due to ventricular fibrillation in coronary patients in the Seattle supervised exercise programs showed an observed attack rate of approximately 1 in 6000 man-hours of medically supervised physical activity (5,6), an incidence that points to the need for immediate availability of trained personnel and equipment to accomplish prompt defibrillation if such persons are to be saved.

The medicolegal implications and malpractice risks to physicians prescribing exercise programs are essentially the same as those elaborated for stress exercise testing. In all instances the physician should make certain that the patient has been apprised of potential risks and hazards, that examination of the patient prior to entrance into the program has been adequate and thorough, that the exercise (whenever possible or feasible) is carried out in facilities totally equipped to handle cardiac arrest, and that the patient and the physical education instructors are thoroughly familiar with the signs and symptoms heralding cardiac catastrophe and requiring immediate cessation of exercise.

JOB PRESCRIPTION

Assent by the physician to the patient's plan to return to specific job or work activity is another part of the myocardial rehabilitation program that has the potential to subject the physician to malpractice liability. Legally, the physician's advice to a patient to return to work or to attempt a specific job constitutes medical treatment. Thus to be protected legally, the physician who gives medical approval to return to work for the post-MI patient must have full understanding of the nature of the work activities the patient proposes to undertake and must not recommend job assignments generally recognized as beyond the patient's physical capacity. A particular malpractice hazard in this area occurs in those situations in which the patient insists on premature return to a job that is beyond the patient's current capacities and obtains medical clearance from the attending physician without fully apprising the physician of the duties entailed.

SUMMARY

Unless the physician involved in the rehabilitation of the post-MI patient keeps in mind certain key legal and insurance factors associated therewith, the physician may unwittingly prevent the patient from obtaining benefits to which the patient is legally entitled, and the physician may very well incur increased risk of being named defendant in medical malpractice litigation should an untoward event occur in this phase of the patient's illness.

The legal and insurance considerations with which the physician should be familiar primarily concern disability benefits (such as those provided by workers' compensation, the Social Security Administration's disability insurance program, and many privately contracted insurance policies), the many legal and insurance considerations that determine an employer's attitude toward rehiring the rehabilitated MI job applicant, and the various medical malpractice pitfalls and risks inherent in medical rehabilitation programs for the post-MI patient.

REFERENCES

1. Weinstock M, Haft JI: The effect of illness on employment opportunities, *Arch Environ Health* 29:79, 1974
2. Explanation for Proposed Informed Consent for Exercise Testing. Memorandum CS 71 524, American Heart Association, New York, June 14, 1971
3. Kavanagh T, Shepherd RH, Pandit V: Marathon running after myocardial infarction. *JAMA* 229:1602, 1974
4. Editorial: Marathon running after myocardial infarction. *JAMA* 229:1637, 1974
5. Bruce RA: Instantaneous and sudden deaths. *JAMA* 226:1229, 1973 (letter)
6. Frederick R: Monthly Report of CAPRI Experience. Seattle Cardiopulmonary Research Institute, Seattle, Wash, January 1974

BIBLIOGRAPHY

Bacorn RW: Legal aspects of exercise stress testing and exercise prescription. In Zohman LR, Phillips RE (eds): *Progress in Cardiac Rehabilitaton: Medical Aspects of Exercise Testing and Training*. Intercontinental Medical, New York, 1973, p 156

Dobrzensky SH: Legal aspects of exercise programs. In Morse RL (ed): *Guidelines for Exercise Programs.* Charles C Thomas, Springfield, Ill, 1972, p 98

Ladimer I: Professional liability in exercise testing. *Am J Cardiol* 20:752, 1972

Rochmis P, Blackburn A: Exercise tests: A survey of procedures, safety, and litigation experience in approximately 170,000 tests. *JAMA* 217:1061, 1971

Sagall EL, Reed BC: *The Heart and the Law—A Practical Guide to Medicolegal Cardiology.* Macmillan, New York, 1968

Sagall EL, Reed BC: *The Law and Clinical Medicine.* JB Lippincott, Philadelphia, 1970

Sagall EL: Malpractice hazards of medically prescribed exercise. In Wecht CH (ed): *Legal Medicine Annual 1975.* Appleton-Century-Crofts, New York, 1975, p 273

The law and cardiac rehabilitation. In Naughton J, Hellerstein HK (eds): *Exercise Testing and Exercise Training in Coronary Heart Disease.* Academic Press, New York, 1973, p 387

APPENDIX: PROPOSED FORM FOR INFORMED CONSENT FOR EXERCISE TESTING OF PEOPLE WITH HEART DISEASE

In order to determine an appropriate plan of treatment to assist in my recovery from my recent heart attack, I hereby consent to voluntarily engage in an exercise test to determine the state of my heart and circulation. The information thus obtained will help to aid my physician in advising me as to the activities in which I may engage.

Before I undergo the test, I will have an interview with a physician. I will also be examined by a physician to determine if I have any condition which would indicate that I should not engage in this test.

The test which I will undergo will be performed on a _____ (describe) with the amount of effort increasing gradually. This increase in effort will continue until symptoms such as fatigue, shortness of breath, or chest discomfort may appear, which would indicate to me to stop.

During the performance of the test, a physician or his trained observer will keep under surveillance my pulse, blood pressure and electrocardiogram. Oxygen intake may also be measured and _____ tests performed.

There exists the possibility of certain changes occurring during the tests. They include abnormal blood pressure, fainting, disorders of heart beat, too rapid, too slow or ineffective, and very rare instances of heart attack. Every effort will be made to minimize them by the preliminary examination and by observations during testing. Emergency equipment and trained personnel are available to deal with unusual situations which may arise.

The information which is obtained will be treated as privileged and confidential and will not be released or revealed to any person without my expressed written consent. The information obtained, however, may be used for a statistical or scientific purpose with my right of privacy retained.

I have read the foregoing and I understand it and any questions which may have occurred to me have been answered to my satisfaction.

Signed   ————————————

Patient

————————————

Witness

————————————

Date

————————————

Physician Supervising the Test

Addendum to Proposed Informed Consent
(to Be Completed When Patient Is Under 21 Years of Age)

(parent)

I am the (legal guardian) of ————————————— ,

Name

the patient who is to engage in the above described exercise test. I have read and understand the foregoing consent form, and I agree to the performance of the test.

Signed   ————————————

Parent
Legal Guardian

13

Vocational Aspects of Rehabilitation After Myocardial Infarction

John Naughton, M.D.

Coronary heart disease (CHD) is a disorder of unknown etiology that begins in early life, progresses insidiously over a number of decades, and manifests itself in middle life and late years as angina pectoris, myocardial infarction, congestive cardiac failure, and sudden death (1). New episodes of myocardial infarction account for approximately 35–40% of the 1.2–1.3 million cardiac events that occur annually throughout the United States. In these 400,000–500,000 first cardiac episodes, 30% of the patients die during the prehospital period, and about 20% of the remainder die either in the coronary care unit or during the first month of recovery. The threat of another episode of myocardial infarction, chronic physical disability, and sudden death lingers as a high probability for all survivors, even though the per annum survival rate for patients with class 1 functional status approaches 95%. The total direct and indirect costs can only be estimated, but they have variously been placed at a low of $17 billion and a high of $30 billion annually. The latter figure is comparable to the peak annual cost of the Vietnam conflict and is of a magnitude sufficient to cause all Americans to pause and ask whether we can afford such a disorder.

Although the outlook for 80% of survivors is quite favorable, it must be appreciated that this life-threatening disease affects all aspects of life-style and that jobs and income are significantly altered for most, if not all, survivors. This chapter will deal with some of the vocational issues that face patients recovered from myocardial infarction.

CARDIAC REHABILITATION

Cardiac rehabilitation is that process by which a patient is restored to and maintained at optimal medical, physiologic, psychologic, social, vocational, and recreational status and during which secondary prevention of the underlying atherosclerotic disease progress is instituted (2).

This process has made significant contributions to the care of cardiac patients during the past generation. These contributions have been made possible by an appreciation of the natural history of myocardial infarction. Specifically, they include the following: introduction of medically supervised and prescribed physical activity during each phase of the recovery, rehabilitation, and maintenance process; refinement of work evaluation; development of educational materials for the patient, spouse, and family. These have resulted in increasing numbers of cardiac patients returning to productive life, as well as a decrease in the average length of hospital stay, acceleration of the restorative process and improvement in all aspects of the quality of life.

A review of the literature reveals that consistent and significant advances have been made in the medical and physiologic aspects of cardiac rehabilitation (3). Some understanding of the psychosocial factors is beginning to develop. Considerable research and development must be carried out if the vocational aspects of cardiac rehabilitation are to approach the levels of development attained in other areas. This author is numbered among those who hope that during the decade ahead emphasis on vocational cardiac rehabilitation will be increased as other advances are incorporated into the so-called usual and customary practice of medicine.

VOCATIONAL HISTORY OF SURVIVORS

Vocational outcome for myocardial infarction survivors has not been thoroughly studied. Stern et al. (4) collected prospective data indicating that of those patients who were working at the time of onset of their illness, 78% returned to work by the end of the first year. In an earlier study, Pell and D'Alonzo (5) reported that even though the 5-year survival rate for patients discharged from hospital care approached 75–80%, far fewer were employed at the end of 5 years. Approximately 50% of salaried patients and 43% of wage earners were employed at 5 years after their infarctions.

If we assume a salvage rate of 250,000–300,000 first cardiac episodes per year, then the unemployment figure per annum due to myocardial infarction could range from 50,000 to 60,000, and the loss in salaries alone could be as high as $750 million. This figure is probably justifiably magnified by the fact that many of the patients who return to work will not be as productive as they were prior to illness, and for many, additional sick days and other side effects will add to the cost.

There are many factors that affect the patient's return to vocational activity. Stern et al. studied "good" and "bad" responders and found that those patients who scored high on *denial* and were free of *anxiety* and *depression* had far better vocational outcomes than did patients who were found to be anxious and/or depressed at 6 weeks after myocardial infarction. This latter group not only had a lower rate of return to work but also failed to make other satisfactory life adjustments. Their findings corroborated those of Cay et al. (6), who reported that the patients who experienced the greatest difficulty, regardless of infarction severity, were those who were anxious and depressed.

The presence or absence of symptoms influences rehabilitation outcome. Hellerstein and Friedman (7) reported that symptom-free patients returned to work and sexual activity at 8 weeks after infarction, but symptomatic subjects did not return to normal activity until 16 weeks after infarction.

The social status and vocation of the patient can have significant effects. For social class I and II subjects, who are characterized as economically, educationally, and vocationally advantaged, the question of return to work often depends only on the desire to do so and the degree of impairment caused by the cardiac condition. Most subjects in these social classes will be either salaried or self-employed and will have jobs that require a minimum of physical effort. They also will have a certain degree of occupational mobility that can be used to adapt to the situation. Only in rare instances (e.g., airline pilots) will their incomes be threatened immediately. In addition, most will be covered by adequate disability insurance that will provide support should illness impair them for 6 months or longer.

Patients at the lower levels of the social-class scale, i.e., III, IV, and V, are not so fortunate. Most are wage earners; they have less formal education; often their jobs are environmentally, physically, and socially stressful; their mobility is quite limited. Obviously it is this population of cardiac rehabilitants for whom much of the social legislation was developed and implemented and to whom greater emphasis must be directed if cardiac rehabilitation as a meaningful care process is to achieve its full potential.

Thus vocational outcome is related to a multitude of factors, and the decision whether a patient can return to the work force is dependent on proper evaluation and integration of all these factors.

DISABILITY

Survivors of myocardial infarction usually are aware that they have a condition that is not only life-threatening but also potentially disabling and crippling. Much of the emotional energy expended during recovery is directed to concerns of performance—on the job, at home, and in recreation. Many of their questions indicate awareness of the need to prepare to deal with lost capacity and future adjustments. Psychologically, these concerns are manifested as anxiety, depression, and loss of ego strength. Fortunately, once the initial threat of death has passed and a patient's condition has stabilized, these concerns can be dealt with constructively, and most survivors can look forward to returning to productive and rewarding life situations.

Nevertheless, physicians, nurses, counselors, employers, and legislators must realize that although overt physical signs are not always present, myocardial infarction is the leading cause of physical disability in the Western world. Like all disabilities, it may be partial or total, temporary or permanent. Unlike many other physical disorders, the disability state is more dynamic than static; this is due to the fact that atherosclerosis is a chronically progressive disorder characterized by subacute episodic illnesses. Thus the cardiac patient's potentials and limitations must be reevaluated as clinical status changes, and in the symptom-free patient they must be reappraised at least annually.

Determination of the degree of disability requires a comprehensive cardiovascular history, adequate physical examination, electrocardiographic and other laboratory evaluation, and performance of an exercise stress test.

History

The historical appraisal should elicit any evidence that cardiac limitation exists. Although the symptoms are myriad, three are paramount: chest pain, shortness of breath, and fatigue. The history should elicit the presence or absence of symptoms at rest, during the performance of routine activity, and during the performance of strenuous or unusual activity. The presence or absence of chest pain provides the most reliable information, but the physician should not forget that dyspnea and/or fatigue are most commonly found in disorders related to loss of myocardial reserve.

Physical Examination

The examiner should look for signs of congestive cardiac failure, abnormal chest wall movements, abnormal cardiac sounds, new murmurs, and a changing heart size.

Electrocardiogram

Specific emphasis should be directed toward detection of heart block, ventricular dysrhythmias, evidence of ventricular aneurysm, and findings of subendocardial ischemia.

Exercise Stress Test (See Also Chapter 8)

A standardized progressive multistage exercise stress test is indicated for those stabilized cardiac patients who are symptom-free at rest. A recommended procedure (8) is to begin with an initial work load that is very low in relation to the subject's anticipated work capacity and gradually increase external stress every 2–3 min. The work loads should be comparable to the various energy requirements encountered in the patient's daily life. Symptoms, physical signs, electrocardiographic changes, blood pressure, heart rate, and work capacity should be measured at each work load.

A test should be stopped at the onset of symptoms, abnormal physical signs, significant electrocardiographic abnormalities, or a decrease in systolic blood pressure; if none of these occurs, the test is stopped when a targeted age-adjusted peak heart rate is reached. The tests of 85–90% of cardiac patients are stopped by the onset of symptoms or electrocardiographic changes or because patients express a subjective need to stop.

If the oxygen requirement at each work load is established, the work threshold of the patient can be described in caloric units or in relation to the oxygen requirements at rest. The latter approach has gained favor in recent years, and metabolic equivalents (mets) have been used to measure patients' performance capacities. A met represents the oxygen requirement at rest, approximately 3.5 ml/kg/min. A severely limited patient might have a work tolerance of 2.0 mets or less; a class 1 or symptom-free patient might be able to handle work loads requiring 7.0 mets or more.

The disability evaluation should integrate the information obtained from the procedures outlined; it should indicate the degree of disability, those factors that may increase the degree of disability, and recommendations to relieve or modify the degree of disability. As is often the situation in medicine, it is the interpretation of the findings on which physicians disagree. In the case of disability evaluation, use of the New York Heart Association's functional status criteria together with the objective information gained from an exercise stress test can minimize the differences between the interpretation of various examiners (9). If one employs these approaches, the following criteria will pertain:

Class 1. Class 1 contains those patients who have heart disease and who are symptom-free when performing routine activities of daily living, including such functions as climbing stairs and prolonged exertion. On an exercise stress test, such a patient should be able to tolerate external work loads of 7 mets (8.0–8.75 kcal/min) or more comfortably. The degree of cardiac impairment for patients in this class ranges from zero to 15%.

Class 2. Class 2 patients are symptom-free at rest and can perform routine daily activities comfortably, but they can become symptom-limited during periods of emotional stress or prolonged physical exertion. Their work tolerances should be in the range of 5–6 mets (5.0–7.25 kcal/min). The degree of cardiac impairment ranges from 20% to 40%.

Class 3. Class 3 patients become symptomatic when performing routine daily activities, and they may have overt signs of congestive cardiac failure that can be relieved by therapy. Their exercise stress tolerance range is 3.0–4.0 mets (3.0–5.0 kcal/min). The degree of cardiac impairment ranges from 50% to 70%.

Class 4. Class 4 patients often are symptomatic at rest; they have evidence of congestive cardiac failure and have stress tolerances of 2.0 mets or less (<2.75 kcal/min). The degree of cardiac impairment ranges from 80% to 95%.

The approach outlined above permits the physician to combine subjective and objective appraisals in the summation and determination of impairment. In many situations a history and physical examination probably will suffice, but there is little doubt that performance of an exercise stress test lends credence to the evaluation. Many "deniers" will pass as class 1 subjects even in the presence of latent congestive heart failure, and many anxious and depressed patients may be overrated as to severity of physical disability. A stress test helps sort out these issues and is of particular help in classifying class 2 and class 3 patients.

If an exercise stress test is designed to include measurement of blood pressure and heart rate in addition to symptoms and electrocardiographic changes, a great deal more can be learned about the nature of the impairment. For instance, many patients will experience a decrease in systolic blood pressure as external stress is increased; such a finding is indicative of diminished myocardial function, and even in the presence of a reasonable level of work tolerance it should be regarded as a poor prognostic sign. Other patients will demonstrate evidence of overt heart failure (their heart rates increase disproportionately at relatively low work loads).

This author's experience as a Social Security evaluator indicates that more and more disability examinations are incorporating exercise stress tests but that examiners are still insufficiently critical when it comes to interpreting the results, characterizing the adaptive responses, and making judgments about the proper level of classification. Our ability to make disability evaluation a rational and respected process will be jeopardized until this is accomplished.

The rating of disability can be partial temporary, partial permanent, total temporary, or total permanent. Myocardial infarction is a disorder in which the ratings can change periodically. Thus there may be a need for reappraisal, particularly when there is a change in the clinical course of a patient who previously was symptom-free.

The determination of disability will vary with the patient's occupational status. Professionals and executives are usually protected by disability insurance that takes effect after 6 months of disability. Their livelihoods and incomes are usually protected during the first 6-month period. The insurance carrier will require a complete evaluation and statement in order to activate disability coverage.

The Social Security Act states that benefits cannot begin before 1 year of disability. The act defines disability as "inability to engage in any substantial gainful activity by reason of any medically determinable physical or mental impairment which can be expected to result in death or which has lasted or can be expected to last for a continuous period of not less than 12 months." The terms of this act may seem somewhat arduous, since most patients requiring these benefits will come from social classes 3, 4, and 5 and will have little fiscal reserve on which to thrive during the first year (9a).

The procedures for applying for Social Security disability, the manner of evaluation, and the criteria for appeals are all specified. Although the medical evaluation is extremely important, so are the vocational and social evaluations. For this reason, judgments regarding qualification often are made in light of whether patients who cannot perform their previous job tasks have the endowment and capacity to be retrained for other jobs, and whether, in fact, such other jobs are available. Obviously it is preferable to return cardiac patients to the working force if this is reasonable and medically possible. There is no greater evidence that work has an important role in a patient's vitality than the evidence encountered in the Social Security system. Their data indicate that the mortality rate for cardiac patients on Social Security disability compensation is twice that for gainfully employed cardiac patients. This is an alarming statistic, unless, of course, inordinate numbers of high-risk patients are placed on disability rolls—a highly unlikely prospect! However, the disability rolls include the more seriously impaired patients.

WORKMEN'S COMPENSATION

Workmen's Compensation represents one of the most significant advances made by modern industrialized Western society. The concept was first advanced in England in 1897; it gained favor in four states in the United States between 1908 and 1911 (10). Today, every state has legislated some form of Workmen's Compensation. The principle is that employment can be a source or cause of injury or illness and that employers must accept blame when an employee is so affected. It may be financed by private insurance or taxation or a combination of both. Only those business units with a limited number of employees, usually less than six, are exempted from providing appropriate coverage.

To be eligible for benefits, the employee or the surviving spouse must be able to demonstrate the job-related nature of the illness or injury. This is easily achieved in situations of resulting physical deformity or industrial accidents. In the area of cardiovascular disease, wherein the specific etiology of the disease state is other than job-related, often it is difficult or impossible to determine whether or not the disorder and the disability associated with it are job-related. This is particularly true for angina pectoris and myocardial infarction. The medical "purist" must argue that the etiology of the underlying condition, atherosclerosis, is unknown and that it is a condition that begins in early life, progressing gradually and insidiously, and that manifestations such as angina pectoris, myocardial infarction, dysrhythmias, and sudden death are natural, expected sequelae, regardless of whether the subject is working, relaxing, or sleeping.

However, Workmen's Compensation legislation was not designed to deal so specifically with the biologic cause of a disease state, and needless to say, it was developed before the complexities of atherosclerosis and coronary heart disease were appreciated. Rather, the legislation was developed to provide economic help for employees whose underlying disease states were aggravated or worsened by specific job circumstances. For cardiac patients, the two areas most often involved in such judgments concern the roles of physical activity and emotional stress. The defendant's physician usually is placed in the uncomfortable position of deciding whether the job requirements or working involvement accelerated manifestations that might have been prevented had working conditions been vastly different. These issues are obviously much more difficult to deal with than is the relationship of atherosclerosis to myocardial infarction.

The American Heart Association created the Committee on the Effect of Strain and Trauma on the Heart and Great Vessels (11) to deal with dilemmas created by Workmen's Compensation legislation. Their most significant recommendation relates to physical effort and suggests that a cardiac event be considered job-related only if the effort performed in association with the development of the condition was excessive or unusual. Many cardiologists have invoked this principle in developing their judgments. In some instances it has been accepted; in others it has been ignored.

We now know (11a) a great deal more about the relationshp of physical activity to the precipitation of cardiac abnormality than we did when the American Heart Association formulated their recommendations in 1962 (11). For instance, middle-aged American men have a physical working capacity or a physical fitness level that is 10–40% below that possessed by healthy European men of the same age. The results of exercise stress testing have demonstrated that many subtle cardiovascular abnormalities, especially ischemic ST-segment depression, can be precipitated during physical activity in so-called healthy workers. The tolerance for activity can be modified by significant changes in the environment (cold, heat, smog), by fatigue, and by the state of physical conditioning. Thus it is conceivable that a given level of physical stress can stimulate vastly different cardiovascular adaptations from day to day and that extreme or unusual exertion may be too narrow a criterion to use in making a proper judgment.

Evaluation of the relationship of emotional stress to the precipitation of cardiovascular abnormality is even more controversial. This is related to the fact that emotional stress, unlike physical stress, has not been quantitated; also, the number of controlled studies documenting the influence of emotionally distasteful events in cardiovascular adaptation is not great. However, there is a sufficient literature documenting that symptoms, dysrhythmias, and cardiac episodes have occurred in relationship to emotionally stressful situations. In the cardiac patient, the use of certain psychologic defense mechanisms may either mask the abnormal adaptation or aggravate it.

Patients who use *denial* as a defense mechanism may appear stable and at ease, but documentation of heart rate responses and cardiac rhythm during the episode may disprove the appearance. This author recalls vividly two case presentations in which denial was manifested. In the first, when I, as the interviewer, suggested that the patient was indeed angry, he denied it, and this denial was accompanied almost instantaneously by an episode of ventricular tachycardia. In the second situation, the patient's denial was directed toward the lack of importance of his wife's role in decisions about his health and life. His heart rate rose precipitously from 76 to 140 beats/min during the denial. In order to establish that these responses were not flukes, the situation of placing the patient in a position that required invoking denial was recreated, and the ventricular tachycardia and sinus tachycardia could be reproduced consistently in the respective subjects.

The anxious patient may not even require a noxious external stimulus to produce abnormal cardiovascular reactions. The patient's own insecurity and discomfiture often are sufficient to produce dysrhythmia, elevation of systemic blood pressure, peripheral vasodilatation with lightheadedness, and any other number of undesirable manifestations.

In modern-day cardiovascular medicine, the physician who becomes involved in Workmen's Compensation cases must be willing to evaluate patients under simulated conditions of physical and/or emotional stress or during actual performance on the job before making an educated judgment of how the individual patient might have responded to the job situation. This approach is, of course, not of much help to a surviving spouse. In these situations, conjecture and best available judgment based on the available data are the only alternatives.

For members of the medical profession, the most frustrating aspect of Workmen's Compensation work has been the manner in which judgments are rendered. In most jurisdictions, the plaintiff's lawyer and the insurance carrier's lawyer present arguments before the presiding judge for and against the conferring of benefits. The physican for the plaintiff is adamant that the job situation played a causal role, and the physician for the carrier is equally certain that the job played no part in the development of the cardiac condition. The judge makes the decision, and there is little doubt that the social and vocational status of the patient or surviving spouse is incorporated into the decision-making process. The adversarial approach has produced a system in which inconsistency and apparent capriciousness have dominated.

Some states, most notably Oregon, Washington, Oklahoma, and Wisconsin, have taken steps to remove the adversarial process and minimize the subjectiveness of judgments by creating panels of cardiovascular experts who review the cases on their merits and forward recommendations to the court for decision. Although the system is not perfected, these states have benefited, and the model probably should be replicated throughout the remaining jurisdictions.

Workmen's Compensation is further complicated by the fact that some states have passed laws specifically granting benefits to civil servants who become ill during the performance of their duties. These special legislations usually apply to firemen and policemen, but they support the concept that cardiovascular disease can be job-related.

A serious social problem created by Workmen's Compensation legislation relates to the reemployability of a cardiac patient. The employer who has lost one judgment obviously does not want to be jeopardized by another cardiac event and therefore attempts to remove the patient from the work force. Certainly this should not happen in an enlightened society with knowledge of the natural history of coronary heart disease. In order to deal with this problem, many industries have changed their position on rehiring cardiac patients, provided the patients sign waivers that absolve employers of all responsibility for subsequent job-related cardiac episodes. The validity of such waivers has been challenged.

VOCATIONAL REHABILITATION

The United States has an elaborate federal-state partnership designed to provide vocational rehabilitation for physically disabled workers. Each state has a Department of Vocational Rehabilitation staffed by counselors who can purchase medical and vocational services designed to return the disabled to the working force. They are also participants in evaluating those clients who apply for Social Security disability benefits.

The Vocational Rehabilitation system has been proved effective in a number of states and in dealing with a multitude of disorders. However, its contribution to impaired cardiac clients has not been considered substantial in that the number of cardiac clients served has been far smaller than was anticipated. This seeming deficiency has raised many questions, most of which are still unanswered.

It is highly probable that the very nature of myocardial infarction may account for the apparent discrepancy. Since most myocardial infarction patients are hospitalized for very short periods of time, usually less than 3 weeks, and so much of their care is transferred to the family, the need for vocational rehabilitation services is not identified. The situation is further aggravated by the knowledge that most survivors should be able to return to their original employment unless other variables are present to delay or obstruct the return.

A second factor relates to the lack of appreciation on the part of many physicians and counselors that myocardial infarction is, indeed, a severe physical impairment. The absence of external signs of physical disability often creates the illusion that a cardiac patient can and will become rehabilitated without any assistance. Obviously this attitude must change, and arrangements for seeking vocational counseling when it is required should be completed prior to hospital discharge.

A third factor that may reduce the number of cardiac clients in the vocational rehabilitation system is the attitude that many counselors and agency supervisors have toward heart disease. The inherent threat of sudden death and other complications, together with inability to assess blame, often makes counselors afraid, and they select clients who have conditions the counselors feel comfortable working with. A concerted professional and public education effort is needed to modify these attitudes, but one must remember that the concept of Workmen's Compensation legislation is diametrically opposed to the concept that a counselor may not be responsible for doing harm to a cardiac client.

The fourth factor that must be considered is the job market with which most rehabilitation agencies and counselors work. The agencies usually are faced with procuring a limited number of career opportunities, and often the jobs are unskilled and physically demanding. In many cases the result is that referring a client for Vocational Rehabilitation services leads to a self-fulfilling prophecy: that the client cannot really be a productive wage earner. This rather depressing prospect can be altered only if rehabilitation agencies avail themselves of a broader job market in which to place clients.

The Vocational Rehabilitation Act of 1973 expanded the tasks of Vocational Rehabilitation agencies remarkably. Specifically, it placed great emphasis on providing services for severely physically disabled clients. It seems that a great challenge has been placed before the cardiovascular medical community to render such services to appropriate cardiac patients.

A number of rehabilitation counselors should be trained as cardiac rehabilitation specialists to work with hospitals, physicians, and industry and business to accelerate and enhance the return of as many cardiac patients as possible to the work force. This process probably would be more productive and rewarding if a few such counselors in every sizable community were prepared to work only in this area and develop the community link necessary to optimize this valuable and necessary service.

OCCUPATIONAL RESTRICTIONS

Theoretically, every stabilized cardiac patient of class 2 cardiovascular status or better should be employable. There are some jobs that might prove too demanding and some that are not appropriate. However, it is important to remember that many jobs are of such nature that additional injury or illness might also cause harm to persons other than the patient. Although a strict list should not be enumerated, the physician must incorporate this factor into the decision to recommend or deny employment. Two jobs that have caused concern are commercial interstate truck driving and commercial piloting. Federal regulations do not militate against a cardiac patient driving a truck, but the general medical practice has been to advise against it. The regulations governing cardiac patients are quite specific, and the Federal Aviation Agency has followed advice and guidelines provided by a committee of experts appointed by the American College of Cardiology.

It is apparent that the goal of rehabilitation is to prevent further injury and acute episodes and to protect the individual patient as well as society. In the years ahead, guidelines will have to be established to aid the physician in making such recommendations more objectively.

UNMET NEEDS

Although substantial advances have been made in enhancing the cardiac patient's return to work and the incidence of return has been increased, there are still many unmet needs.

In the area of medical care for the patient with angina pectoris or myocardial infarction there is a need to bridge care from the time of hospital discharge until return to work. At the present time this phase of care is left to the patient and family, and attempts at reinforcement of the recovery and rehabilitation process often go amiss. It has been suggested that this gap in care could be bridged by activities such as "Heart Clubs" or by developing and staffing day-care centers to care for the patient and family. Although appropriate definitive studies are lacking, Aldes et al. (12) reported that intensive rehabilitation care for a vocationally unemployed group of 45 patients led to identifying 20 patients as medically nonrehabilitative and to returning 17 of the remaining 25 to productive jobs. Since upwards of 20% of survivors are in need of vocational services, it appears that the unemployment pool might be reduced from that figure to a more acceptable one ranging from 10% to 13%.

Croog et al. (13) published a scholarly review of the vocational problems facing the cardiac survivor in 1968. Although the review was exhaustive, its conclusion was rather simple and straightforward: namely, there was a paucity of creditable studies on which to base educated judgments in this area. It is hoped that this significant contribution to our lack of knowledge will lead to meaningful change in the years ahead (see Chapter 11).

The Rehabilitation Services Administration of the Department of Health, Education, and Welfare has provided funding to this area. In their attempts to combine research with demonstration they have funded a five-center study of the effects of medically supervised and prescribed physical activity on rehabilitation outcomes of male survivors of myocardial infarction between the ages of 30 and 64 years. This study is known as the National Exercise and Heart Disease Project. Its results will be available in late 1980 or early 1981.

The National Heart, Lung, and Blood Institute has created a Task Force on Cardiac Rehabilitation (1). It has not yet formally funded efforts in cardiac rehabilitation, but its Advisory Committee is reviewing the role that this institute should play in eliminating the unmet needs.

REFERENCES

1. Report of the Task Force on Cardiovascular Rehabilitation, National Heart and Lung Institute: *Needs and Opportunities for the Coronary Heart Disease Patient.* Department of Health, Education and Welfare Publication (NIH) 75-750, Washington, D.C., December, 1974

2. Supplement: Exercise in the prevention, the evaluation, and the treatment of heart disease. *J SC Med Assoc* 65:87, 1969

3. Naughton J, Hellerstein H (eds): *Exercise Testing and Exercise Training in Coronary Heart Disease.* Academic Press, New York, 1973

4. Stern MJ, Pascale L, Ackerman A: Life adjustment post myocardial infarction: Determining predictive variables. *Arch Intern Med* 137:1680, 1977

5. Pell S, D'Alonzo C: Immediate mortality and five year survival of employed men with a first myocardial infarction. *N Engl J Med* 270:915, 1964

6. Cay E, Vetter N, Phillip A, et al: Psychological status during recovery from an acute heart attack. *J Psychosom Res* 16:422, 1972

7. Hellerstein H, Friedman E: Sexual activity and the post-coronary patient. *Arch Intern Med* 44:1028, 1970

8. Patterson J, Naughton J, Pietras R, et al: Treadmill exercise in the assessment of functional capacity of cardiac patients. *Am J Cardiol* 30:757, 1972

9. Sagall E, Reed B (eds): *The Heart and the Law,* Appendix V, Guides to the evaluation of cardiac disability. Macmillan, New York, 1968

9a. Hollingshead AB, Redlion FC: *Social Class and Mental Illness.* Wiley, New York, 1959

10. Sagall E, Reed B (eds): *The Heart and the Law,* Chapter 1, Workmen's compensation. Macmillan, New York, 1968, p 5

11. Report of the Committee on the Effect of Strain and Trauma on the Heart and Great Vessels. *Circulation* 26:612, 1962

11a. Report of the Committee on Stress, Strain and Heart Disease, American Heart Association, *Circulation* 55:825A, 1977

12. Aldes JH, Stein SP, Grotin S: A program to effect vocational restoration of "unemployable" cardiac cases. *Chest* 54:32, 1968

13. Croog SH, Levine S, Lurie Z: The heart patient and the recovery process. A review of the directions of research in social and psychological factors. *Soc Sci Med* 2:111, 1968

14

Community Resources for Rehabilitation of the Myocardial Infarction Patient

Nanette Kass Wenger, M.D.

The goal of the rehabilitative approach to the patient with myocardial infarction (MI) is early resumption of a normal or near-normal life-style. Therefore the plan of care must be designed to help the patient achieve optimal physiologic improvement, attain optimal self-care and a useful activity level in the home and work environment, return to a former occupation or retrain for a more appropriate one if indicated, and minimize the impact of the illness on patient, family, and community. The important components of post-MI rehabilitative programs include progressive physical activity, patient and family education, and psychosocial and vocational counseling. An ideal rehabilitation program is one that is incorporated into the plan of care during hospitalization for the acute problem, one that involves the patient's family and social environment as a support system, and one that continues in the office of the patient's physician and/or in a variety of community facilities. The responsibility for restoration of the coronary patient to productive life or to independent living, and therefore the initiation and coordination of the rehabilitative effort, are the province of the patient's primary physician; however, the physician may and often should utilize the knowledge, skills, techniques, and services of a variety of medical consultants and health care personnel to implement the actual rehabilitative processes.

Much of the capability to effect rehabilitation should be available within the local community—in the community hospital, in the office of the primary physician, and through private, governmental, public, and voluntary health care agencies and facilities. In some cases all that is necessary to incorporate the rehabilitation process into the medical care system is some retraining of available personnel, redirection of attitudes and expectations, and more nearly optimal use of already trained personnel and available facilities. Nevertheless, some MI patients with more complex diagnostic problems may require newer evaluative techniques: exercise stress testing, ambulatory electrocardiographic monitoring,

295

myocardial scintigraphy, cardiac catheterization and coronary angiography, etc. Some patients may require specialized surgical management, e.g., myocardial revascularization. Other patients with more severe impairment may benefit from detailed psychologic or psychiatric evaluation or vocational assessment or from institution of programs and efforts designed to enhance any of a variety of areas of function: physiologic, psychologic, social, vocational, educational. When such consultative services are not available in the community, it may be necessary for the physician to refer patients to specialized cardiac centers staffed by personnel with particular knowledge and training and equipped with elaborate and often expensive diagnostic and therapeutic facilities. Nevertheless, patients referred for these services must eventually be returned to the care of their primary physicians and to the services and facilities in their local communities.

PHASES OF ILLNESS

Rehabilitative efforts for the MI patient are best discussed in relation to the phase of the illness; the MI patient's need for care by various members of the health team and the facilities needed for delivery of these services vary considerably with each stage of the illness.

Phases I and II encompass the period of acute illness; phase I is the time in the intensive care unit or coronary care facility, and phase II is the remainder of the hospitalization. In the United States the current average duration of hospitalization for patients with uncomplicated MI is 10–14 days. Phase III, the convalescent period, generally takes place at home and may vary considerably in duration, but it is usually 2–8 weeks. Phase IV is best designated a recovery-maintenance phase; its particular concerns include a wide variety of efforts to enhance function, to decrease coronary risk factors, and to prevent recurrence or progression of the disease process.

At each phase of the illness the primary physician must formulate a plan to manage and assess the patient's problems, modifying this plan according to the patient's response to therapy. This plan of care must include evaluation of function (severity of disease, complications, emotional response to illness, etc.), monitoring of desired effects and adverse effects of all therapeutic maneuvers, and periodic reassessment of function in the several spheres as function is changed by therapy.

Phase I

The currently accepted standard of care for the patient with acute MI involves admission to a hospital with the equipment and personnel for continuous electrocardiographic monitoring and with appropriately trained staff for intensive cardiac care. The primary physician is responsible for arranging immediate admission of MI patients to such a facility. In the coronary care unit or intensive care unit physicians and nurses with specialized training in acute cardiac care have the greatest responsibility; the physician immediately involved may or may not be the primary-care physician. Initial emphasis is appropriately on prevention and control of dysrhythmias and management of chest pain, heart failure, and/or shock.

However, major emotional reactions of varying severity (typically anxiety and depression) that are characteristic concomitants of MI occur during this phase and require attention. The immediate threat of dying produces anxiety, and the patient may respond to the anticipated invalidism and life-style restrictions with depression. Provision of preliminary information about MI and its management and structured plans for return toward normal living (initiation of a progressive ambulation program) afford the patient and family tangible and realistic reassurance and help avert or decrease emotional complications. With this approach, only rarely will specific psychotherapy be required. Blue-collar workers who sustain MI tend to have less facility in understanding complex monitoring equipment and coronary care unit procedures than their white-collar counterparts; thus particular attention must be devoted to detailed and repeated explanations of the immediate modalities of care and plans for future care. Special attention, too, is required to prepare patients for transfer out of the intensive care unit or coronary care unit, which is associated with changes in staff, in intensity of surveillance, and in complexity of equipment.

Because rehabilitative components must be incorporated into the acute care phase, all hospitals admitting patients with MI should have the personnel and facilities to assist the primary physician in providing or implementing rehabilitative services for coronary patients. In a small community hospital, the primary physician and a coronary care unit nurse may readily fulfill all the functions of a rehabilitation team, with aid from a hospital dietitian or social worker when appropriate. Larger medical centers with larger patient populations may have far more elaborate health care teams that include nurses, nurse educators, dietitians, social workers, physical and occupational therapists, and sometimes psychologists and rehabilitation counselors. But it is the responsible physician who must institute, direct, and determine the extent of early ambulation activities, although these activities may be implemented by a nurse, a therapist, a physician assistant, or even family members if they are properly supervised. The more complex and extensive the rehabilitation team, the more extensive the coordination required of the primary physician. Family and friends must always be considered and involved in the rehabilitation process, and their roles are best delineated by the primary physician. The responsible physician also must determine the content of the education/information program provided to the patient and family, must guide the rehabilitation counselor in replying to early questions from the patient's employer, and must coordinate these health care components with the traditional concerns of medical care.

Phase II

During the remainder of the hospital stay, phase II, as the intensity of physiologic monitoring, arrhythmia surveillance, and therapy diminishes, the roles and responsibilities of the nurse, nurse educator, nutritionist, social worker, occupational and physical therapists, and vocational counselor increase.

Progressive levels of physical activity remain under the direction of the responsible physician, as is the case with other prescriptive forms of therapy. Simple calisthenics and walking require no specialized equipment or facilities and are readily performed in the patient's room or hospital corridor. Telemetry, when available, may be used for selected patients, or direct electrocardiographic recording may be performed during activity; however, in most cases measurements of heart rate and blood pressure responses suffice.

The physician-designed, and usually nurse-implemented, educational program helps to define the patient's responsibility and role in the management of the illness, particularly as it relates to response to symptoms and adherence to prescribed therapy—diet, drugs, activity, etc. Nurse–patient bedside conferences in a small community hospital are just as effective as the class or conference sessions for groups of patients that may be led by nurse educators, dietitians, social workers, etc., in larger urban hospital centers. Family counseling may be done effectively by a variety of health care specialists; it may even be the direct responsibility of the primary physician in a small rural hospital. Family counseling should consider the life-style adjustments to be anticipated during convalescence, both in the family setting and subsequently in the community, and it should focus on averting overprotection of the MI patient.

Again, it must be kept in mind that patients in the lower socioeconomic groups tend to ask fewer questions (and thus acquire inadequate information) about planning for convalescence, rehabilitation, resumption of physical activities, sexual activity, return to work, etc. Particular attention must be directed toward providing the requisite information and encouraging requests for advice and help. The information must be presented by the physician and other members of the health care team in terms, values, concepts, and language that are understandable and acceptable to the patient and family. Cultural and ethnic differences in family structure and roles, as well as community health beliefs, attitudes toward work, etc., must be considered in counseling the post-MI patient and family.

For patients with more severe physiologic impairment, teaching energy-conserving techniques in self-care and in daily living activities constitutes an important role for the nurse or therapist. Again, the responsible physician initiates and coordinates these patient care activities; referral to more specialized care centers may be necessary for selected patients.

A system for detailed communication must be instituted to ensure continuity of care when different responsible physicians provide care in the hospital and in a distant community for the long-term ambulatory phase, as well as when patients with more complex problems are referred to larger medical centers for more specialized care following the acute hospitalization.

Phase III

Phase III, the convalescent period, is characterized by lessening roles for the physician and hospital-based nurses as the patient leaves the hospital environment and returns to the community. During this phase, rehabilitative efforts are designed to restore the physical, emotional, and social status of the patient in preparation for resumption of pre-illness activities, including return to work. However, in the United States there is no formal organization of convalescent/rehabilitative care (as contrasted with the highly structured and routinized rehabilitative efforts in many European countries); this results in extreme variability in the rehabilitative services offered. There is progressively greater involvement of the family and friends, as well as community-based public health or visiting nurse, dietitian, social worker, vocational counselor, employer, and other individuals and/or groups within the community, and all their efforts should be designed to enhance the function, adjustment, and self-sufficiency of the patient. The patient, too, actively assumes more responsibility for health care.

In smaller communities and for patients with uncomplicated clinical courses, the primary physician, at times with the help of a community nurse, may provide all requisite management, guidance, and counseling. As was the case during hospitalization, the more complex the clinical presentation of the illness, and the greater the degree of functional impairment, and the larger the patient population, then the more elaborate the composition and interrelationships of the rehabilitation team become. Communication among the health professionals is of extreme importance to ensure continuity of care and to maintain uniformity in the instructions and advice given the patient and family.

Nevertheless, it is during convalescence that the primary physician (aided by consultants, if necessary) must be prepared to assess the patient's physical performance (clinically and by exercise function testing, as indicated), the coronary risk factors warranting modification, and the need for specific pharmacologic and/or surgical intervention. The latter may require long-term ambulatory monitoring, multilevel exercise stress testing, coronary angiography, etc. When these assessments cannot be performed in the local community, referral to larger cardiac centers must be made.

The primary physician is also responsible for assessing the patient's knowledge about the disease, the therapy, and the plans for health care; and for determining patient and family needs for additional counseling and therapy regarding emotional adjustments to 'illness and altered level of function, return to sexual activity, life-style changes, family relationships, etc. A large variety of patient-family educational materials are available from the in-hospital rehabilitation programs and from many professional, voluntary, and governmental health agencies: the American Heart Association, the Diabetes Association, the American Medical Association, the National Heart, Lung, and Blood Institute, the National High Blood Pressure Education Program, to name a few. State, county, and city health departments and neighborhood health centers have trained personnel and educational materials to aid the physician in the community phase of patient-family education and information; personnel in these facilities may also help guide the patient to other governmental and voluntary health resources in the community, some of which may offer financial assistance (e.g., welfare departments, United Community Services, old age assistance programs, workmen's compensation programs, social security disability programs) and/or direct rehabilitation services or consultations. The services of community-based programs such as Weight-Watchers, antismoking groups, etc., may prove valuable, as may employee health education groups in industry. All factors relating to return to work, particularly the necessity for job retraining, when required, must be evaluated during phase III. These areas involve the total functional capacity of the patient, and their assessment by the responsible physician determines the need for additional specialized services. As was previously stated, when these additional specialized personnel and facilities are not available within the local community, referral may be required to larger cardiac centers, many of which are affiliated with medical graduate teaching and training institutions.

Phase IV

In phase IV, the recovery-maintenance phase, the scope of rehabilitation programming (and therefore the personnel, facilities, and services involved) becomes even more diverse. Although the primary physician must continue to coordinate rehabilitative care, the emphasis must be directed toward decreasing undue dependence of the patient on the physician and on the strictly medical care aspect of the illness and increasing the patient's realistic adaptation to illness and return to a normal or near-normal life-style and role in the community.

Therefore the vocational counselor, the employer, and the industrial physician and nurse often assume dominant roles, as must family, friends, fellow workers, etc. Appropriately, this health maintenance phase of the illness also includes important roles for individuals involved with community programming in areas such as exercise training programs (cardiac conditioning), educational programs (including vocational retraining), and recreational-social programs.

During this phase of the illness, a patient's cardiovascular status often has improved sufficiently to allow a return to prior levels of occupational or daily living activities. Nearly half of all MI survivors have mild uncomplicated illness without significant residual cardiovascular disability. Indeed, well over 85% of patients employed at the onset of illness return to work within 2–4 months after uncomplicated MI, characteristically returning to the same jobs. This group requires little in the way of vocational rehabilitative efforts, as over two-thirds of these patients are likely to work for at least 5 years. They may be considered rehabilitation successes without formal rehabilitation intervention, although it is impossible to gauge the supportive effects of positive and optimistic attitudes of the health care personnel, family, and friends during the acute illness and recovery. For this group of patients, the primary physician's continued medical management involves surveillance of dietary and drug therapy, as required, and institution of additional measures designed to enhance cardiac function. An important component is individualized prescriptive physical activity with the goals of enhancing cardiopulmonary function and promoting a sense of well-being. This prescriptive physical activity requires prior multistage exercise stress testing to ensure the safety and accuracy of exercise prescription; subsequently the patient may carry out an individual home exercise program or participate in a supervised community cardiac conditioning program. In some instances the primary physician may have the skills and equipment/facilities for the performance of both exercise testing and training; multilevel bicycle ergometer or treadmill exercise stress testing with appropriate equipment for electrocardiographic and blood pressure monitoring and for emergency care, if needed, may be available in the office of the physician or in the community hospital. Similarly, a gymnasium or large room (with trained supervisory personnel and emergency care equipment) may be available in a community hospital, in a local school, in community service club facilities, in the YMCA, in a Jewish Community Center, in an industrial complex, or as a privately owned facility. Elaborate or expensive exercise equipment is not required for cardiac conditioning programs; simple calisthenics and a walk-run sequence often are the major activity components. However, the health professionals at these facilities must be knowledgeable about exercise physiology, care of cardiac patients, and emergency cardiac care;

and emergency cardiac care equipment must be at hand. Alternatively, referral may be made within the community to cardiac consultants and their staff of nurses, exercise physiologists, physical therapists, physical educators, etc. For patients in communities with limited resources and for patients with more severe impairment, referral may be necessary to more specialized or cardiac rehabilitation centers. When appropriate, even for the patient who has returned to a productive role, the primary physician must consider surgical intervention (myocardial revascularization) to relieve chest pain symptoms and enhance cardiac function; and referral may be required to appropriate local or distant diagnostic and therapeutic facilities.

The importance of the rehabilitative approach for an "intermediate" group of patients must be stressed. Physical conditioning to enhance function, vocational counseling and minor occupational adjustments to match the physical requirements of the job with the patient's cardiac capabilities, and psychosocial support and counseling may avert cardiac invalidism and reenforce the concept of return to normal or near-normal life-style.

For the patient with more extensive physiologic, psychologic, or vocational impairment, the primary physician frequently will require consultative services. Indeed, the report of the Joint Working Party of the Royal College of Physicians of London and the British Cardiac Society recommends that "any myocardial infarction patient who has not returned to work at three months from the onset of his illness should be referred . . . for assessment of his physical and psychosocial state." The timing and scope of this referral are the responsibilities of the primary physician.

What referral services are necessary and appropriate? Which should be readily available? Physical (physiologic) status can be assessed by clinical and laboratory evaluation, usually including exercise (cardiac function) testing, with cardiac catheterization and coronary arteriography often being indicated, particularly for the more severely impaired patient. Efforts designed toward restoration and enhancement of function may include prescription of pharmacologic and/or exercise therapy; in some cases surgical intervention with myocardial revascularization, aneurysmectomy, and/or valve replacement may be warranted. The rehabilitative approach is equally important and appropriate after myocardial revascularization procedures. The consultants involved may thus include the cardiologist, the cardiovascular surgeon, and/or the rehabilitation specialist (whose training may be in internal medicine/cardiology, in cardiology, in rehabilitation medicine, etc.). Facilities include a hospital center with diagnostic and cardiovascular surgical capabilities and a variety of community cardiac conditioning (exercise training) centers that may be hospital-based, privately owned, industry-related or run under the auspices of voluntary agencies such as the YMCA, Jewish Community Center, etc.

Psychosocial and vocational status assessment requires the skills of psychologists, psychiatrists, social workers, vocational counselors, work physiologists, etc., whose services may be available in specialized cardiac care and rehabilitation facilities, work evaluation centers or units, or governmental or private rehabilitation agencies. Prominent among the latter are the work evaluation units related to local heart associations and the state vocational rehabilitation agencies. Services available include comprehensive occupational evaluation and a wide range of individual and group counseling and placement services. These become particularly important when patients with physiologic impairment possess only manual skills and have little formal education, thus limiting the vocational scope. Special training schools, sheltered industrial workshops, and on-the-job evaluations may be required to enhance vocational function.

The services of consultants and referral facilities may be required for widely varying periods of time. However, provision must always be made for the return of the patient to the local community: to the care of the primary physician, to the use of local services and facilities (e.g., community exercise programs, counseling services, discussion groups, therapy and educational programs, rehabilitation service agencies, Coronary Clubs or Mended Hearts groups, etc.), and to the social support system of family and friends.

SUMMARY

Invalidism is often unnecessarily and unduly prolonged after MI because of misinformation and unjustified fears about the natural history of the illness and because of psychosocial problems; indeed, impairment of function appears to be more often related to these difficulties than to actual physiologic limitations. To help correct or avert these problems, the rehabilitative approach must be begun at the onset of illness and remain as a continuing feature in the long-term care of the patient; rehabilitation must be the responsibility of the patient's primary physician, who may be a general physician, an internist, or a practicing cardiologist. Cardiovascular rehabilitation services should be designed to restore the patient, to a productive, active, and satisfying life as rapidly as possible.

For patients with significant residual cardiac damage or particular psychologic, social, or vocational problems, conventional medical management often is insufficient to ensure reintegration into society and return to a productive lifestyle. The clinician should appreciate this problem early in the course of the illness and institute referral for specialized consultant assessment and management. However, all aspects of long-term care and rehabilitation of the patient after MI must remain under the aegis of the primary physician, ultimately utilizing the personnel, facilities, and services of the local community.

REFERENCES

1. A Programme for the Physical Rehabilitation of Patients with Acute Myocardial Infarction, Freiburg, West Germany, Freiburg Working Group, EURO 5030 (1), 1968
2. Inter-Society Commission for Heart Disease Resources: Resources for the optimal care of patients with acute myocardial infarction. *Circulation* 43:A-171, 1971
3. Wenger NK, Hellerstein HK, Blackburn H, et al: Uncomplicated myocardial infarction. Current physician practice in patient management. *JAMA* 224:511, 1973
4. Semple T, Blackburn H, et al: *Myocardial Infarction. How to Prevent. How to Rehabilitate.* ISC Handbook. Boehringer, Mannheim, West Germany, 1973
5. Wenger NK: Coronary Care—Rehabilitation After Myocardial Infarction. Prepared for the Coronary Care Committee, Council on Clinical Cardiology and the Committee on Medical Education, Dallas, American Heart Association, 70-002C, 1973

6. Naughton J, Hellerstein H (eds): *Exercise Testing and Exercise Training in Heart Disease*. Academic Press, New York, 1973

7. Report of Task Force on Cardiovascular Rehabilitation, National Heart and Lung Institute: Needs and Opportunities for Rehabilitation for the Coronary Heart Disease Patient, December 15, 1974, Washington, DC, Department of Health, Education, and Welfare publication (NIH) 75-750, 1974

8. Hackett TP, Cassem NH: Coronary Care—Patient Psychology. Prepared for the Coronary Care Committee, Council on Clinical Cardiology and the Committee on Medical Education, Dallas, American Heart Association, 70-029-A, 1975

9. Joint Working Party of the Royal College of Physicians of London and the British Cardiac Society: Cardiac rehabilitation 1975. *J R Coll Physicians Lond* 9:281, 1975

Glossary

Acclimatization.   Physiological adjustments brought about through continued exposure to a particular environmental stress, such as changes in climate.

Acidosis.   The situation in which the acid-base balance shifts to the acid side, due either to increased levels of unbuffered acids in blood or to a reduction in blood bicarbonate.

Actin.   Thin protein filament that acts with the protein filament myosin to allow muscle contraction.

Actomyosin.   Result of the interaction of actin and myosin protein filaments in muscle.

Adenosine diphosphate (ADP).   One of the chemical products of the breakdown of adenosine triphosphate (ATP) for energy during muscle contraction.

Adensine triphosphate (ATP).   A high-energy compound from which the body derives energy.

Adipose tissue.   Fat tissue.

Adrenal glands.   Endocrine glands directly above each kidney, composed of the medulla (secreting the hormones epinephrine and norepinephrine) and the cortex (secreting cortical hormones).

Adrenaline (epinephrine).   A chemical liberated from the adrenal medulla and from sympathetic nerve endings. Important effects include cardiac stimulation and constriction of blood vessels with a consequent rise in blood pressure.

Aerobic.   Living, active, or occurring only in the presence of oxygen.

Aerobic exercise.   Exercise during which the energy needed is supplied by inspired oxygen.

Aerobic power (max $\dot{V}O_2$).   The maximal volume of oxygen consumed per unit of time, also known as maximal oxygen uptake or maximal oxygen consumption.

Age-predicted maximal heart rate.   Mean highest heart rate attained during effort by individuals at various ages.

Alactic acid oxygen debt.   Part of the oxygen debt that is not accompanied by an increase in lactic acid in the blood.

Alkalosis.   The situation in which the acid-base balance shifts to the alkaline, or basic, side.

Anaerobic.   Living or active in the absence of oxygen.

305

Anaerobic endurance.   The ability to persist in physical activities of short duration that require high rates of energy expenditure. These high rates of energy expenditure cannot be met solely by aerobic metabolism.

Anaerobic exercise.   Exercise during which the energy needed is provided without utilization of inspired oxygen.

Anaerobic threshold.   That point where the metabolic demands of exercise cannot be met totally by available aerobic sources and at which an increase in anaerobic metabolism occurs, as reflected by an increase in blood lactate.

Aneurysm.   A spindle-shaped or saclike bulging of the wall of a blood-filled vein, artery, or ventricle.

Angina pectoris.   Pain or discomfort in the chest, and often in the left arm and/or the shoulder, due to an inadequacy of the blood supply to meet the oxygen needs of the heart muscle. Commonly results from activity or emotion when the coronary arteries are narrowed by atherosclerosis.

Angiography.   An invasive technique for diagnosing cardiovascular disease involving x-ray examination of the heart and blood vessels to visualize the course of a fluid opaque to x-rays that has been injected into the bloodstream.

Anoxia.   Literally, absence of oxygen. Often used to indicate inadequate blood or tissue oxygen. See also *Hypoxia.*

Anthropometry.   The measurement of the size and proportions of the human body.

Anticoagulant.   A drug that inhibits clotting of the blood.

Antihypertensive agents.   Drugs used to lower arterial blood pressure.

Arrhythmia.   Alteration in the normal rhythm of the heartbeat. See also *Dysrhythmia.*

Arteriosclerosis.   Loss of elasticity or hardening of the arteries. A precursor to various cardiovascular diseases.

Arteriovenous oxygen difference (A-V O_2 difference).   The difference between the oxygen content of arterial and venous blood.

Asystole.   Absence of contraction of the atria and/or of the ventricles.

Atheroma (plural, *atheromata).*   A deposit of fatty and other substances in the inner lining of the artery wall, characteristic of atherosclerosis.

Atherosclerosis.   A form of arteriosclerosis characterized by localized accumulations of lipid-containing material within or beneath the intimal surfaces of arteries.

Athlete's heart.   An enlarged heart, typically found in endurance athletes, due primarily to hypertrophy of the left ventricle. It is no longer considered to be a disease.

ATP.   See *Adenosine triphosphate.*

Atrial tachycardia.   Repetitive rapid cardiac contractions arising from an ectopic focus in the atrium.

Atrioventricular block (A-V block).   Impairment of normal electrical conduction between the atria and the ventricles.

Atrioventricular bundle (Bundle of His, A-V bundle).   A bundle of specialized muscle fibers. The only known direct muscular connection between the atria and the ventricles. Conducts impulses for rhythmic cardiac contraction from the atrioventricular node to the ventricular muscle.

Autonomic nervous system.   Part of the nervous system that innervates smooth and cardiac muscle and glandular tissue. Governs more or less automatic or involuntary activity.

A-V O$_2$ difference.   See *Arteriovenous oxygen difference.*

Basal metabolic rate (BMR).   The lowest level of energy expenditure, determined when the body is at complete rest.

Bigeminy.   Paired cardiac contractions, the second of the pair from an ectopic pacemaker, occurring in a recurring pattern.

Blood pressure.   The driving force that moves blood through the circulatory system. Systolic blood pressure is the blood pressure when the ventricular muscle contracts (systole); diastolic blood pressure is the blood pressure when the ventricular muscle is relaxed between beats (diastole). Blood pressure is generally expressed by two numbers (e.g., 120/80 mm Hg), the first representing the systolic pressure and the second the diastolic pressure.

Bradycardia.   Abnormally slow heart rate, generally, one below 60 beats per minute.

Bundle branch block.   Prolongation of duration of ventricular activation (QRS complex) due to delay in conduction in one or more bundle branches or fascicles.

Bundle of His.   See *Atrioventricular bundle.*

CAD.   Abbreviation for coronary artery disease, generally used to indicate coronary atherosclerotic heart disease.

Calorie.   A unit of work or energy equal to the amount of heat required to raise the temperature of 1 g of water 1° C. A large calorie or kilocalorie is a unit of heat energy required to raise the temperature of 1 kg of water 1° C under specified conditions. In physiology it is used as a measure of work and energy; calories per minute is a measure of power (or rate of energy utilization). Metabolically, 1 cal is the equivalent of approximately 200 ml of oxygen consumption.

Cardiac arrest.   Cessation of cardiac function, with disappearance of arterial blood pressure.

Cardiac catheterization.   Passage of a catheter through a vein or an artery into the cardiac chambers; used to diagnose intracardiac abnormalities.

Cardiac cycle.   One total heartbeat, i.e., one complete contraction (systole) and relaxation (diastole) of the heart.

Cardiac index.   Cardiac output per square meter of body surface area, expressed as liters per M^2 BSA.

Cardiac output.   The volume of blood pumped from a ventricle of the heart per unit of time; cardiac output is the product of heart rate and stroke volume (CO = HR × SV).

Cardiogenic shock.   Shock resulting from diminution of cardiac output, as in myocardial infarction.

Cardiomegaly.   Enlargement of the heart.

Cardiorespiratory endurance.   The ability of the lungs and heart to take in and transport adequate amounts of oxygen to the working muscle, allowing activities that involve large muscle masses (e.g., running, swimming, bicycling) to be performed over long periods of time.

Carotid sinus.   A slight dilatation where the internal carotid artery arises from the common carotid artery, which supplies blood to the head and neck. The carotid sinus contains special nerve end organs that respond to changes in blood pressure by causing a change in the heart rate. External pressure on the carotid sinus, stimulating nerves in the sinus, can cause slowing of the heart rate.

Catecholamines.   Compounds secreted by the adrenal medulla; a class of chemicals that includes adrenaline and noradrenaline (epinephrine and norepinephrine).

Catherization.   See *Cardiac catheterization.*

CHD.   Abbreviation for coronary heart disease, generally used to indicate coronary atherosclerotic heart disease.

Cholesterol.   A lipid or fatty substance essential for life and found in various tissues and fluids. Elevated levels in the blood have been associated with an increased risk of coronary atherosclerosis.

Chronotropic.   Affecting time or rate, especially of the heartbeat.

Circuit training.   Selected exercises or activities performed in sequence.

Claudication.   Pain and limping caused by inadequate circulation of the blood in the arteries of the limbs.

Collateral circulation.   Circulation of the blood through nearby smaller vessels when a main vessel has been narrowed or occluded.

Concentric contraction.   Contraction of a muscle resulting in shortening of the muscle.

Conditioning.   Augmentation of the energy capacity of muscle through an exercise program.

Congestive heart failure.   Impairment of the heart's ability to maintain an adequate flow of blood to the tissues. Fluid retention typically occurs. See also *Myocardial insufficiency.*

Continuous work.   Exercise performed to completion without rest periods.

Convection.   The transfer of heat from one place to another by the motion of a heated substance.

Coronary arteries.   Those arteries that supply the heart muscle or myocardium.

Coronary atherosclerosis.   Commonly called coronary heart disease. An irregular thickening of the inner layer of the walls of the coronary arteries whose lumen becomes narrowed with a resultant reduction in the blood and oxygen supply to the heart muscle. See also *Atherosclerosis.*

Coronary occlusion.   An obstruction in a branch of one of the coronary arteries that hinders the flow of blood to part of the heart muscle. This muscle may die because of lack of blood and oxygen supply (myocardial infarction). Sometimes called a coronary heart attack or heart attack.

Coronary thrombosis.   Formation of a clot in a branch of one of the arteries which supply blood to the heart muscle (coronary arteries). A form of coronary occlusion. See *Coronary occlusion.*

CP.   See *Creatine phosphate.*

Creatine phosphate (CP).   Phosphocreatine. An energy-rich compound that plays a critical role in providing energy for muscular contraction.

Cross-bridges.   The linkages between actin and myosin filaments during muscle contraction.

Defibrillator.   Any agent or measure, such as an electric shock, that stops an incoordinated contraction of the heart muscle and restores a normal heartbeat.

Density.   The mass per unit volume of an object.

Depolarization.   The process of activation of automatic, conductile, and contractile elements from the resting or polarized state. The QRS complex of the electrocardiogram represents ventricular depolarization.

Diastole.   The relaxation (resting) phase of each cardiac cycle, immediately following the contraction, or systolic, phase.

Diastolic (blood) pressure.   See *Blood pressure.*

Digitalis.   A drug that augments the contraction of the heart muscle, slows the rate of conduction of cardiac impulses through the atrioventricular node, and by improving the efficiency of heart function may promote the elimination of excess fluid from body tissues.

Diuretic.   A medicine that enhances the urinary excretion of fluid.

Double product.   See *Rate pressure product.*

dP/dt.   Expression, used in kinetics, of the rate of change of pressure with time.

Dynamometer.   A device for measuring muscular strength.

Dyspnea.   Difficult or labored breathing.

Dysrhythmia.   An abnormal rhythm of the heartbeat.

Eccentric contraction.   Lengthening of the muscle under tension, as when lowering a heavy object.

ECG.   See *Electrocardiogram.*

Ectomorphy.   One of three categories of the somatotype in which the body is characterized by linearity, fragility, and delicacy of body structure.

Ectopic.   Abnormal origin (as of a heartbeat).

Efficiency.   The ratio of work output to work input.

Ejection fraction (EF).   The difference between LV (left ventricular) end diastolic volume and LV end systolic volume.

EKG.   See *Electrocardiogram.*

Electrocardiogram (ECG, EKG).   A graphic record of the electrical activity of the heart, obtained with an electrocardiograph.

Electrolyte.   Any substance that, in solution, is capable of conducting electricity by means of its atoms or groups of atoms, and in the process is broken down into positively and negatively charged particles. Examples are sodium and potassium.

Embolism.   See *Embolus.*

Embolus (plural, *emboli*).   A clot or other plug of material transported by the blood from a larger vessel into a smaller one, thus obstructing circulation.

Endomorphy.   One of three categories of the somatotype in which the body is characterized by roundness, softness, and excess fat.

Endothelium.   The thin inner lining of blood vessels.

Endurance.   The ability to resist fatigue. Includes muscular endurance, which is a local or specific endurance, and cardiovascular endurance, which is a more general, total body endurance.

Energy.   The capacity to perform work.

Enzyme.   A complex organic substance capable of speeding specific biochemical processes in the body.

Epicardium.   The outer layer of the heart wall. Also called the visceral pericardium.

Epidemiology.   The science dealing with the factors that determine the frequency and distribution of a disease in a community.

Epinephrine.   See *Adrenalin.*

Ergometer.   An apparatus or device, such as a treadmill, a stationary bicycle, or steps, used for measuring the physiological effects of exercise.

Essential hypertension.   Sometimes called primary hypertension and commonly known as high blood pressure. An elevated blood pressure not caused by kidney or other evident disease.

Evaporation.   The loss of heat through the conversion of the water in sweat to a vapor.

Exercise prescription.   Individualized exercise program involving the duration, frequency, intensity, and mode of exercise.

Extrasystole.   A contraction of the heart, originating in an ectopic focus, that occurs prematurely and interrupts the normal rhythm.

False negative.   A test or an examination indicating that a condition or disease is not present when it is in fact present.

False positive.   A test or an examination indicating that a condition or disease is present when in fact it is not.

Fast twitch muscle fiber.   One of several types of skeletal muscle fibers that have low oxidative capacity and high glycolytic capacity, and are associated with speed or power activities.

Fat weight.   Absolute amount of body fat. Fat weight plus lean body weight equals total body weight.

Fibrillation.   The condition of being twitched or finely and rapidly contracted; exceedingly rapid contractions or twitchings of muscular fibrils, but not of the muscle as a whole. Commonly occurs in atria or ventricles of the heart as well as in recently denervated skeletal muscular fibers.

Flexibility.   The range of motion of the body's joints.

Frank-Starling effect.   The increased contraction of the heart muscle caused by stretching of the muscle fibers upon increased filling of the cardiac chambers.

Gallop rhythm.   An extra (third or fourth) heart sound that resembles a horse's gallop when the heart rate is fast.

Ganglionic blocking agent.   A drug that blocks the transmission of a nerve impulse at the nerve center (ganglia). Such a drug may be used in the treatment of high blood pressure.

Glycogen.   The storage form of carbohydrates in the body, found predominantly in the muscles and the liver.

Glycogen loading.   Manipulating exercise and diet to optimize the total amount of glycogen stored in the body.

Glycolysis.   The breakdown of glucose to pyruvic or lactic acid. Also, sometimes used to describe the breakdown of glucose into carbon dioxide and water.

Heart block.   Interference with conduction of electrical impulses from the atria to the ventricles which can be partial or complete. This can result in dissociation of the rhythms and contractions of the atria and the ventricles.

Heat cramp.   Severe cramping of skeletal muscles due to excessive dehydration and associated salt loss.

Heat exhaustion.   A disorder due to excessive heat load on the body, characterized by breathlessness, extreme tiredness, dizziness, and rapid pulse, and usually associated with a decrease in sweat production.

Hemodynamics.   The study of the flow of blood and the forces involved.

Hemoglobin.   The oxygen-carrying iron pigment of red blood corpuscles. When it has absorbed oxygen in the lungs, it is bright red and called oxyhemoglobin. After it has given up its oxygen in the tissues, it is purple in color and is called reduced hemoglobin.

Humidity.   Pertaining to the moisture in the air.

Hypercholesterolemia.   An excess of cholesterol in the blood. See also *Cholesterol.*

Hyperlipidemia.   Abnormally high concentration of lipids in the blood.

Hyperlipoproteinemia. An increase in the concentration of the three fatty substances of the blood: cholesterol, phospholipid, and triglyceride.

Hyperplasia. An increase in the number of cells in a tissue or organ.

Hypertension. Commonly called high blood pressure. A transient or persistent elevation of blood pressure above the normal range, which may eventually lead to heart, kidney, and brain damage.

Hyperthermia. An elevated body temperature.

Hyperthyroidism. A condition in which the thyroid hormone secretion is excessive. This increases body metabolism and may result in tachycardia.

Hypertrophy. An increase. in the size of a cell or organ.

Hyperventilation. Excessive ventilation of the lungs caused by increased depth and frequency of breathing above levels necessary for normal function and usually resulting in elimination of carbon dioxide.

Hypoglycemia. Low blood sugar.

Hypotension. Commonly called low blood pressure. Blood pressure below the normal range. Most commonly used to describe an acute fall in blood pressure, as occurs in shock.

Hypothermia. The lowering of the body temperature in order to slow the metabolic processes, as during heart surgery. In this cooled state body tissues require less oxygen.

Hypoxia. Inadequate supply of oxygen in the blood or tissues due to a reduced partial pressure of oxygen.

Incidence. The number of new cases of a disease developing in a given population during a specified period of time, such as a year.

Infarction (infarct). An area of a tissue that is damaged or dies as a result of not receiving a sufficient blood supply. Myocardial infarct refers to an area of heart muscle damaged or killed by an insufficient flow of blood and oxygen through the coronary arteries that normally supply it.

Inotropic. Affecting force or energy of muscular contraction.

Intercoronary anastomoses. So-called collateral circulation, which consists of small arterial channels that develop, circumventing coronary artery obstructive lesions, to enhance blood supply to hypoxic areas of the myocardium.

Intermittent work. Exercises performed with alternate periods of rest, as opposed to continuous work.

Interval training. A training program that alternates bouts of heavy or very heavy work with periods of rest or light work.

Intima. The innermost layer or lining of a blood vessel.

Intramyocardial tension. Pressure multiplied by stress.

Ischemia. A local, usually temporary, deficiency of blood supply to some part of the body, often caused by a constriction or an obstruction of the blood vessel supplying the area.

Isometric (static) contraction.   A muscular contraction in which there is no change in the angle of the involved joint(s) and little or no change in the length of the contracting muscle. Tension is developed but no mechanical work is performed.

Isoproterenol.   A sympathomimetic drug possessing the inhibitory properties, the cardiac excitatory actions, but not the vasoconstrictor actions of epinephrine.

Isotonic (dynamic) contraction.   Contraction of a muscle occurring when equal tension on the muscle is maintained while the length of the muscle is decreased during the performance of work or exercise.

Isotope.   A term applied to one or two elements, chemically identical, but differing in some other characteristic, such as radioactivity. Radioactive isotopes are often used in medicine to trace the fate of substances in the body.

Kcal.   See *Kilocalorie.*

Ketone bodies (substrate).   Any organic compound containing the carbonyl group.

Kilocalorie (Kcal).   The heat required to raise the temperature of 1 kg of water 1° C under specified conditions.

Kilogram meters per minute.   See *Kilopond meters per minute.*

Kilopond meters per minute (kpm/min).   In a normal gravitational field these are identical with kilogram meters per minute. This is a measure of power and is usually used to describe the external work load. Alternatively, this external load may be expressed in watts. Approximately 50 watts equals 300 kpm/min, or 100 watts is equivalent to 600 kpm/min. Conversely, 1 watt equals about 6 kpm/min. 1.78 ml of oxygen are required for 1 kpm/min of work. The bicycle ergometer is usually calibrated in kilopond meters per minute, but some electrically braked units may be calibrated in watts.

Krebs cycle.   A series of chemical reactions occurring in mitochondria in which carbon dioxide is produced and hydrogen ions and electrons are removed from carbon atoms (oxidation). Also referred to as the tricarboxyclic acid cycle (TCA) or citric acid cycle.

Lactic acid (lactate).   A fatiguing metabolite of the lactic acid system resulting from the incomplete breakdown of glucose. The end product of glycolysis or anaerobic metabolism.

Lactic acid oxygen debt.   The portion of the oxygen debt that is associated with a rise in blood lactic acid.

Lean body mass.   The body mass that does not include fat tissue.

Lean body weight.   The difference between the total body weight and the fat weight. The weight of the body that is not fat, e.g., bone, muscle, skin, organ weights, etc.

Left bundle branch block.   Blockage or delay of conduction in the left bundle branch of the heart.

Left ventricular stroke work index (LVSWI).   Index of left ventricular mechanical work per stroke = (LVSPm − LVED) × SI × 1.36/100 kg meters/beat/M². (LVSP = left ventricular systolic pressure, LVED = left ventricular end diastolic pressure, SI = stroke index.)

Left ventricular volume (LVV).   Volume of blood contained in the left ventricle, usually at end diastole.

Lipids.   Any of various substances including fats, waxes, phosphatides, cerebrosides, and related and derived compounds, that with proteins and carbohydrates constitute principal structural components of living cells.

Lipoprotein.   A complex of fat and protein molecules.

Maximal oxygen uptake ($\dot{V}O_2$ max).   The maximal rate at which oxygen can be consumed per minute. The best physiological index of total body endurance. Also referred to as aerobic power, maximal oxygen intake, maximal oxygen consumption, and cardiovascular endurance capacity.

Mesomorphy.   One of three categories of the somatotype in which the body is of muscular build.

met.   The name for a resting metabolic unit, independent of body weight. One met is the equivalent of approximately 1.2 cal/min. The oxygen equivalent of 1 met is 3.5 to 4.0 ml/kg/min. The term met is now preferred for energy requirement or utilization.

Metabolism.   The sum total of the energy-producing and -absorbing processes in the body, i.e., the energy used by the body.

Mitochondria.   Subcellular energy-producing structures located within the cells. Mitochondria contain the enzymes responsible for the generation of adenosine triphosphate by aerobic mechanisms.

Morbidity rate.   The ratio of the number of cases of a disease to the number of well people in a given population during a specific period of time, such as a year. The term morbidity involves two separate concepts: a) Incidence is the number of new cases of a disease developing in a given population during a specific period of time, such as a year. b) Prevalence is the number of cases of a given disease existing in a given population at a specified moment in time.

Mortality rate, cause specific.   The ratio of deaths from a specific cause to total population during a given period of time, such as a year.

Muscle fiber.   The structural unit of a muscle. A single cell with multiple nuclei composed of a number of smaller units called myofibrils.

Muscular endurance.   The ability of a muscle or muscle group to perform repeated contractions for an extended period of time.

$M\dot{V}O_2$.   Myocardial oxygen uptake, usually expressed as ml O_2/100 gm LV/min.

Myocardial infarction (myocardial infarct).   Damage or death of an area of heart muscle (myocardium) resulting from a reduction of the blood and oxygen supply reaching that area.

Myocardial insufficiency.   Inability of the heart muscle (myocardium) to maintain normal circulation (See also *Congestive heart failure*).

Myocardium.   The muscular wall of the heart. The thickest of the three layers of the heart wall, it lies between the inner layer (endocardium) and the outer layer (epicardium).

Myofibril.   The small elements that comprise the muscle fiber, composed of the contractile proteins actin and myosin.

Myoglobin.   Oxygen-binding protein in skeletal muscle.

Myoneural junction.   The junction between the muscle fiber and its nerve.

Myosin.   Contractile protein in muscle. Myosin molecules make up the thick filaments in muscle. Myosin acts with actin to allow the muscle to contract.

Necrosis.   Death of a cell or group of cells in contact with living tissue.

Net oxygen cost.   The amount of oxygen, above resting values, required to perform a given amount of work. Also referred to as net cost of exercise.

Nitrites.   A group of chemical compounds, many of which cause dilation of the small blood vessels, and thus lower blood pressure. They are vasodilators. Examples are amyl nitrite, sodium nitrite, etc.

Nitroglycerin.   A drug (one of the nitrates) that relaxes the muscles in the blood vessels. It is one of the vasodilators. Often used to relieve angina pectoris.

Noradrenaline (norepinephrine).   A hormone secreted by sympathetic nerve endings and by the adrenal medulla. Noradrenaline causes vasoconstriction and increases blood pressure.

Norepinephrine.   See *Noradrenaline*.

Normotensive.   Characterized by normal blood pressure.

Obesity.   An excessive amount of body fat. The state of being overweight as a result of excess fat.

Overload.   Stressing the body or parts of the body to levels above that normally experienced.

Oxidation (oxidizing).   To combine or cause to combine with oxygen. Loss of one or more electrons from an element or a compound.

Oxidative phosphorylation.   The production of adenosine triphosphate dependent on oxidative processes in the electron transport system of the mitochondria.

Oxygen debt.   The quantity of oxygen above normal resting levels used in the period of recovery after any specific exercise or muscular activity.

Oxygen deficit.   The difference between the theoretical oxygen requirement of a physical activity and the oxygen actually used during the activity.

Oxygen pulse.   The amount of oxygen removed from the blood per heartbeat. Calculated by dividing the oxygen intake by the heart rate over a given period of time.

Oxygen transport system ($\dot{V}O_2$).   Composed of the stroke volume (SV), the heart rate (HR), and the arterial-mixed venous oxygen difference (A-V O_2 diff). Mathematically, it is defined as $\dot{V}O_2 = SV \times HR \times$ A-V O_2 diff.

Oxygen uptake.   The oxygen used by the mitochondria of all body cells.

Oxyhemoblobin (HbO_2).   Hemoglobin chemically combined with oxygen.

Pacemaker.   Also called sino-atrial node, or S-A node, of Keith-Flack. A small mass of specialized cells in the right atrium which generates the electrical impulses that initiate contraction of the heart. The term pacemaker, or more exactly electric cardiac pacemaker, also applies to an electrical device that can substitute for a defective natural pacemaker.

Palpitation.   A fluttering sensation of the heart or abnormal rate or rhythm of the heart experienced by the person.

Papillary muscles.   Small bundles of muscles in the wall of the ventricles to which the cords leading to the cusps of the atrioventricular valves (chordae tendinae) are attached. When the valves close, these muscles contract and tighten the cords that hold the valves firmly shut.

Parasympathetic nervous system.   A part of the autonomic or involuntary nervous system. Stimulation of various parasympathetic nerves causes the pupils of the eye to contract, makes the heart beat more slowly, and produces other nonvoluntary reactions.

Paroxysmal tachycardia.   A period of rapid heartbeat that begins and ends suddenly.

Peripheral resistance.   The resistance offered by the arterioles and capillaries to the flow of blood from the arteries to the veins. An increase in peripheral resistance causes a rise in blood pressure.

Phlebitis.   Inflammation of a vein, often in the leg. Sometimes a blood clot forms in the inflamed vein.

Phosphocreatine (PC).   A chemical compound stored in muscle which when broken down aids in manufacturing ATP.

Physical work capacity.   The capacity to perform physical work. Usually measured in oxygen consumption or in kilopond meters per minute while at a specific heart rate (e.g., PWC_{150} or PWC_{170}).

Polyunsaturated fat.   A fat capable of absorbing additional hydrogen. These fats are usually liquid oils of vegetable origin, such as corn oil or safflower oil. A diet high in polyunsaturated fats tends to lower the blood cholesterol. These fats are substituted for saturated fat in a diet in an effort to lessen the hazard of fatty deposits in blood vessels.

Power.   Work performed per unit time.

Premature atrial contraction (PAC).   Disorder of rhythm and contraction, caused by abnormal foci in the atrium that discharge impulses earlier or more frequently than those from the S-A node.

Premature ventricular contraction (PVC).   A disturbance of rhythm, arising from ectopic foci in the ventricles.

Pressor.   A substance that raises the blood pressure.

Primary hypertension.   Sometimes called essential hypertension and commonly known as high blood pressure. An elevated blood pressure not caused by kidney or other evident disease.

Procainamide.   A drug used to treat abnormal rhythms of the heartbeat.

Progressive overload.   Gradually increasing the training stimulus in a systematic manner.

Progressive resistance exercise (PRE).   The resistance used in training is progressively increased systematically as the body adapts to the training stimulus.

Propranolol.   A beta-adrenergic blocking agent, used to treat angina pectoris, hypertension, dysrhythmias, etc.

Pulmonary wedge pressure.   Pressure measured by a catheter wedged in a small branch artery of the pulmonary arterial tree. A reflection of left atrial and left ventricular end diastolic pressure.

Pulse.   Periodic expansion of the artery resulting from the systole of the heart.

Pulse pressure.   The mathematical difference between the systolic and diastolic blood pressures.

Pulsus alternans.   A pulse in which there is a regular alternation of weak and strong beats, evidence of severe left ventricular failure.

Pyruvic acid (pyruvate).   The end product of aerobic glycolysis; the precursor of lactic acid (lactate).

Quinidine.   A drug used to treat abnormal rhythms of the heartbeat.

Rate pressure product (RPP).   An index of myocardial oxygen consumption. There is a close correlation between myocardial oxygen consumption and the product of heart rate and mean systolic blood pressure. Sometimes called double product.

Rehabilitation.   The return of a person disabled by accident or disease to the optimal attainable physical, mental, emotional, social, and economic usefulness, and if employable, an opportunity for gainful employment.

Relative body fat.   The ratio of fat weight to total body weight, expressed as a percentage.

Relative humidity.   A ratio expressing the degree of moisture in the air.

Repolarization.   The reestablishment of resting membrane potential following depolarization. This is represented by the ST-T components of the electrocardiogram.

Reserpine.   An antihypertensive agent.

Residual volume.   The volume of air remaining in the lung following a maximal expiration. Vital capacity plus residual volume equals total lung capacity.

Respiratory exchange ratio (R).   Also called the respiratory quotient (RQ). The ratio of the amount of carbon dioxide produced to the amount of oxygen consumed ($\dot{V}CO_2/\dot{V}O_2$).

Right bundle branch block.   Delay or blockage of conduction in the right bundle branch of the heart.

Sarcomere.   The functional contractile unit of muscle, which is a part of the myofibril.

Sarcoplasm.   The cytoplasm of a muscle fiber.

Sarcoplasmic reticulum.   A network of channels extending throughout the muscle fibers that serves to regulate the availability of calcium to the troponin molecules of the thin filaments.

Saturated fat.   A fat not capable of absorbing any more hydrogen. These fats are usually the solid fats of animal origin such as in milk, butter, meat, etc.

Sclerosis.   Hardening, usually due to an accumulation of fibrous tissue.

Secondary hypertension.   An elevated blood pressure caused by specific diseases.

Second wind.   A phenomenon characterized by a sudden transition from an ill-defined feeling of distress or fatigue during the early portion of prolonged exercise to a more comfortable, less stressful feeling later in the exercise.

Serum enzymes.   Enzymes such as creatine phosphokinase (CPK) and serum glutamic oxalacetic transamine (SGOT) that are released into the circulation from myocardial muscle when cell death takes place. Also called cardiac enzymes.

Serum glutamic-oxalacetic transaminase (SGOT).   An enzyme that catalyzes the intermolecular transfer of an amino group from glutamic acid to oxalacetic acid. An elevated level of the enzyme in the blood occurs with myocardial infarction.

SGOT.   See *Serum glutamic-oxalacetic transaminase.*

Slow-twitch fibers.   One of several types of skeletal muscle fibers characterized by high oxidative capacity and low glycolytic capacity; associated with endurance-type activities.

Somatotype.   The characterization of the body physique in an objective and systematic manner.

Specificity of training.   The principle underlying the construction of a training program for a specific activity or skill and the primary energy systems involved during performance.

Sphygmomanometer.   An instrument for measuring blood pressure in the arteries. An indirect means of measuring blood pressure.

Spirometer.   An instrument used to measure lung volumes and dynamic lung function.

Steady-state.   Pertaining to the time period during which a physiological function (such as $\dot{V}O_2$) remains at a constant (steady) value.

Stenosis.   Constriction or narrowing of a passage or orifice.

Strength.   The ability to exert muscular force briefly.

Stroke volume (SV).   The amount of blood pumped out of the ventricles with each contraction (systole).

Submaximal exercise.   Exercise at less than maximal intensity; also refers to exercise of less than maximal duration.

Sympathetic nervous system.   A part of the autonomic nervous system or involuntary nervous system that regulates tissues not under voluntary control, e.g., glands, heart, and smooth muscle. See also *Parasympathetic nervous system.*

Syncope.   A transient loss of consciousness due to inadequate blood flow to the brain.

Systole.   The contraction phase of the heartbeat. Atrial systole is the period of the contraction of the atria. Ventricular systole is the period of the contraction of the ventricles.

Systolic ejection period (SEP).   The time during which blood is ejected during ventricular systole.

Systolic (blood) pressure.   See *Blood pressure.*

Tachycardia.   Abnormally fast heart rate; generally, a rate faster than 100 beats/min.

Tension time index (TTI).   Determinant and approximate equivalent of myocardial oxygen consumption (LVSPm × HR × SEP). (LVSPm = left ventricular mean systolic pressure, HR = heart rate, SEP = systolic ejection period.)

Thrombophlebitis.   Inflammation and blood clotting in a vein.

Thrombosis.   Formation of a clot in a blood vessel.

Thrombus.   The formation or presence of a blood clot (thrombus) in a blood vessel or a heart chamber. When dislodged, a thrombus becomes an embolus.

Tidal volume (TV).   The volume of air inspired or expired per breath.

Total lung capacity (TLC).   The sum of the vital capacity and the residual volume.

Training.   An exercise program to improve performance.

Triglycerides.   A triester of glycerol with one, two, or three acid molecules.

Vagus nerves.   Two of the nerves of the parasympathetic nervous system that extend from the brain through the neck and thorax into the abdomen.

Valsalva maneuver.   Making an expiratory effort with the glottis closed, resulting in increased intra-abdominal and intrathoracic pressures.

Vasoconstriction.   A decrease in the diameter and cross-sectional area of a blood vessel caused by a contraction of the smooth muscle cells in the walls of the vessel.

Vasoconstrictor.   a) Vasoconstrictor nerves are a part of the involuntary nervous system. When stimulated, they cause the muscles of the arterioles to contract, increasing the resistance to blood flow and raising the blood pressure. b) Chemical substances that stimulate the muscles of the arterioles to contract are called vasoconstrictor agents, or vasopressors. An example is adrenalin.

Vasoconstrictor nerves.   Part of the involuntary nervous system. When stimulated, they cause the muscles of the arterioles to contract, increasing the resistance to blood flow and raising the blood pressure. Chemical substances that stimulate the muscles of the arterioles to contract are called vasoconstrictor agents, or vasopressors. An example is adrenalin.

Ventilation.   The movement of air into and out of the lungs.

Ventricular fibrillation.   Fibrillary twitches of the ventricular muscle without effective contraction.

Vital capacity.   The greatest volume of air that can be expired following maximal inspiration.

Watt.   See *Kilopond meters per minute.*

Wenckebach phenomenon.   A form of second degree A-V block consisting of progressive lengthening of PR intervals in consecutive cardiac cycles until interrupted by a blocked sinus beat.

Work.   The product of force and distance.

Work load 150 (WL 150).   Work performance or work tolerance as an index of fitness measured as the power (kg meters/min) at which a subject's heart rate (HR) reaches or would be expected to reach 150 beats/minute.

SOURCES

The various definitions in the Glossary were obtained from the following sources:

Golding, LA, Bos, RR: *Scientific Foundations of Physical Fitness Programs.* Burgess, Minneapolis, 1967

Lamb, DR: *Physiology of Exercise Responses and Adaptations.* Macmillan, New York, 1978

Mathews, DK, Fox, EL: *The Physiological Basis of Physical Education and Athletics.* W. B. Saunders, Philadelphia, 1976

Naughton, JP, Hellerstein, HK (eds): *Exercise Testing and Exercise Training in Coronary Heart Disease.* Academic Press, New York, 1973

Wilmore, JH: *Athletic Training and Physical Fitness: Physiological Principles and Practices of the Conditioning Process.* Allyn and Bacon, Boston, 1977

Wilson, PK (ed): *Adult Fitness and Cardiac Rehabilitation.* University Park Press, Baltimore, 1975

Zohman, LR, Phillips, RE (eds): *Medical Aspects of Exercise Testing and Training.* Intercontinental Medical Book Corp., New York, 1973

Index

Aerobic capacity, 134, 138-141, 166-169
Age, *see* Risk factors, age
Ambulation therapy, early:
    patient selection, 56-57
    physiologic basis, 55-56
    prototype program, 57-61
    results, 61-63
    walking program, 60-61
American Heart Association, educational materials,
        123-124, 130, 249
Aneurysm, ventricular, 25, 33
        resection, 25
Angina pectoris, 11-12, 14, 35
    exercise therapy, 42-44
    treatment, 40-44
Angiography, 13, 36
Anxiety, definition, 243
    and early ambulation, 54, 56
    psychotropic drugs for, 249
    relaxation techniques, 252
Arrhythmias, diagnosis, 39
    exercise and, 176, 210
    ventricular ectopic, 32
Arteriography, 13
Aspirin therapy, 75
Atherosclerosis, 3-4

Bed rest therapy, 53-56. *See also* Ambulation
        therapy, early
Behavior, characterization for diagnosis, 89-90
Behavior modification, 76, 90, 93-95
Birth control pills, *see* Risk factors, birth control pills
Blood pressure, lowering program, 9, 75. *See also*
        Heart rate; Risk factors, hypertension

Cardiac failure, 32, 44
Cardiac rupture, 26
Catheterization, cardiac, 36-39
Chair treatment, 54
Cholesterol, *see* Serum cholesterol
Chronotropic capacity, 165
Coronary artery disease, 35
Coronary bypass surgery, 14, 44, 47
Coronary Drug Project (CDP), research results,
        68-71, 74, 76

Coronary heart disease, 1-3, 12
    deaths, 26, 29
    incidence, 1-3, 29
    prognosis, 68-72

Denial as defense, post infarction, 244, 247-248,
        284
Depression after infarction, definition, 243
    diagnosis, 244
    homecoming depression, 245, 249
    prevention, 250
Diet, cholesterol, 83-85
    eating behavior change, 86-87
    history measurement, 79, 107-110
    lipid lowering, 74-75, 82-83
    nutrition program, 80-82, 122
    polyunsaturated fats, 84-85
    sodium restrictions, 44, 81
Digitalis, 44, 46
Diuretics, 44, 45
Doctor, *see* Physician

Early ambulation therapy, *see* Ambulation therapy,
        early
Echocardiography, 37
Electrocardiography, ambulatory, 37, 39
    for prognosis, 13, 70-76, 169
    quantitative exercise, 169-176
Electrography, intracardiac, 39
Employment, energy expenditures for, 147-148,
        154-155
    heart laws, 272-273
    return to work problems, 261-263, 274-275,
        284-285, 292
Energy requirements of selected activities, 149, 195,
        214-215
Ergometer, 158, 163, 194
Ergometer tests, *see* Exercise tests
Exercise physiology, cardiovascular control, 142
    heart rate, 141-142, 144
    maximum exercise effects, 141
    maximum oxygen uptake, 138-141
    myocardial oxygen demand, 145-146, 167-169
    skeletal muscle, *see* Skeletal muscle physiology
    stroke volume, 142-143

Exercise tests:
  arm ergometer, 158
  classification, 152-156
  general rules for, 156
  handgrip, 161
  during hospitalization, 163-165
  hyperventilation, 162
  isometric, 161-162
  liability of prescribing physician, 276-281
  non-steady state, 156-157
  objectives, 150
  realistic, 150-151, 153-156
  standardized versus non-standardized, 147, 149
  steady state, 157
  symptom-limited, 152
  Valsalva Maneuver, 161-162, 207
Exercise therapy:
  adherence to program, 192
  arm versus leg work, 158-160, 190-191, 206-207
  complications during, 212
  consent form, 230
  contraindications, 151-152, 164, 193-194, 198, 204,
    208, 220-222, 228
  cooling off period, 191, 227
  as depression prevention, 250
  diagnosis, 177-179, 194-195, 203-205
  duration of exercise, 184, 210
  evaluation of program, 196-197, 225-226
  frequency of exercise, 185, 210
  history, 53-55
  illustrated exercises, 231-241
  individualization of program, 203-205
  intensity of exercise, 184, 207-210
  phases of program, 48-50, 203-204, 213-219
  phases of session, 177-179
  program outline, 58-60, 120-121, 213-219
  questionnaires and forms, 111-113, 218
  sports participation, 192, 219-223
  supervised program organization, 223-229
  supervised versus unsupervised, 212
  target heart rate, 179-182
  types of exercise, 186-189, 206-207

Family role changes after infarction, 259-261

Glucose intolerance, see Risk factors, glucose
    intolerance

Heart attack, see Myocardial infarction
Heart block, 27
Heart failure, see Cardiac failure
Heart rate, target, 179-182, 208-210, 216
  training, 183, 211
Heart rate monitors, 217
Heberden, William, 11, 53
Herrick, J. B., 12, 53
Hypercholesterolemia, see Risk factors,
    hypercholesterolemia
Hypertension, see Risk factors, hypertension

Hyperuricemia, see Risk factors, hyperuricemia
Hypnosis for convalescence, 252

Ileal bypass surgery, 75, 85
Intervention program, 91-93
  dealing with failure, 95
Ischemia, myocardial, 19-20, 21
    control of size, 34
    transient, 27
Isometric exercise, 57, 147, 161, 207

Karvomen test method, 183, 208

Lipid lowering therapy, 5-8, 74-75, 85

Marriage problems after infarction, 260
Mets requirements for activities, 195, 214-215
MI, see Myocardial infarction
Mitral regurgitation, 33
Mobilization, see Ambulation therapy; Exercise
    therapy
Myocardial infarction:
  atrial, 21, 27
  complications, 23-24, 32-34
  control of size, 34
  definition of, 12, 269-270
  definition of phases, 48-50, 296-302
  evaluation methods, 35-39
  left ventricle damage, 32-33
  myths about, 248, 262
  pathologic changes, 21-27
  rehabilitation, see Rehabilitation after
    myocardial infarction
  right ventricle, 20-21
  risk factors, see Risk factors
  scar formation, 21-22
  subendocardial, 20
  see also Reinfarction
Myocardium, aerobic impairment, 169
  oxygen demands, 34, 41, 167-169
  rupture, 33

Necrosis, extent, 24-25
  influence of site on, 26-27
Nitroglycerin, 41
Nuclear cardiology, 39
Nurse, role in patient education, 123-124, 126,
    251-252
Nutrition, see Diet

Obesity, see Risk factors, obesity
Oxygen demand, 145-146, 167-169
Oxygen uptake, maximal, 138-141, 166-169

Pacemaker, cardiac, 32
Papillary muscle rupture, 26-27
Patient, employment situation problems post-MI,
    261, 284-285, 292
  family problems post-MI, 259-261
  insurance and Workmen's Compensation,
    270-274, 288-291

physician communication, 258
population description, 30-31
psychologic adaptation to illness, 118, 245-248
psychologic response by social class, 245, 258-259
psychotropic drug use, 249
unwarranted invalidism, 246
Patient education, 117-119, 123-131, 248-249
audiovisual, 123-124
exercise prescription, 120-121, 250
group classes, 124-126, 251
learning objectives, 118
medication instructions, 122
Physician, influence on adherence, 256-258
malpractice considerations, 275-276
legal testimony, 272
liability for exercise tests, 276-281
liability problems, 269-281
patient communication, 258
Prasozin, 47. *See also* Vasodilator drugs
Propranolol, 147
Psychosocial risk factors, *see* Risk factors, psychosocial

Rehabilitation after myocardial infarction:
adherence problems, 95, 192-193, 210-211, 256-258
degree of disability determination, 285-288
exercise therapy, *see* Exercise therapy
individualization of patient management, 30, 34, 203-205
institutional help, 123, 263-266, 291-292
legal problems, 269-281
psychologic aspects, 243-253
rationale, 29-33
social influences, 255-268
Reinfarction, prevention, 77-97
risk factors, 68-72
risk reduction programs and materials, 73-77, 91-93, 100-106
Risk factors, 2-4, 8-11
age, 4
birth control pills, 87
glucose intolerance, 4-5
hypercholesterolemia, 5-8, 77-79, 83-85

hypertension, 8, 87
hyperuricemia, 5
and mortality rate, 4-11, 69-70
obesity, 5, 85-87
psychosocial, 71-72
reinfarction, 68-72
smoking, 5-7, 76, 113-115
cessation, 87-89, 122
Risk profile, 72-73
Risk reduction, learning materials, 100-106
rationale, 40, 77

Salt free diet, *see* Diet, sodium restrictions
Self-help techniques for behavior change, 93-95
Serum cholesterol, dietary, 6-8, 83-85
measurement, 77-79
Sexual activity in post-MI patient, 49, 121
Shock, cardiogenic, 33, 35
Skeletal muscle physiology, 134-137
anaerobic metabolism, 136-137
fiber types, 137
glycogen content, 136
Smoking, *see* Risk factors, smoking
Social Security disability program, 273
Sphygmomanometers, 154-155, 161
Sports for post-MI patient, 192, 219-223
Stress management, 87, 89, 247-248
ST-T displacement, 169-176
Surgery methods, 14, 47
coronary bypass, 14, 44, 47
ventricular resection, 25

Thrombo-embolism prevention, 33-34
Transcendental meditation, 252

Valsalva Maneuver, *see* Exercise tests, Valsalva Maneuver
Vasodilator drugs, 46-47
Ventricles, aneurysms, 25, 33
improving function, 46-47
Ventriculography, 25

Wenckebach-type heart block, 27
Work, occupation, *see* Employment
Workmen's Compensation, 270-274, 288-291